theclinics.com

SURGICAL ONCOLOGY CLINICS OF NORTH AMERICA

Surgical Management of Pelvic Malignancy

GUEST EDITOR
Harold J. Wanebo, MD, FACS

CONSULTING EDITOR
Nicholas J. Petrelli, MD

April 2005 • Volume 14 • Number 2

SAUNDERS

An Imprint of Elsevier, Inc.
PHILADELPHIA LONDON TORONTO MONTREAL SYDNEY TOKYO

W.B. SAUNDERS COMPANY
A Division of Elsevier Inc.

The Curtis Center • Independence Square West • Philadelphia, PA 19106–3399

http://www.theclinics.com

SURGICAL ONCOLOGY CLINICS OF NORTH AMERICA
April 2005
Editor: Catherine Bewick

Volume 14, Number 2
ISSN 1055-3207
ISBN 1-4160-2787-4

Surgical Oncology Clinics of North America (ISSN 1055–3207) is published quarterly by W.B. Saunders Company. Corporate and editorial offices: The Curtis Center, Independence Square West, Philadelphia, PA 19106–3399. Accounting and circulation offices: 6277 Sea Harbor Drive, Orlando, FL 32887–4800. Periodicals postage paid at Orlando, FL 32862, and additional mailing offices. Subscription prices are $165.00 per year (US individuals), $244.00 (US institutions) $83.00 (US student/resident), $188.00 (Canadian individuals), $295.00 (Canadian institutions), $113.00 (Canadian student/resident), $225.00 (foreign individuals), and $295.00 (foreign institutions) $113.00 (foreign student/resident). Foreign air speed delivery is included in all *Clinics* subscription prices. All prices are subject to change without notice. POST-MASTER: Send address changes to *Primary Care: Clinics in Office Practice*, W.B. Saunders Company. Periodicals Fulfillment. Orlando, FL 32887–4800. **Customer Service: 1-800-654-2452 (US). From outside the United States, call 1-407-345-4000. E-mail: hhspcs@harcourt.com.**

Reprints. For copies of 100 or more, of articles in this publication, please contact the Commercial Reprints Department, Elsevier Inc., 360 Park Avenue South, New York, New York 10010-1710. Tel. (212) 633-3813 Fax: (212) 462-1935 email: reprints@elsevier.com.

Surgical Oncology Clinics of North America is covered in *Index Medicus and EMBASE/Excerpta Medica, Current Contents/Clinical Medicine, and ISI/BIOMED.*

Printed in the United States of America.

CONSULTING EDITOR

NICHOLAS J. PETRELLI, MD, MBNA Endowed Medical Director, Helen F. Graham Cancer Center, Newark, Delaware; and Professor, Department of Surgery, Jefferson Medical College, Philadelphia, Pennsylvania

GUEST EDITOR

HAROLD J. WANEBO, MD, FACS, Professor of Surgery, Boston University School of Medicine, Boston, Massachusetts; and Adjunct Professor of Surgery, Brown University School of Medicine, Providence; and Chairman Emeritus, Department of Surgery; Program Director, Surgical Oncology Fellowship, Roger Williams Medical Center, Providence, Rhode Island

CONTRIBUTORS

TAKAYUKI AKASU, MD, Head, Department of Surgery, National Cancer Center Hospital, Tokyo, Japan

HERVY E. AVERETTE, MD, Professor, Department of Obstetrics and Gynecology, Division of Gynecologic Oncology, Jackson Memorial Hospital, Sylvester Comprehensive Cancer Center, University of Miami, Miami, Florida

DIMITRA G. BARABOUTI, MD, Clinical Research Fellow, Colorectal Service, Memorial Sloan-Kettering Cancer Center, New York, New York

GIOVANNI BEGOSSI, MD, Surgical Resident, The University of Massachusetts Medical Center, Worcester, Massachusetts

DENNIS S. CHI, MD, Assistant Attending Surgeon, Gynecology Service, Department of Surgery, Memorial Sloan-Kettering Cancer Center, New York, New York

FEDERICO A. CORICA, MD, Chief Resident in Urology, Medical University of South Carolina, Charleston, South Carolina

E. DAVID CRAWFORD, MD, Professor, Departments of Surgery and Radiation Oncology, Head, Urologic Oncology, University of Colorado Health Sciences Center, Denver, Colorado

DAMIAN E. DUPUY, MD, Professor of Diagnostic Imaging, and Director of Ultrasound, Department of Diagnostic Imaging, Brown Medical School, Rhode Island Hospital, Providence, Rhode Island

VICTOR W. FAZIO, MD, MS, FRCS, FRACS, R.W. Turnball Professor and Chairman, Department of Colorectal Surgery, Cleveland Clinic Foundation, Cleveland, Ohio

SHIN FUJITA, MD, PhD, Head, Department of Surgery, National Cancer Center Hospital, Tokyo, Japan

JOEL GOLDBERG, MD, Fellow, Division of Colon and Rectal Surgery, Department of Surgery, University of Minnesota Medical School, Minneapolis, MN

MARY GORDINIER, MD, Assistant Professor, Gynecologic Oncology, Brown University; and The Program in Women's Oncology, Department of Obstetrics and Gynecology, Women's and Infant's Hospital of Rhode Island, Providence, Rhode Island

CORNELIUS O. GRANAI, MD, Director, The Program in Women's Oncology, Department of Obstetrics and Gynecology, Women's and Infant's Hospital of Rhode Island; and Associate Professor, Brown University, Providence, Rhode Island

ALEXANDER G. HERIOT, MD, MA, FRCS(Gen), FRCSEd, Colorectal Fellow, Department of Colorectal Surgery, Cleveland Clinic Foundation, Cleveland, Ohio

FRANCIS J. HORNICEK, MD, PhD, Associate Professor, Orthopaedic Oncology Service, Massachusetts General Hospital, Harvard Medical School, Boston, Massachusetts

THOMAS E. KEANE, MB, FRCSI, Professor and Chairman, Department of Urology, Medical University of South Carolina, Charleston, South Carolina

ROBERT KIM, MD, Fellow, Division of Gynecologic Oncology, Department of Obstetrics and Gynecology, Cleveland Clinic Foundation, Cleveland, Ohio

ELIECER KURZER, MD, MPH, Clinical Fellow, Division of Endourology and Laparoscopy, Department of Urology, University of Miami School of Medicine, Miami, Florida

NICHOLAS C. LAMBROU, MD, Assistant Professor, Department of Obstetrics and Gynecology, Division of Gynecologic Oncology, Jackson Memorial Hospital, Sylvester Comprehensive Cancer Center, University of Miami, Miami, Florida

RAYMOND J. LEVEILLEE, MD, Associate Professor and Chief, Division of Endourology and Laparoscopy, Department of Urology, University of Miami School of Medicine, Miami, Florida

LLOYD A. MACK, MD, FRCSC, Surgical Oncologist, Tom Baker Cancer Centre; and Research Associate, Departments of Oncology and Surgery, University of Calgary, Calgary, Alberta, Canada

HENRY J. MANKIN, MD, Edith M. Ashley Professor Emeritus, Orthopaedic Oncology Service, Massachusetts General Hospital, Harvard Medical School, Boston, Massachusetts

MURUGESAN MANOHARAN, MD, FRCS(Eng), FRACS, Director, Neobladder and Urostomy Center; and Assistant Professor of Urology, Department of Urology, University of Miami School of Medicine, Miami, Florida

PAUL D. MARONI, MD, Resident, Division of Urology, Department of Surgery, University of Colorado Health Sciences Center, Denver, Colorado

WAYNE A. McCREATH, MD, Attending Physician, Obstetrics and Gynecology Division, Crystal Run Healthcare, Middletown, New York

ANDERS MELLGREN, MD, PhD, Adjunct Associate Professor, Division of Colon and Rectal Surgery, Department of Surgery, University of Minnesota Medical School, Minneapolis, Minnesota

YOSHIHIRO MORIYA, MD, PhD, Chief, Department of Surgery, National Cancer Center Hospital, Tokyo, Japan

J. MATT PEARSON, MD, Fellow, Department of Obstetrics and Gynecology, Division of Gynecologic Oncology, Jackson Memorial Hospital, Sylvester Comprehensive Cancer Center, University of Miami, Miami, Florida

ANTONELLA RESTIVO, MD, Fellow, Gynecologic Oncology, The Program in Women's Oncology, Women's and Infant's Hospital of Rhode Island; and Clinical Teaching Fellow, Brown University Department of Obstetrics and Gynecology, Providence, Rhode Island

PETER G. ROSE, MD, Section Head, Section of Gynecologic Oncology; Professor, Reproductive Biology, Surgery and Gynecology, Case Western Reserve University, Cleveland, Ohio

DAVID A. ROTHENBERGER, MD, Professor, Divisions of Colon and Rectal Surgery and Surgical Oncology, Department of Surgery, University of Minnesota Medical School; and Associate Director of Clinical Research, University of Minnesota Cancer Center, Minneapolis, MN

EMERY SALOM, MD, Clinical Assistant Professor and Gynecologic Oncology Fellow, Department of Obstetrics and Gynecology, University of Miami, Jackson Memorial Hospital, Miami, Florida

CAROLINE J. SIMON, MD, Research Fellow, Department of Diagnostic Imaging, Brown Medical School, Rhode Island Hospital, Providence, Rhode Island

WALLEY J. TEMPLE, MD, FRCSC, FACS, Professor of Surgery and Oncology, University of Calgary; and Chief, Division of Surgical Oncology, Tom Baker Cancer Centre, Calgary, Alberta, Canada

HARI S.G.R. TUNUGUNTLA, MD, MCh (Urol), Fellow in Female and Reconstructive Urology, Department of Urology, University of Miami School of Medicine, Miami, Florida

KIMBERLY A. VARKER, MD, Post-Doctoral Research Fellow (NRSA), Department of Surgery, The Ohio State University, Columbus, Ohio

HAROLD J. WANEBO, MD, FACS, Professor of Surgery, Boston University Medical School, Boston, Massachusetts; Adjunct Professor, Brown University, Providence, Rhode Island; and Chairman Emeritus, Department of Surgery; Program Director, Surgical Oncology Fellowship, Roger Williams Medical Center, Providence, RI

W. DOUGLAS WONG, MD, FACS, FRCS, Chief, Colorectal Service, Memorial Sloan-Kettering Cancer Center, New York, New York; and Professor of Surgery, Cornell University Medical College, New York, New York

SEIICHIROU YAMAMOTO, MD, Staff, Department of Surgery, National Cancer Center Hospital, Tokyo, Japan

CONTENTS

FORTHCOMING ISSUES

July 2005

Cancer Screening
Thomas Weber, MD, *Guest Editor*

October 2005

The Evolution of Radical Surgery in Oncology
Marvin J. Lopez, MD, *Guest Editor*

January 2006

Melanoma
Anton Bilchik, MD, PhD, *Guest Editor*

RECENT ISSUES

January 2005

Breast Cancer
Stephen B. Edge, MD, *Guest Editor*

October 2004

Adjuvant Therapy of Pancreatic Adenocarcinoma
John P. Hoffman, MD, *Guest Editor*

July 2004

Palliative Surgical Oncology
Lawrence D. Wagman, MD, *Guest Editor*

April 2004

Multidisciplinary Approach to Anal Cancer
Morton S. Kahlenberg, MD and
Charles R. Thomas, Jr, MD, *Guest Editors*

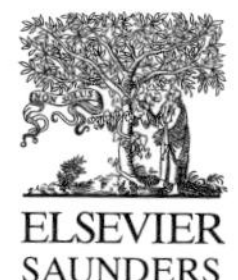

ELSEVIER
SAUNDERS

Surg Oncol Clin N Am
14 (2005) xv–xvi

SURGICAL
ONCOLOGY CLINICS
OF NORTH AMERICA

Foreword

Surgical Management of Pelvic Malignancy

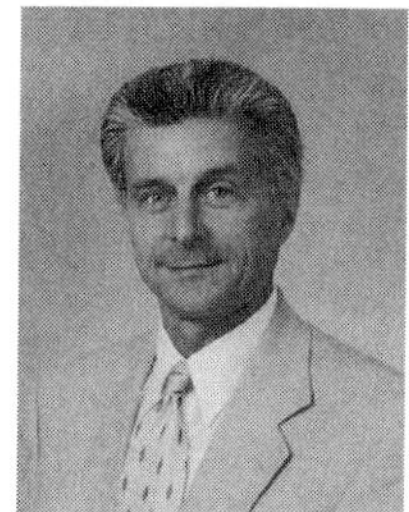

Nicholas J. Petrelli, MD
Consulting Editor

This issue of the *Surgical Oncology Clinics of North America* presents Harold J. Wanebo, MD, as Guest Editor. Dr. Wanebo is Chief of the Division of Surgical Oncology at the Roger Williams Medical Center in Providence, Rhode Island, and is a member of the Department of Surgery at Brown University School of Medicine and the Boston University School of Medicine. This issue is devoted to the surgical management of pelvic malignancies, of which one could describe Dr. Wanebo as an expert in this field. There are five sections devoted to rectal cancer, gynecologic malignancies, urologic oncology, musculoskeletal sarcomas, and ablative techniques.

All of the articles in this issue are outstanding. They demonstrate the importance of expertise in the surgical management of pelvic malignancies. The overview of extended abdominoperineal resection and abdominosacral resection by Dr. Wanebo is outstanding and obviously described by an individual who probably has the most experience with this technique anywhere in the country. The article by Dr. Douglas Wong on total mesorectal excision is a must-read for surgeons in training. The "wake-up call" concerning local excision for rectal cancer is an outstanding discussion by Dr. David Rothenberger.

The articles on gynecologic malignancies and urologic oncology are by individuals with experience and a track record to be modeled. Also, details described by Dr. Wally Temple from the University of Calgary concerning

1055-3207/05/$ - see front matter
doi:10.1016/j.soc.2005.01.002

extended pelvic resections for sarcoma and visceral tumors invading the musculoskeletal pelvis are aptly described.

I congratulate Dr. Wanebo and his colleagues for an extremely informative issue of the *Surgical Oncology Clinics of North America*. I am sure readers will enjoy this issue as much as I have.

Nicholas J. Petrelli, MD
Helen F. Graham Cancer Center
4701 Ogletown-Stanton Road, Suite 1213
Newark, DE 19713, USA
Department of Surgery
Thomas Jefferson University
College Building, 1025 Walnut Street
Philadelphia, PA 19107, USA

E-mail address: npetrelli@christianacare.org

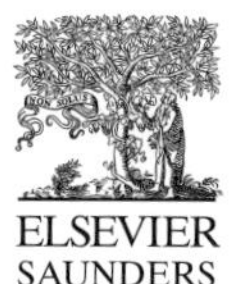

ELSEVIER
SAUNDERS

Surg Oncol Clin N Am
14 (2005) xvii–xviii

SURGICAL
ONCOLOGY CLINICS
OF NORTH AMERICA

Preface

Surgical Management of Pelvic Malignancy

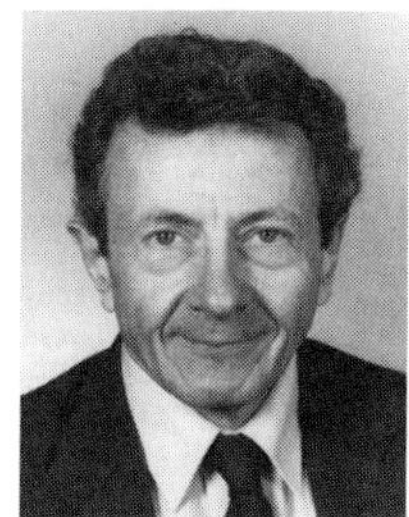

Harold J. Wanebo, MD, FACS
Guest Editor

The goal of this issue is to bring together experts in the major disciplines involved in treating pelvic cancer, and to exemplify the areas of commonality as well as unique differences among these disciplines. Years ago, when I was a young fellow in training at Memorial Sloan Kettering, there was a concept of a "pelvic ring rotation" in which the fellows spent time in the Rectum and Colon Service, the Gynecology Service, and the Urology Service. It was a marvelous opportunity to learn the major elements, philosophies, and surgical techniques in the management of cancers of the pelvis. Each of the disciplines had something unique to offer, and there was surprising commonality among the differences in these disciplines. We have attempted to capture this type of experience in this issue of the *Surgical Oncology Clinics of North America*, in which we have brought together experts in colorectal surgery, gynecologic oncology, urologic oncology, and participants who come from different disciplines such as musculoskeletal oncology and surgical oncology. The initial outline for this issue as offered to the publisher was quite broad and probably unrealistic, so I was required to shorten it to bare-bone presentations. I would consider this a first step in developing a common scientific and philosophical database among the disciplines involved.

The authors have done yeoman's job in synthesizing the data and philosophies for their respective articles. We are thankful to Elsevier for

1055-3207/05/$ - see front matter
doi:10.1016/j.soc.2005.01.001

allowing us to include the numerous figures and tables required to adequately present the author's viewpoint. I trust that readers will enjoy and learn as much as I did in reviewing these excellent articles.

Harold J. Wanebo, MD, FACS
Department of Surgery
Boston University School of Medicine
Boston, MA, USA
Division of Surgical Oncology
Department of Surgery
Roger Williams Medical Center
825 Chalkstone Avenue
Providence, RI 02908-4735, USA

E-mail address: hwanebo@rwmc.org

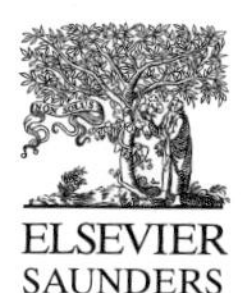
ELSEVIER
SAUNDERS

Surg Oncol Clin N Am
14 (2005) 137–155

SURGICAL
ONCOLOGY CLINICS
OF NORTH AMERICA

Current Management of Rectal Cancer: Total Mesorectal Excision (Nerve Sparing) Technique and Clinical Outcome

Dimitra G. Barabouti, MD[a],
W. Douglas Wong, MD, FACS, FRCS[a,b,*]

[a]*Colorectal Service, Memorial Sloan-Kettering Cancer Center, 1275 York Avenue, C-1067, New York, NY 10021, USA*
[b]*Cornell University Medical College, 525 East 68th Street, New York, NY 10021, USA*

Over the last two decades, total mesorectal excision (TME) has brought a dramatic improvement in the outcome of surgery for rectal cancer. The impressively low local recurrence rates seen with TME, and the major improvements in survival, sphincter preservation, and preservation of autonomic pelvic nerve function, have been consistent and reproducible in many trials, setting new quality standards in rectal cancer surgery. This article reviews the studies that set the background for TME, describes the present authors' surgical technique, and discusses the impact of TME on cancer recurrence and survival, sphincter preservation, and autonomic nerve preservation. Finally, the article reviews TME-based trials that investigate the role of radiation and chemotherapy in the treatment of rectal cancer.

Background

The goal of TME is the excision of the rectum along with its blood vessels and surrounding lymph nodes within an intact visceral fascial envelope. Preserving the integrity of the mesorectal fascial envelope and obtaining a negative circumferential (radial) margin are the key elements in minimizing pelvic recurrence.

* Corresponding author. Colorectal Service, Memorial Sloan-Kettering Cancer Center, 1275 York Avenue, C-1067, New York, NY 10021.

E-mail address: wongd@mskcc.org (W.D. Wong).

1055-3207/05/$ - see front matter
doi:10.1016/j.soc.2004.11.003

Many theories have attempted to explain the mechanism of local (pelvic) recurrence of rectal cancer, including the implantation of shed tumor cells at the anastomosis [1] and the up-regulation of tumor growth at the anastomosis [2]. In 1963, however, Bussey Morson showed that local recurrences after surgery for rectal cancer were stage-related, associated with mural penetration, nodal involvement [3]. Other risk factors for pelvic recurrence are vascular, lymphatic, or perineural invasion [4]. These factors suggest that the cause of pelvic recurrence is the inadequate clearance of the regional mesorectal disease or inadequate resection.

In 1982, Heald et al [5] first reported the presence of non-nodal foci of metastatic disease (mesorectal deposits) in the distal mesorectum of rectal cancer specimens. Reynolds et al [6] showed a widespread distribution of these deposits, detecting them in the mesorectum deep to the tumor, but also in the distal mesorectum as far as 5 cm below the mural tumor. These studies indicated that failure to perform TME carries the risk of leaving residual disease in the distal mesorectum or at the circumferential margin and predisposes the patient to local recurrence.

Conventional surgery uses blunt dissection for the mobilization of the rectum. The rectosacral fascia is encountered at the level of S4, anchoring the rectum to the sacral curvature. Blunt dissection will frequently violate the mesorectum at this level, leaving lymph node– or metastatic deposit–containing fat attached to the pelvic sidewall, sacrum, or pelvic floor [7]. On coronal section of the mesorectum, this persistent residual disease (positive lateral margin) can be documented; it serves as the nidus for local recurrence, which becomes clinically evident approximately 18 months later.

In 1986, Quirke et al [8] showed a direct correlation between the status of the circumferential margin and the risk of local recurrence in a clinical pathologic study of the specimens from 52 patients, with a follow-up period of 2 years. All patients had undergone conventional resections using standard blunt pelvic dissection. Significant concave portions of the mesorectum were missing from what would be the normal convex contour of the mesorectal fat. Whole-mount sections of the entire operative specimen were examined by transverse slicing. Previously unsuspected involved lateral resection margins were identified in 14 (27%) of the specimens. Approximately 85% of these patients with positive margins (12 of 14) developed a pelvic recurrence. There were no local recurrences in patients who had undergone curative resection and who had negative lateral margins (34 of 34), as compared with four of five patients (80%) with curative resections and involved margins.

Further studies corroborated these findings. Ng et al [9] reported on 80 patients undergoing proctectomy for cancer, with a median follow-up period of 26.6 months. The lateral resection margins were positive in 20% of cases among those undergoing curative resections; the pelvic recurrence rate was 17% in patients with uninvolved margins and 60% in those with involved margins ($P < 0.001$).

Adam et al [10] reported a prospective study of 190 patients undergoing conventional surgery for rectal cancer with a median follow-up period of 5 years. They measured the closest point where any tumor (ie, nodal disease, non-nodal implants, or venous invasion) approached the lateral margin and defined any margin of less than 1 mm as a positive margin. Positive lateral margins were identified in 36% of cases and in 25% of the patients who underwent curative resections. The local recurrence rate was 64% in patients with positive circumferential margins versus 9% in those with negative margins overall. This rate was 66% versus 8%, respectively, in those undergoing curative resection. Similarly, the overall 5-year survival rate was only 15% in those with involved margins versus 66% in those with uninvolved margins (24% versus 74% in curative resections). The authors advocated that pelvic recurrence was directly related to inadequate surgical resection with involved circumferential (lateral) margins.

The technique of TME was introduced by Heald at the North Hampshire Hospital in Basingstoke, England in 1979 [11]. Heald and Ryall's [12] first series of 112 curative anterior resections showed an unprecedented cumulative risk of local recurrence at 5 years of 2.7% and an overall 5-year survival rate of 87.5%, with a tumor-free survival rate of 81.7%. These were the best reported results in rectal cancer treatment up to that time.

The results of the initial TME clinical studies [11–13], with the findings of the clinical pathology studies by Quirke [8], Ng [9], Adam [10], and Reynolds [6], constitute the foundation for the practice of TME.

Anatomy of the mesorectum

Embryologically, the mesorectum originates from a circular multilayer concentrate of mesenchymal cells, which form lamellae of rectal adventitia filled with fatty tissue during development. The outer lamellae of the rectal adventitia condense to form a fascial sheath known as the visceral fascia of the mesorectum [14,15]. The visceral mesorectal fascia envelopes the rectum with its mesorectum. In addition, there is the parietal endopelvic fascia, extending downward in the pelvis from the retroperitoneum. This fascia extends along the pelvic walls and overlies the piriformis, coccygeal and levator ani muscles, the anterior surface of the sacrum and coccyx, the anococcygeal ligament, and the presacral venous plexus.

Posteriorly, the visceral and the parietal fascial layers are separated by a thin layer of loose areolar tissue. This layer is easily entered to open the retrorectal space. Caudally, the retrorectal space ends at the anal sphincter, whereas cranially, the visceral fascia thins out over the sacral promontory. At the level of S4, the retrorectal space is interrupted with a more or less strong condensation of fibers running in a craniocaudal direction from the parietal fascia to the visceral fascia. This fascia has been referred to as the rectosacral fascia.

Anteriorly, the rectum and mesorectum are separated from the seminal vesicles and prostate by Denonvilliers' fascia. This fascia was originally described in men, but in women, an equivalent, although thinner, rectovaginal fascia exists. Posterior to Denonvilliers' fascia, the mesorectum is covered by the visceral fascia. Surgical planes exist anterior and posterior to Denonvilliers' fascia [16,17]. Either plane may be developed during the mobilization of the rectum.

Laterally and below the peritoneal reflection, the lateral ligaments of the rectum are encountered as condensations of the visceral fascia. The ligaments connect to the parietal fascia on the pelvic sidewall. The nature of the lateral ligaments has been debated in the literature. Many authors regard them as a clinical or a surgical term [7,18], whereas others regard them as a real anatomic structure [19–21]. The importance of the lateral ligament to local recurrence was recognized as early as the 1950s with the work of Sauer and Bacon [22,23], who identified in their operative specimens lymph nodes with metastasis along the lateral ligament.

Pelvic autonomic nerves

The pelvic sympathetic nerve fibers originate from splanchnic branches from T12 through L2. These fibers pass distally by means of preaortic nerve branches and form the superior hypogastric plexus near the sacral promontory. This plexus gives rise to the right and left hypogastric nerves, which are found along the posterolateral pelvic brim just below the course of the ureters. The hypogastric nerves lie in the areolar tissue plane between the visceral and the parietal fascia. The plane between these two fascial layers is very thin at the level of the pelvic brim, making the hypogastric nerves seem adherent to the visceral fascia of the mesorectum. The relation of the hypogastric nerve to the mesorectum and visceral fascia has been a subject of discussion. Havenga et al [7,24], in their cadaver dissections, identified the hypogastric nerve anterior to the visceral fascia, on the posterior surface of the mesorectal fat. Bissett et al [25], however, have described the hypogastric nerve medial, posterior, and unattached to the visceral fascia (fascia propria of the rectum) in their clinical studies. Takahashi et al [18] emphasized that the hypogastric nerve is situated very close to the visceral endopelvic fascia. In the current authors' experience, the hypogastric nerve is found in close proximity and posterior to the visceral endopelvic fascia. With careful dissection, the mesorectum enveloped by the visceral fascia can be mobilized, leaving the intact hypogastric nerves behind.

The parasympathetic pelvic nerves (nervi erigentes) are anterior branches of the S2–4 nerve roots; they run laterally, caudad, and anteriorly along the pelvic wall over the piriformis muscle, covered by the parietal fascia. At the pelvic side wall, the nervi erigentes join the hypogastric nerve to form the inferior hypogastric plexus, otherwise known as the pelvic autonomic nerve plexus (Fig. 1). Rectal branches of the inferior hypogastric plexus run

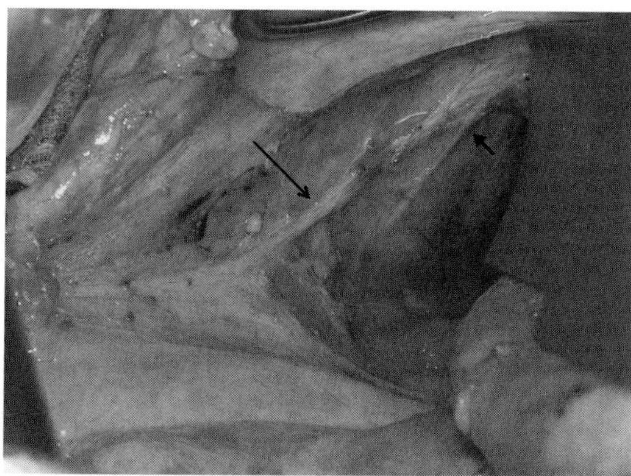

Fig. 1. The left hypogastric nerve (*long arrow*) joins the left nervi erigentes (*short arrow*) at the pelvic side wall to form the inferior hypogastric plexus.

medially, entering the mesorectum, with terminal branches of the middle hemorrhoidal vessels. Genitourinary branches of the inferior hypogastric plexus continue to the anterior visceral compartment (ie, the bladder and either the prostate and seminal vesicles or the uterus and vagina) [7].

Technique

TME is a "specimen-oriented" surgery: the examination of the mesorectum for completeness of the excision predicts local recurrence and survival [8–10]. An often used analogy is the excision of a sebaceous cyst: recurrence is more likely if the wall of the cyst is incompletely excised or if the cyst is perforated. In a similar concept, the goal of TME is the excision of the rectum with blood vessels and surrounding pararectal lymph nodes within an intact visceral fascial envelope and the en bloc resection of lymph nodes along the superior rectal and inferior mesenteric arteries [26].

The operation begins with exploration of the abdomen, placement of a wound protector and a self-retaining retractor, and exposure of the sigmoid colon. The peritoneal line of Toldt is incised and the sigmoid and descending colon are mobilized from lateral to medial. The splenic flexure is taken down, if necessary, for a tension-free anastomosis. The gonadal vessels and the ureter are identified and preserved. The pelvic peritoneum is divided to the level just above the cul-de-sac. The preaortic nerves and the superior hypogastric plexus are also left behind in the retroperitoneum, covering the aortic bifurcation and the area between the common iliac vessels just above the sacral promontory. The sigmoid is tented up, thus delineating the superior rectal vessels. The peritoneum is then divided medially, following the curvature of the vessels. The dissection of the superior rectal and inferior mesenteric vessels can also be done from right to left, and this method is more commonly applied during the laparoscopic approach.

The proximal resection bowel margin is usually determined by choosing healthy sigmoid or descending colon for a low anastomosis. In the absence of palpable proximal mesenteric lymph nodes, the vascular pedicle is divided just below the left colic branch, if the sigmoid is to be used for the anastomosis, or above the left colic branch, if the distal descending colon is to be used. The bowel is divided with a linear cutting stapler. The proximal colon is then packed away in the left upper quadrant. Gentle retraction on the rectal stump facilitates exposure during the pelvic dissection.

The pelvic dissection begins with the posterior dissection of the mesorectum. The retrorectal space is entered at the level of the sacral promontory and the filmy areolar tissue in the plane between the visceral mesorectal fascia and the parietal endopelvic fascia is sharply divided using electrocautery. At this time, the right and left hypogastric nerves are identified along the posterolateral pelvic brim. Because the nerves are often adherent to the visceral fascia, they may be lifted with the mesorectum. Care has to be taken to divide any attachments between the hypogastric nerves and the mesorectum. The dissection is carried medial to the nerves. The parietal endopelvic fascia is left intact, covering presacral vessels in the midline and internal iliac vessels and endopelvic muscles laterally.

Anteriorly, the crease between the seminal vesicles or the vagina and the rectum is identified, the peritoneum overlying the cul-de-sac is incised, and the prerectal space is opened. The anterior dissection plane is best found just posterior to the seminal vesicle or the vagina. If the tumor is anterior, the dissection is kept anterior to Denonvilliers' fascia; if the tumor is posterior, the Denonvilliers' fascia is divided and the dissection is carried posterior to this fascial layer. Instead of incising the cul-de-sac peritoneum, Heald's group dissects a cuff of it off the seminal vesicles or upper vagina en bloc with the mesorectum.

The anterior dissection is alternated with the lateral mobilization of the rectum. Medial, superior, and counter traction are applied to delineate the lateral ligaments. The dissection is directed from anterior to posterolateral. The lateral ligaments are divided using electrocautery. To date, there is no published study of nerve injury in relation to quantity (amperage and duration) of electrocautery. During this step, however, excessive medial traction on the mesorectum may tent the pelvic autonomic nerve plexus inward, placing it at risk for injury, especially if the surgeon were to use clamping or stapling. To avoid such injury, it is the current authors' practice to strictly avoid clamping or stapling during this step of the procedure. Electrocautery is sufficient because the proper planes are relatively avascular.

As the anterior dissection proceeds below the seminal vesicles, the correct plane is exposed by applying gentle retraction on the prostate or the vagina using a St. Mark's retractor, while the rectum is being pushed down with a sponge stick. Small rectoprostatic or rectovaginal vessels are often encountered during this step and can usually be sealed with cautery;

however, prolonged cautery on the posterior vaginal wall should be avoided, because it may contribute to a fistula.

The dissection is then directed again posteriorly, following the curvature of the mesorectum, anterior to the presacral fascia to protect the nervi erigentes. The mesorectum, rectum, and sacrum curve anteriorly at the level of the parasympathetic nerves, so the angle of dissection follows this curve and proceeds in an anterior direction to the pelvic floor. During the entire dissection, the mesorectum is inspected periodically to ensure it is intact.

The nervi erigentes are not routinely viewed during this dissection because they are covered by the posterolateral endopelvic parietal fascia. The location of the nervi erigentes behind the endopelvic fascia may be indicated by a gentle upward (anterior) tugging of the hypogastric nerves, giving the impression of vertical pillars laterally on the pelvic sidewall from the sacrum to the junction of the hypogastric nerves and inferior hypogastric plexus [26]. Knowledge of their location prevents inadvertent injury. Dissection too wide of the endopelvic fascia laterally can cause injury of the nerves.

At the level of S4, the rectosacral fascia is encountered posteriorly. Again, the rectosacral (Waldeyer's) fascia is the endopelvic parietal fascia reflecting from the levators and covering the distal rectal tube and anorectal junction. The rectosacral fascia is divided sharply. Blunt dissection should be strictly avoided because it will tear the mesorectum at the level of the attachment of the rectosacral fascia. The division of the rectosacral fascia will allow the complete mobilization of the distal rectum. The puborectalis sling is now exposed. The rectal muscular tube past the distal edge of the mesorectum is cleaned circumferentially. This is the distal resection margin for mid- and lower rectal tumors.

Consideration should be given to shedding of intraluminal tumor cells during the resection. Viable tumor cells can be found in the lumen of the rectum and anal canal distal to the tumor. Various techniques have been used in an attempt to minimize the potential for implantation of these intraluminal malignant cells, which could cause cancer recurrence. The current authors' practice is to place a stapler below the tumor without closing it. A right-angle bowel clamp is then placed across the rectum below the tumor but above the stapler. The rectum is irrigated with water, saline, or betadine. After the washout, the stapler is closed and fired, and the rectum is divided along the stapler.

For a midrectal cancer, the distal resection margin is below the distal edge of the mesorectum, with a margin of at least 2 cm below the tumor [27,28]. For a distal rectal cancer treated with preoperative radiation, the current authors accept a distal resection margin of 1 cm below the tumor at the bared rectal tube [29]. For a distal rectal cancer not invading the sphincters, dissection into the intersphincteric plane is sometimes needed to acquire a 1-cm distal margin. This dissection extends in the plane of the bared rectal tube beneath Waldeyer's and within the upper external anal sphincter formed by the puborectalis sling. In women, who have a short anal canal, the anterior circular fibers of the external sphincter may be revealed with further dissection in the anterior intersphincteric plane.

Whether TME is needed for an upper rectal cancer has been a subject of much debate. Pathologic examination of upper rectal cancer specimens has not identified metastases to lymph nodes in the mesorectum more than 5 cm distal to the cancer [30,31]. Specifically, Hida et al [30] performed a retrospective examination of 198 specimens resected over a 10-year period, evaluating distal intramural spread and lymph node involvement. Intramural spread was seen in 10.6% of patients, extending distally up to 2 cm from proximal rectal cancers and 1 cm from distal rectal tumors. Intramural spread was not identified for T1 or T2 tumors. Distal mesorectal nodal metastases were identified in 20% of patients with stage T3 disease, with the greatest distance to a lymph node metastasis being 4 cm. In 12 patients (24%), the mesorectum distal to the tumor was involved by cancer. The maximum distance from the primary carcinoma to a metastatic focus was more than 2 cm in 5 of these 12 individuals and was 5 cm in 1 patient.

It seems that for an upper rectal cancer, a tumor-specific mesorectal excision with a distal 5-cm margin is most likely sufficient to remove all pararectal lymph nodes with the potential to contain metastases. In this case, the distal mesorectal margin should be resected at a 90° angle to the long axis of the rectum. This way, the surgeon avoids "coning" distally into the mesorectum, which carries the risk of leaving involved lymph nodes or metastatic deposits behind.

Quality of the total mesorectal excision specimen

The quality of the TME is assessed by examining the specimen at the back table. The intact visceral mesorectal fascia has a bilobed, smooth surface, with a glistening reflection, and is often described as "a baby's bottom."

Quirke's group [8] suggested three grades of mesorectal fascial envelope quality that have been shown to correlate with the likelihood of local recurrence: poor quality, with deep clefts into the mesorectal fat that expose the bared muscularis of the rectal wall; intermediate quality, with merely superficial clefts into the mesorectal fat that do not expose the muscularis; and good quality, evincing a mesorectal fascial envelope that is intact circumferentially.

A specimen graded as poor quality is considered an incomplete mesorectal excision and is associated with a local recurrence rate of approximately 75%, which is similar to local recurrence rates when excised specimens are examined and found to test positive for microscopic malignant tissue at the radial margins. Intermediate- and good-grade specimens can probably be considered complete mesorectal excisions, associated with a local recurrence rate of less than 30%, similar to that in patients whose excisions test negative at the radial margins. Furthermore, survival is predicted by intactness of the mesorectal fascial envelope. The patient survival rate associated with complete mesorectal specimens is approximately 80%; with incomplete specimens, this rate is approximately 60%. Also, the higher local recurrence rates seen with rectal cancers within 10 cm from the anal verge have been associated with the increased incidence of incomplete TME observed in such specimens [32,33].

Reconstruction

After TME, reconstruction requires a coloanal or a very distal rectal anastomosis. The current authors routinely create a colonic J-pouch when the distance from the anal verge to the anastomosis is less than 6 cm. The colonic J-pouch has been shown to produce improved functional outcome compared with the straight coloanal anastomosis for low-lying lesions [34], with these results lasting at least 2 years [35]. Prospective, randomized trials comparing 5-cm with 10-cm J-pouches have shown increased incidence of evacuation difficulties with the 10-cm pouch [34,36].

The techniques of coloplasty [37] and end-to-side anastomosis also have been used to address the loss of the reservoir function of the rectum and improve functional outcome after TME. For the method of anastomosis, the use of the stapler is appropriate to the level of the anorectal junction. Care must be taken not to incorporate the puborectalis muscle or the vagina into the stapler. An anastomosis to the dentate line, however, requires a transanal hand-sewn anastomosis.

Problems

TME is technically challenging because of the confinements of the bony pelvis and the need to preserve the autonomic nerve plexus and to resect the rectum and mesorectum as an intact envelope. Although initial reports of TME indicated prolonged operations and increased blood loss, current experience has indicated an operative time for TME of less than 4 hours, with fewer than 15% of patients requiring transfusion.

The fact that TME leaves a "bared" rectal tube free of mesorectum and the high leak rates (10%–20%) in the initial TME reports [38,39] raised concerns regarding the vascular supply to the anastomosis. Increased experience has currently led to anastomotic leak rates of 5% or less [40]. The current authors' institution uses fecal diversion with a loop ileostomy selectively.

Oncologic outcomes

In studies of conventional surgery for rectal cancer (involving blunt dissection), local recurrence rates have averaged 30%, with 5-year survival rates ranging from 27% to 42%. Since it was introduced, there have been several series evaluating TME with minimal use of adjuvant therapy that report local recurrence rates of 4% to 8% and cancer-specific survival rates of 70% to 80% at 5 years [41,42].

Heald and Ryall [12] presented their first series of 112 curative anterior resections in 1986, showing an impressive local recurrence rate at 5 years of 2.7% and an overall corrected 5-year survival rate of 87.5%, with a tumor-free survival rate of 81.7%. Many investigators have raised concerns about patient case mix and analytic techniques, unclarified selection process, and incorrect use of definitions [43,44]. Heald's group updated their results in 1998 with a report of 519 rectal cancer resections; this report included patients with tumors situated up to 15 cm from the anal verge, with an average follow-up period of 8.3 years [45]. Few patients with locally advanced disease (9%) received preoperative radiation, and approximately 6% received chemotherapy postoperatively. The overall local recurrence rate, with or without distant metastasis, was 6% at 5 years and 8% at 10 years. Patients undergoing low anterior resections had much better outcomes than those who required abdominoperineal resections (5% local recurrence at 5 y and 10 y versus 17% and 36%, respectively). The local recurrence rates were unrelated to Dukes' stage or to the level of the anastomosis. The overall recurrence rates for low anterior resections and abdominoperineal resections combined were 19% at 5 years and 22% at 10 years. The 5- and 10-year cancer-specific survival rates were 68% and 66%, respectively, and 80% and 78%, respectively, for those undergoing curative resections.

MacFarlane et al [46] reported on a group of 135 "high-risk" patients with T3 or T4 lesions or lymph node metastases, but with no distant metastases. All patients had tumors with distal margins located 12 cm or less from the anal verge. Patients deemed "incurable" were excluded from their analysis of local recurrence and survival. The median follow-up period was 7.7 years. The local recurrence rate was 5% at 5 years. The overall recurrence rate at 5 years was 22%; it was 32% in the Dukes' C subgroup. This rate was affected by stage of disease, extramural vascular invasion, and tumor differentiation. The recurrence-free, cancer-specific 5-year survival rate was calculated to be 78%.

In 1995, Enker et al [47] reported on 246 consecutive patients with curable Dukes' B and C tumors, with tumors situated 0 to 12 cm from the anal verge, who underwent resection between 1979 and 1993. Seventy patients (28.5%) had received perioperative radiation with or without chemotherapy. Only 18 tumors (7.3%) recurred locally. Pelvic recurrences without distant metastatic disease were seen in 5.7% of patients. Overall local recurrence rates correlated with nodal status and perineural invasion, but not with tumor height or with the type of resection (low anterior resection versus abdominoperineal resection). The rate of distant failure without local recurrence was 23.6%. The overall 5-year survival rate in this group of high-risk patients was 74.2%, which correlated with stage, nodal status, and type of operation (anterior resection versus abdominoperineal resection). In an update in 2000 on 544 patients, these results persisted, with an actuarial 5-year local recurrence rate of 5.2% and a 5-year cancer-related survival rate of 73.5% [42].

The excellent results of TME on local control and survival have been reproduced in single-surgeon and in multisurgeon series. In Aitken's [48] series in 1996 of 64 patients who underwent curative resection with TME, with at least 24 months' follow-up, only one patient (1.6%) developed a local recurrence. In a multisurgeon study, Arbman et al [49] evaluated outcomes in Östergötland, Sweden. They compared 230 patients who had undergone TME resections between 1990 and 1992 (the TME group) with 211 control subjects (conventional operations performed between 1984 and 1986). Only one control and three TME patients underwent radiotherapy, and none received chemotherapy. All the resections were curative. The local recurrence rate was 6% in the TME group and 14% in the conventional surgery group.

Kockerling et al [50] evaluated 1581 curative resections performed in Erlangen, Germany, between 1985 and 1991, at the time of the introduction of TME. These patients were compared with historical controls who underwent resection between 1974 and 1984. No patient received adjuvant therapy. The mean follow-up period was 13.1 years (minimum, 4 y). The local recurrence rates decreased from 39.4% to 9.8% over the study period ($P < 0.0001$), and the 5-year survival rate increased from 50% to 71% ($P < 0.0001$).

Havenga et al [51] reported on 691 consecutive patients undergoing curative TME resections by TME-trained surgeons at three specialized centers and 720 patients undergoing curative conventional surgery. All patients had stage II or III rectal cancer within 12 cm of the anal verge. This prospective study compared the results of two separate groups of surgeons, one performing only TME and one conventional surgery. The 95% confidence interval for the local recurrence rate was 4% to 9% in the TME group, as compared with 32% to 35% in the conventional group—an absolute difference of 25% in local recurrence rates. The 5-year overall and cancer-specific survival rates in the two groups were 62% to 75% and 75% to 80% versus 42% to 44% and 52%, respectively.

A large, multicenter, randomized trial evaluating the use of preoperative radiotherapy in conjunction with TME-based surgery was presented in 2001 by the Dutch Colorectal Cancer Group. TME-trained surgeons from 84 Dutch hospitals, 13 Swedish hospitals, and 11 other European and Canadian centers participated in the study. They achieved a local recurrence rate in the TME-only group of 8.2% with a 2-year overall survival rate of 82%. The local recurrence rate decreased to 2.4% in the radiotherapy group [52,53].

Heald's group recently published their outcomes on node-positive patients [54]. In their study, 470 patients underwent curative anterior resection with TME. Of those, 170 patients were node-positive. The overall local recurrence rate was 4.5%, and the systemic recurrence rate was 24%. The local recurrence rate was 2% for patients with Dukes' A tumors, 4% for Dukes' B, and 7.5% for patients with Dukes' C disease. The systemic recurrence rate was 8% for Dukes' A, 18% for Dukes' B, and 37% for patients with Dukes' C disease. These results reconfirm the appropriateness of TME for the treatment of rectal cancer and emphasize the role of the surgeon in achieving local control.

Sphincter preservation

TME is a far superior technique to conventional surgery in mobilizing the rectum and achieving a dissection down to the level of the anorectal junction. This capability has enhanced the feasibility of mobilization of mid- and lower rectal tumors from above. The acceptance of the 2-cm distal margin (or 1 cm for distal tumors treated with preoperative radiotherapy) was also a significant step toward the establishment of sphincter-preserving surgery for rectal cancer [27,29]. Rectal cancer responds to preoperative chemoradiotherapy (CRT), with a 10% to 20% pathologic complete response rate. The combination of TME and preoperative CRT has significantly reduced the abdominoperineal resection (APR) rate for T3 mid- and lower rectal cancers without compromising the oncologic outcome [55,56].

Although a large percentage of the patients treated with sphincter-sparing surgery report satisfactory sphincter function, several functional problems have been documented postoperatively in this population. The "anterior resection syndrome" is a term commonly used and is characterized by frequency, urgency, and some degree of incontinence. These symptoms become more evident as the level of anastomosis becomes lower [57]. They seem to be associated with alterations in the reservoir function of the neorectum.

There is considerable evidence suggesting that radiotherapy also has a potential adverse effect on sphincter function, which is dose-dependent. Preoperative radiation given in the Swedish Rectal Cancer Trial impaired continence and increased urgency and stool frequency, as reported in a retrospective survey [58]. The Memorial Sloan-Kettering Cancer Center group compared the long-term functional results of 109 patients who received preoperative radiotherapy, postoperative radiotherapy, or no radiotherapy in conjunction with low anterior resection and a straight coloanal anastomosis [59]. The postoperative radiotherapy group had significantly higher rates of clustering and frequency of defecation compared with the preoperative radiotherapy or no radiotherapy group. The authors attributed these differences to the irradiation of the neorectum.

Gervaz et al [60] studied the effects of pre- and postoperative CRT on the function of the colonic J-pouch. They observed that chemoradiation not only increased the incidence of anal incontinence but contributed to difficulties in pouch evacuation. As the potential effects of radiotherapy on sphincter function are recognized, radiation oncologists are focusing on new advances in technology to produce regimens that minimize the dose delivered to nontarget structures, including the anal sphincter.

Pelvic autonomic nerve preservation

In the mid-1970s, Tsuchiya and Ohki [61], in Yokohama, Japan, were the first to develop an autonomic nerve–preserving technique for rectal cancer surgery. Deliberate tracking and preservation of the autonomic nerves in conjunction with TME (TME-ANP) was introduced by Enker et al [47] in 1991. In 1996, Havenga et al [62] reported on sexual and urinary functional results in a group of 136 patients (82 men and 54 women) who underwent TME-ANP. The ability to achieve a spontaneous erection was maintained by 86% of the patients younger than 60 years and by 67% of patients aged 60 years and older. Approximately 87% of male patients maintained their ability to achieve orgasm. Retrograde ejaculation was encountered in 7.5% of patients before the operation and in 20% to 40% of patients after the operation. A diminished ejaculation was reported by two thirds of patients. The type of surgery (abdominoperineal resection compared with low anterior resection) and an age of 60 years or older were significantly associated with male sexual dysfunction. Of the female patients, 85% were able to experience arousal with vaginal lubrication and 91% could achieve orgasm. Most patients had few or no complaints related to urinary function. The incidence of neurogenic bladder was zero.

Maurer et al [63] compared sexual function after TME-ANP with historical control patients who underwent conventional surgery in the same institute before introduction of TME-ANP. In the group of patients who underwent conventional surgery, 75% of male patients were able to achieve an erection before the operation compared with 6% after the operation. In the group of patients who underwent TME-ANP, 58% of patients were able to achieve an erection before the operation and 26% of patients could do so after the operation.

Radiation may affect the vasa nervosa of the autonomic nerves, leading to fibrosis and dysfunction. It may also be associated with smooth muscle fibrosis, causing vasculogenic impotence. Moreover, patients with rectal cancer may have pre-existing, benign prostatic hypertrophy or stress incontinence. Because of their average age, they may have comorbidities, such as coronary artery disease, peripheral vascular disease, and diabetes mellitus, or use medications to treat these conditions, which all may influence sexual function. The causes of sexual and urinary dysfunction after surgery for rectal cancer are complex. TME with attention to autonomic nerve preservation is feasible, however, and has been clearly shown to improve functional outcomes in rectal cancer surgery.

Total mesorectal excision and adjuvant treatment

The major studies that influenced the guidelines for the adjuvant treatment of rectal cancer in the past were based on the results of conventional surgery [64–66]. As TME emerged as the new gold standard, producing local recurrence rates lower or comparable to the combination of conventional surgery, radiation, and chemotherapy, the question was whether adjuvant therapy is warranted for all patients undergoing TME. This question is particularly important when the potential toxicity of this therapy is taken into account. Another point of discussion is whether the combined treatment should consist of the standard treatment or a modified regimen.

TME now forms the basis of large randomized clinical trials in which the role of adjuvant therapy is being re-examined. The Dutch Colorectal Cancer Group study was the first to evaluate the efficacy of preoperative radiation on local recurrence and survival should the patients undergo standardized TME [52]. The rate of local recurrence at 2 years was 2.4% in the radiotherapy-plus-surgery group and 8.2% in the surgery-only group ($P < 0.001$). Survival was similar in the two groups.

Sauer et al [67] recently presented the results of the German Rectal Cancer Study, a phase 3 trial that compared preoperative and postoperative CRT for patients with locally advanced rectal cancers who underwent TME-based resection. The study randomized 823 patients, 24 of whom were ineligible. With a median follow-up period of 40 months, the local recurrence rate was 6% in the preoperative CRT group and 13% in the postoperative CRT group ($P < 0.006$). There was no difference in the incidence of distant metastases, the disease-free survival, or the overall survival. There was a statistically significant decrease in the acute and chronic toxicity of CRT in the group treated with preoperative combined-modality therapy. Preoperative CRT also improved sphincter preservation for distal rectal cancers. The investigators concluded that preoperative CRT should be the new standard adjuvant treatment for locally advanced rectal cancer.

The specific indications for adjuvant therapy in combination with TME are also a subject of debate and ongoing research. Merchant et al [68] reported on 95 patients with stage T3 N0 M0 rectal cancer treated with TME without adjuvant therapy. With a median follow-up period of 53 months, the 5-year actuarial rate of local failure was 12% (crude, 9%) and the overall survival rate was 75%. The only statistically significant risk factor for local recurrence was lymphovascular invasion. The authors suggested that select patients with T3 N0 M0 rectal cancer may not require adjuvant therapy for local control.

The recently published results from Basingstoke on node-positive patients (discussed previously) also challenge the indications of preoperative radiotherapy [54]. From their results, the authors advocate that with careful TME, the local recurrence rate can be dramatically reduced in these high-risk patients. They currently support the use of radiotherapy preoperatively for very low tumors or fixed and tethered tumors and only selectively for node-positive tumors. As noted by Rothenberger [69] in the accompanying invited commentary, however, the highly selected subgroup of patients used in the study rates raises some concerns. These were only the 170 node-positive patients treated with anterior resection and TME in whom clear margins were achieved in surgery. Patients treated with APR, mesorectal transection, or Hartmann's resection were excluded from the study. Moreover, 159 patients treated by anterior resection with TME were excluded because they had residual macroscopic disease at the time of surgery. The exclusion of this last group may significantly increase the risk of bias favoring outcomes achieved by TME alone. These patients may actually be the ones that would benefit from preoperative CRT to achieve a curative resection.

Laparoscopic total mesorectal excision

Many trials reporting on laparoscopic intestinal resection for malignancy, including the Clinical Outcomes of Surgical Therapy Study Group trial, have included no or very few cases of rectal cancer. In skilled hands, abdominoperineal resection, where the cancer dissection and removal of the specimen are performed by means of the perineum, has been considered the ideal starting point for laparoscopic surgery for rectal cancer [70]. In 2000, Weiser and Milsom [71] published their preliminary results from 21 laparoscopic rectal resections with TME for low rectal adenocarcinoma. Half of the patients had T3 lesions or nodal disease and underwent neoadjuvant therapy. The results were encouraging and showed the safety of the procedure, with acceptable operative time, blood loss, and morbidity.

It seems that the benefits of laparoscopic rectal resection are similar to those of colon resection, including reduced length of stay, reduced narcotic use, and improved pulmonary function. In addition, there is the potential for improved visualization provided by the laparoscope deep in the pelvis. The fact that the entire laparoscopic team can have a clear and close view of deep pelvic dissections is likely to accelerate the teaching of rectal cancer surgery.

Education

Training on the TME-ANP technique is necessary for every surgeon operating on patients who have rectal cancer. Martling et al [72] showed that local recurrence rates decreased by more than 50% as a result of a surgical teaching initiative in the county of Stockholm. The Dutch study showed consistent, reproducible results of TME in a multi-institutional setting, with surgeons trained on the technique by experienced consultants.

Major educational programs have been undertaken in many European countries. In the United States, TME is considered the standard of care in the treatment of rectal cancer and is an essential part of the colon and rectal surgery training.

Summary

The clinical results initially reported for TME-based operations have been reproduced in series with sufficiently large patient cohorts. The long-term follow-up indicates that the results observed at 5 years are durable and associated with cancer cure and not delayed time to recurrence. This increase in cure and local control has been accompanied by dramatic increases in sphincter, sexual, and urinary function preservation. TME-based operations are now established as the standard of care for rectal cancer and form the basis for trials investigating the role of adjuvant therapy. Educational efforts are currently focused on spreading the technique of TME-ANP, and improvements in technology are leading TME into the era of minimally invasive surgery.

References

[1] Gordon-Watson C. Origin and spread of cancer of the rectum in surgical treatment. Lancet 1983;1:239–45.
[2] Williamson RCN, Davis PW, Bristol JB, Wells M. Intestinal adaption and experimental carcinogenesis after partial colectomy: increased tumour yields are confirmed to the anastomosis. Gut 1982;23:316–25.
[3] Bussey HJR, Morson BC. General results of surgical treatment of rectal cancer at St. Mark's Hospital, 1928–1952. Acta Unio Int Contra Cancrum 1963;19:1510–3.
[4] Gastrointestinal Tumor Study Group. Prolongation of the disease-free interval in surgically treated rectal carcinoma. N Engl J Med 1985;312:1465–72.
[5] Heald RJ, Husband EM, Ryall RD. The mesorectum in rectal cancer surgery—the clue to pelvic recurrence? Br J Surg 1982;69(10):613–6.
[6] Reynolds JV, Joyce WP, Dolan J, Sheahan K, Hyland JM. Pathological evidence in support of total mesorectal excision in the management of rectal cancer. Br J Surg 1996;83:1112–5.
[7] Havenga K, DeRuiter MC, Enker WE, et al. Anatomical basis of autonomic nerve-preserving total mesorectal excision for rectal cancer. Br J Surg 1996;83:384–8.
[8] Quirke P, Durdey P, Dixon MF. Local recurrence of rectal adenocarcinoma due to inadequate surgical resection. Lancet 1986;I:996–9.
[9] Ng IOL, Luk ISC, Yuen ST, et al. Surgical lateral clearance in resected rectal carcinomas: a multivariate analysis of clinicopathological features. Cancer 1993;71:1972–6.
[10] Adam IJ, Mohamdee MO, Martin IG, et al. Role of circumferential margin involvement in the local recurrence of rectal cancer. Lancet 1994;344(8924):707–11.
[11] Heald RJ. A new approach to rectal cancer. Br J Hosp Med 1979;22:277–81.
[12] Heald RJ, Ryall RD. Recurrence and survival after total mesorectal excision for rectal cancer. Lancet 1986;1:1479–82.
[13] Enker WE, Philipsen SJ, Heilweil ML, et al. En bloc pelvic lymphadenectomy and sphincter preservation in the surgical management of rectal cancer. Ann Surg 1986;203:426–33.
[14] Fritsch H. Development of the rectal fascia. Anat Anz 1990;170:273–80.

[15] Church JM, Raudkivi PJ, Hill GL. The surgical anatomy of the rectum—a review with particular relevance to the hazards of rectal mobilization. Int J Colorectal Dis 1987;2: 158–66.
[16] Lindsey I, Guy RJ, Warren BF, et al. Anatomy of Denonvilliers' fascia and pelvic nerves, impotence, and implications for the colorectal surgeon. Br J Surg 2000;87:1288–99.
[17] van Ophoven A, Roth S. The anatomy and embryological origins of the fascia of Denonvilliers: a medico-historical debate. J Urol 1997;157:3–9.
[18] Takahashi T, Ueno M, Azekura K. Lateral ligament: its anatomy and clinical importance. Semin Surg Oncol 2000;19:386–95.
[19] Rutegard J, Sandzen B, Stenling R, et al. Lateral rectal ligaments contain important nerves. Br J Surg 1997;84:1544–5.
[20] Nano M, Lanfranco G, Dal Corso H, et al. The lateral ligaments of the rectum: myth or reality? Chir Ital 2000;52:313–21.
[21] Sato K, Sato T. The vascular and neuronal composition of the lateral ligament of the rectum and the rectosacral fascia. Surg Radiol Anat 1991;13:17–22.
[22] Sauer I, Bacon HE. Influence of lateral spread of cancer of the rectum on radicability of operation and prognosis. Am J Surg 1951;81:111–20.
[23] Sauer I, Bacon HE. A new approach for excision of carcinoma of the lower portion of the rectum and anal canal. Surg Gynecol Obstet 1952;95:229–42.
[24] Havenga K, Enker WE. Autonomic nerve preserving total mesorectal excision. Surg Clin N Am 2002;5:1009–18.
[25] Bissett IP, Chau KY, Hill GL. Extrafascial excision of the rectum: surgical anatomy of the fascia propria. Dis Colon Rectum 2000;43:903–10.
[26] Phang PT. Total mesorectal excision: technical aspects. Can J Surg 2004;47(2):130–7.
[27] Paty PB, Enker WE, Cohen AM, et al. Treatment of rectal cancer by low anterior resection with coloanal anastomosis. Ann Surg 1994;219:365–73.
[28] Shirouza K, Isomoto H, Kakegawa T. Distal spread of rectal cancer and optimal margin of resection for sphincter-preserving surgery. Cancer 1995;76:388–92.
[29] Moore HG, Riedel E, Minsky B, et al. Adequacy of 1-cm distal margin after restorative rectal cancer resection with sharp mesorectal excision and preoperative combined-modality therapy. Ann Surg Oncol 2003;10(1):80–5.
[30] Hida J, Yasutomi M, Maruyama T, Fujimoto K, Uchida T, Okuno K. Lymph node metastases detected in the mesorectum distal to carcinoma of the rectum by the clearing method: justification of total mesorectal excision. J Am Coll Surg 1997;184:584–8.
[31] Scott N, Jackson P, al-Jaberi I, Dixon MF, Quirke P, Finan PJ. Total mesorectal excision and local recurrence: a study of tumour spread in the mesorectum distal to rectal cancer. Br J Surg 1995;82:1031–3.
[32] Nagtegaal ID, van de Velde CJH, van der Worp E, Kapiteijn E, Quirke P, van Krieken JHJM, for the Dutch Colorectal Cancer Group. Macroscopic evaluation of rectal cancer resection specimen: clinical significance of the pathologist in quality control. J Clin Oncol 2002;20:1729–34.
[33] Phang PT, MacFarlane J, Taylor RH, et al. Effects of positive resection margin and tumor distance from anus on rectal cancer treatment outcomes. Am J Surg 2002;183:504–8.
[34] Hida J, Yasutomi M, Maruyama T, et al. Enlargement of colonic pouch after proctectomy and coloanal anastomosis: potential cause for evacuation difficulty. Dis Colon Rectum 1999; 42:1181–8.
[35] Lazorthes F, Chiotasso P, Gamagami RA, et al. Late clinical outcome in a randomized prospective comparison of colonic J-pouch and straight coloanal anastomosis. Br J Surg 1997;84:1449–51.
[36] Lazorthes F, Chiotasso P, Gamagami RA, et al. Prospective, randomized study comparing clinical results between small and large colonic J-pouch following coloanal anastomosis. Dis Colon Rectum 1997;40:1409–13.

[37] Fazio VW, Mantyh CR, Hull TL. Colonic "coloplasty": novel technique to enhance low colorectal or coloanal anastomosis. Dis Colon Rectum 2000;43:1448–50.
[38] Karanjia ND, Corder AP, Bearn P, Heald RJ. Leakage from stapled low anastomosis after total mesorectal for carcinoma of the rectum. Br J Surg 1994;81:1224–6.
[39] Carlsen E, Schlichting E, Guldvog I, Johnson E, Heald RJ. Effect of the introduction of total mesorectal excision for the treatment of rectal cancer. Br J Surg 1998;85:526–9.
[40] Enker WE, Merchant N, Cohen AM, et al. Safety and efficacy of low anterior resection for rectal cancer: 681 consecutive cases from a specialty service. Ann Surg 1999;230(4): 544–54.
[41] Harnsberger JR, Vernava VM, Longo WE. Radical abdominal lymphadenectomy: historic perspective and current role in the surgical management of rectal cancer. Dis Colon Rectum 1994;37:73–87.
[42] Murty M, Enker W, Martz J. Current status of total mesorectal excision and autonomic nerve preservation in rectal cancer. Semin Surg Oncol 2000;19:321–8.
[43] Isbister WH. Basingstoke revisited. Aust N Z J Surg 1990;60:243–6.
[44] Marsh PJ, James RD, Schofield PF. Definition of local recurrence after surgery for rectal carcinoma. Br J Surg 1995;82:465–8.
[45] Heald RJ, Moran BJ, Ryall RD, et al. Rectal cancer—the Basingstoke experience of total mesorectal excision, 1978–1997. Arch Surg 1998;133:894–9.
[46] McFarlane JK, Ryall RD, Heald RJ. Mesorectal excision for rectal cancer. Lancet 1993;341: 457–60.
[47] Enker WE, Thaler HT, Cranor ML, Polyak T. Total mesorectal excision in the operative treatment of carcinoma of the rectum. J Am Coll Surg 1995;181:335–46.
[48] Aitken RJ. Mesorectal excision for rectal cancer. Br J Surg 1996;83:214–6.
[49] Arbman G, Nilsson E, Hallböök O, Sjödahl R. Local recurrence following total mesorectal excision for rectal cancer. Br J Surg 1996;83:375–9.
[50] Kockerling F, Reymond M, Altendor-Hofmann A, et al. Influence of surgery on metachronous distant metastases and survival in rectal cancer. J Clin Oncol 1998;16:324–9.
[51] Havenga K, Enker WE, Norstein J, et al. Improved survival and local control after total mesorectal excision or D3 lymphadenectomy in the treatment of primary rectal cancer: an international analysis of 1411 patients. Eur J Surg Oncol 1999;25:368–74.
[52] Kapiteijn E, Marijnen CA, Nagtegaal ID, et al. Preoperative radiotherapy combined with total mesorectal excision for resectable rectal cancer. N Engl J Med 2001;345:638–46.
[53] Kapiteijn E, Van de Velde C. The role of total mesorectal excision in the management of rectal cancer. Surg Clin N Am 2002;82(5):995–1007.
[54] Cecil T, Sexton R, Moran B, Heald R. Total mesorectal excision results in low local recurrence rates in lymph node-positive rectal cancer. Dis Colon Rectum 2004;47:1145–50.
[55] Wagman R, Minsky BD, Cohen AM, et al. Sphincter preservation in rectal cancer with preoperative radiation therapy and coloanal anastomosis: long term followup. Int J Radiat Oncol Biol Phys 1998;42:51–7.
[56] Ota DM. Rectal cancer: the sphincter-sparing approach. Surg Clin North Am 2002;82(5): 983–93.
[57] Paty PB, Enker WE, Cohen AM, et al. Long-term functional results of coloanal anastomosis for rectal cancer. Am J Surg 1994;167:90–5.
[58] Dahlberg M, Glimelius B, Graf W, Pahlman L. Preoperative radiation affects functional results after surgery for rectal cancer. Dis Colon Rectum 1998;41:543–51.
[59] Nathanson DR, Espat NJ, Nash GM, et al. Evaluation of preoperative and postoperative radiotherapy on long-term functional results of straight coloanal anastomosis. Dis Colon Rectum 2003;46(7):888–94.
[60] Gervaz P, Rotholtz N, Belin B, et al. Colonic J-pouch function in rectal cancer patient's impact of adjuvant chemo-radiation therapy. Dis Colon Rectum 2001;44:1667–75.
[61] Tsuchiya S, Ohki S. Radical surgery for rectal cancer with preservation of pelvic autonomic nerves. Taipei, Taiwan: Republic of China Surgical Society; 1992.

[62] Havenga K, Enker WE, McDermott K, et al. Male and female sexual and urinary function after total mesorectal excision with autonomic nerve preservation for carcinoma of the rectum. J Am Coll Surg 1996;182:495–502.
[63] Maurer CA, Z'Graggen K, Renzulli P, et al. Total mesorectal excision preserves male genital function compared with conventional rectal cancer surgery. Br J Surg 2001;88:1501–5.
[64] Swedish Rectal Cancer Trial. Improved survival with preoperative radiotherapy in resectable rectal cancer. N Engl J Med 1997;336:980–7.
[65] Krook JE, Moertel C, Gunderson L, et al. Effective surgical adjuvant therapy for high-risk rectal carcinoma. N Engl J Med 1991;24:709–15.
[66] Thomas PR, Lindblad ER. Adjuvant postoperative radiotherapy and chemotherapy in rectal carcinoma: a review of the Gastrointestinal Tumor Study Group experience. Radiother Oncol 1988;13:245–52.
[67] Sauer R, Becker H, Hohenberger W, et al. German Rectal Study Group. Preoperative versus postoperative chemoradiotherapy for rectal cancer. N Eng J Med 2004;351:1731–40.
[68] Merchant NB, Guillem J, Paty P, et al. T3N0 rectal cancer: results following sharp mesorectal excision and no adjuvant therapy. J Gastrointest Surg 1999;3:642–7.
[69] Rothenberger DA. Invited commentary. Dis Colon Rectum 2004;47:1149–50.
[70] Seow-Choen F, Eu KW, Hoy H, et al. A preliminary comparison of a consecutive series of open versus laparoscopic abdominoperineal resection for rectal adenocarcinoma. Int J Colorectal Dis 1997;12:88–90.
[71] Weiser M, Milsom JW. Laparoscopic total mesorectal excision with autonomic nerve preservation. Semin Surg Oncol 2000;19:396–403.
[72] Martling AL, Holm T, Rutqvist LE, et al, for the Stockholm Colorectal Cancer Study Group and the Basingstoke Bowel Cancer Research Project. Effect of a surgical training program on outcome of rectal cancer in the county of Stockholm. Lancet 2000;356(9224):93–6.

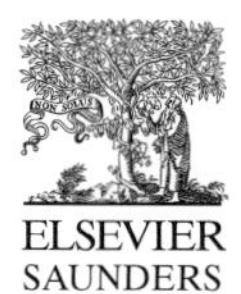
ELSEVIER
SAUNDERS

Surg Oncol Clin N Am
14 (2005) 157–181

SURGICAL
ONCOLOGY CLINICS
OF NORTH AMERICA

Proctectomy with Coloanal Anastomosis

Victor W. Fazio, MD, MS, FRCS, FRACS*,
Alexander G. Heriot, MD, MA, FRCS(Gen), FRCSEd

Department of Colorectal Surgery, Cleveland Clinic Foundation, 9500 Euclid Avenue, Cleveland, OH 44118, USA

Surgical management tends to evolve over time as a result of contributions from multiple physicians. The management of carcinoma of the rectum is a good example of this. Developments in understanding of the pathology and spread of the tumor, combined with technical advances, have altered significantly the surgical approach, from radical ablative surgery at the start of the twentieth century to restorative sphincter-preserving surgery at the start of the twenty-first century [1]. This is combined with increased awareness of the value of functional outcome and oncologic outcome.

In 1908, radicality was considered the key, and Ernest Miles proposed abdominoperineal resection (APER) as the appropriate approach to rectal cancer, based on Halstead's principles of radical surgery to excise potential areas of lymph node spread, which he considered to be proximal and distal to the tumor [2]. Despite high morbidity and mortality associated with APER, the procedure was supported by William Mayo [3], who believed that sphincter preservation increased morbidity. APER remained the approach of choice for the next 30 years and replaced the posterior approach to rectal tumors that had been advocated by Kraske [4]. Restorative resection for rectal cancer was first performed in the United States by Balfour in 1910 but gained increasing popularity from the 1940s onwards. It was initially applied only to rectosigmoid tumors, with some units still performing APER for rectal tumors into the 1960s. Developments in pathology with respect to the limits of distal rectal cancer spread supported reduction of resection margin distal to the tumor.

Because of the need for a permanent colostomy with APER, along with genitourinary dysfunction, numerous techniques for colorectal and coloanal anastomosis were described during the twentieth century. The pull-through

* Corresponding author.
E-mail address: faziov@ccf.org (V.W. Fazio).

1055-3207/05/$ - see front matter
doi:10.1016/j.soc.2004.11.008

technique described by Hochenegg in 1900 [5] of abdominoperineal proctosigmoidectomy with sphincter preservation was reported by several renowned surgeons, including Babcock [6], Bacon [7], Black [8], Dixon [9], Turnball and Cuthbertson [10], and Cutait and Figlioni [11]. Bacon reported survival equivalent to APER but with lower morbidity [7]. Techniques for endoanal low rectal anastomosis first were described by Parks in 1972 [12], although in relation to benign rectal resections. Direct anastomoses using a posterior approach were described by Localio et al [13] and Mason [14] in the 1970s, without and with sphincter division, respectively. In 1982, Parks and Percy [15] reported coloanal anastomosis for low rectal cancer, with excision of the distal rectal mucosa and hand-sewn endoanal anastomosis, which is the modern technique. The technical developments in stapling devices over the last 30 years have increased the attractiveness and availability of low anastomoses, resulting in most coloanal anastomoses being stapled, usually using a double stapling technique developed by Knight and Griffen in 1980 [16]. The trend of restorative procedures after proctectomy with increasingly distal anastomosis rather than nonrestorative procedures has continued throughout the twentieth century up to the current position of rates of APER of less than 10% [17].

Despite the trend of using distal anastomosis, there is no precise definition for coloanal anastomosis [18,19]. A cancer in the lower third of the rectum that is proximal to the distal 1 cm of the rectum may be excised by low anterior resection and colorectal anastomosis. Tumors lower than that area require proctectomy with rectal division at the level of the levator ani muscle and anastomosis to the proximal anal canal with coloanal anastomosis at the top of the anal canal [19]. The anastomosis can be placed lower in the anal canal, down to the level of the dentate line, after transanal mucosectomy and hand-sewn anastomosis. The concept of complete removal of the rectum and associated mesorectum with an anastomosis at some position along the length of the anal canal remains consistent, however, regardless of which technique is applied.

Anatomy

The rectum is enveloped by its own fascial envelope, the fascia propria, which is continuous with the parietal endopelvic fascia that covers the pelvic floor, and great care is taken during rectal mobilization for malignant disease to avoid breaching this "package." The lower part of the rectum is attached to the sacrum by Waldeyer's fascia, which covers the presacral fascia and must be divided to mobilize the rectum. Anteriorly, the fascial envelope is continuous with the rectovesical fascia of Denonvilliers. This thickened fascia extends from the peritoneal reflection to the urogenital diaphragm and forms part of the rectovaginal septum. Fascia also may be condensed lateral to the rectum to form the lateral rectal ligaments [20].

The anal canal commences at the anorectal ring, where the rectum passes through the pelvic floor and passes to the anal verge. It is approximately 4 cm long in men and 2.5 to 3 cm in women, and it passes back and down from the rectum from a point at which the rectum is pulled forward by the sling-like puborectalis muscle [21]. The anal canal sits like a tube within a funnel, the sides of the funnel being formed by the levator ani muscle, with the stem of the funnel formed by the external sphincter. The latter is a continuous, circumferential band of striated muscle—up to 10 mm thick—that encircles the anal canal. It attaches to the perineal body anteriorly and the coccyx posteriorly via the anococcygeal raphe, and the ischiorectal fossae lie laterally. Superiorly, the fibers of the external sphincter blend with the puborectalis muscle, which is the most caudal part of the levator ani muscle. The internal sphincter lies within the external sphincter and is formed by thickening of the circular smooth muscle fibers of the rectum. Proctectomy and coloanal anastomosis include division of this circular muscle ring at some point between the level of the caudal limit of the mesorectum and the level of the dentate line—either via the pelvis or transanally—and reanastomosis with the colon.

Distal resection margin and oncologic outcome

The principle of complete oncologic resection has remained foremost in consideration of rectal cancer resection. Developments in pathology with respect to the distal spread of rectal tumors provided stimulus for the distal migration of resection, combined with clinical evidence of no deterioration in oncologic outcome despite reduced distal resection margins. Westhues [22] and Dukes [23] reported limited distal tumor spread in the 1930s, which encouraged the application of restorative resection for rectal tumors over APER. In the 1950s, Dukes [23] and Grinnell [24] reported distal tumor spread over 2 cm to be rare, other than in patients with poorly differentiated tumors, and they recommended distal resection margins of 2.5 cm with well-differentiated tumors but 6 cm in poorly differentiated tumors. Goligher et al [25], in a classic study in 1951, reported distal spread beyond the main body to the tumor in only 98 (6.5%) of 1500 rectal cancers and commented that a distal margin of 1 in would have cleared 68 of these. Two percent of tumors extended more than 2 cm beyond, however, which led to the suggestion of 5 cm as a safe distal resection margin.

Technical advances in anastomosis led to reappraisal of the extent of margin required as strict application of the "5-cm rule," which severely limited the proportion of cases amenable to restorative resection. In a study of 334 patients who underwent curative resection for rectal cancer, Pollet and Nicholls [26] reported that a distal margin of 2 cm did not compromise survival or local recurrence. The National Adjuvant Breast and Bowel Project reported no difference in survival between a margin of 2 cm and a margin more than 3 cm [27]. Williams et al [28] assessed 50 APER and identified no distal spread in 76% of cases. In five cases with distal spread of 1 cm or more, all were poorly differentiated Dukes C tumors and the patients died from metastatic disease. The concept of distal spread being limited to advanced poorly prognostic lesions has been echoed by other reports [29,30]. Karanjia et al [31] reported no increase in local recurrence with distal margins of 1 cm, although Phillips et al [32] reported an increased recurrence after anterior resection when the margin was less than 1 cm. There is a point at which local recurrence is increased by reduction in distal margin. Hermanek [33] reported that the risk of local recurrence increases as the distal margin becomes less than 20 mm, and a balance must be made between striving for reanastomosis by reducing the distal resection margin and compromising the oncologic outcome for the patient. Reported oncologic outcome for coloanal anastomosis is comparable to that achieved for low anterior resection (Table 1).

Tumors that are positioned just above the anorectal ring or extend into the upper part of the anal canal require partial excision of the internal sphincter to obtain adequate clearance and preserve the option of an anastomosis. Several studies have reported oncologic outcome to be similar to that of tumors positioned more proximal in the rectum that can be removed without internal sphincter division, although the total number of patients reported is small [34–36]. Rullier et al [36] reported 16 patients (5 T2 and 11 T3 stage tumors) who underwent intersphincteric resection with partial or complete excision of the internal sphincter, 12 of whom received preoperative radiotherapy. At a median follow-up of 44 months, there was no local recurrence and the 5-year survival rate was 75%. This approach has been used for T4 tumors, combined with preoperative chemoradiotherapy and excision of the adjacent levator muscles [37]. There was no local recurrence, and at a median follow-up of 58 months, all six patients were disease free.

Downstaging with adjuvant therapy for sphincter preservation

Preoperative radiotherapy may result in shrinkage of a primary rectal cancer. Researchers have proposed that this approach may allow a sphincter-saving resection to be performed in a case that would otherwise necessitate an APER. Concern over the oncologic outcome has resulted in

Table 1
Oncologic outcome after proctectomy and coloanal anastomosis for rectal cancer

Author	No. patients	Local recurrence (%)	5-y survival rate (%)
Hautefeuille [97]	35	22	64
Paty et al [59]	134	11	73
Cavaliere [98]	117	7	69
Gamagami [99]	174	7.9	78
Berger [100]	154	13	68.8

the concept that the decision over choice of operation should be made before any adjuvant therapy, however. Rouanet et al [38] reported a series of 27 patients with distal rectal cancer in whom it was believed that APER was required for resection. After preoperative radiotherapy, 17 patients underwent proctectomy with coloanal anastomosis, with no evidence of decrease in survival or increase in local recurrence. The opinion of whether the patients originally required APER remains a potential area of dispute. Grann et al from Memorial Sloan Kettering Hospital [39] reported a similar series, with 17 of 20 patients able to undergo restorative resection for rectal cancer rather than an APER, as was proposed on their initial assessment, after preoperative chemoradiotherapy. Rullier et al [40] reported a series of 43 advanced low rectal cancers (40 T3 and 3 T4), 70% of which were within 2 cm of the anal sphincter. All patients received long-course preoperative chemoradiotherapy and underwent proctectomy with sphincter preservation, with 25 patients undergoing intersphincteric resection. Eighteen of the patients were downstaged on pathology (T0, T1, T2) and the authors concluded that the preoperative chemotherapy and downstaging allowed sphincter preservation. Whether this result would have been feasible without the preoperative adjuvant therapy is not proven, however.

Functional and physiologic outcome of straight coloanal anastomosis

Proctectomy has a significant functional impact on a patient. Conservation of the sphincter complex and avoidance of a permanent stoma seems to limit the reduction in quality of life compared with a permanent stoma [41,42], which has been shown to be true for patients who undergo high anterior resection [43,44]. Low anterior resection, however, has a greater functional impact on urgency, frequency, and degrees of soiling and incontinence [45–47]. Lewis et al [48] reported on function in 11 patients 1 year after straight coloanal anastomosis. Five patients had urgency, 8 had soiling, and the median frequency of evacuation was 4 per day. In a review, Camilleri-Brennan and Steele [49] reported that the quality of life after ultra-low anastomosis varied. Frequency and urgency have been attributed to loss of the rectal reservoir [45,50]. Researchers also have reported that "anterior resection syndrome" may be associated with damage to the inferior mesenteric ganglia and the hypogastric plexus [51]. Matzel et al [52] assessed function with respect to the level of the anastomosis and reported that daily stool frequency ranged from 5.2 to 2.8 to 2.1, and the residual rectum ranged from 0.5 cm to 5.1 cm to 8.9 cm, respectively. Functional variation was matched by physiologic outcome. Maximum tolerated volume ranged from 50 mL to 77 mL to 171 mL, and rectal compliance ranged from 2.6 mL/mm Hg to 3.7 mL/mm Hg to 6.5 mL/mm Hg, respectively.

Low anastomoses also impact on sphincter function. Molloy et al [53] reported a significant resting pressure after coloanal anastomosis, with a greater reduction with hand-sewn compared with stapled anastomosis. Preoperative resting pressure predicts patients who are likely to have postoperative continence problems [54]. Use of transanal staplers can result in internal sphincter damage, with 18% of patients showing persistent anterior anal sphincter defects and defects increasing in frequency as the diameter of the stapler increased [55]. The rectoanal inhibitory reflex is present in 94% of patients preoperatively but only 17% of patients postoperatively. The reflex only recovers in 25% of patients [56]. Anal sensation is also reduced [56]. Resection of the superior portion of the anal canal to obtain tumor clearance also can impact continence. Gamagami et al [57] showed that if less than 1 cm of anal canal is excised, more than 80% of patients remain fully continent, but if 1 cm to 1.25 cm is resected, less than 50% of patients were fully continent at 2 years. Intersphincteric dissection seems to have less impact, however, despite partial resection of the internal sphincter, with 97 of 110 patients fully continent after intersphincteric tumor resection [58]. There is a spectrum of functional outcome after straight coloanal anastomosis. Paty et al [59] assessed function in 81 patients after straight coloanal anastomosis and reported function as excellent in 28%, good in 28%, fair in 32%, and poor in 12%, with frequency and evacuation problems being the major complaints. Patients with larger maximum tolerated volume, lower rectal sensation, and a longer high-pressure zone preoperatively have better early evacuatory function postoperatively [60], but some improvement over time may result from a dilatation of the neorectum [48,61,62].

Colonic reservoirs

J pouch

Functional outcome

The use of a colonic pouch after low colorectal or coloanal anastomosis was first reported in 1986 by Lazorthes et al [63] and Parc et al [64]. Lazorthes et al [63] reported a series of 65 patients after ultra-low anterior resection, 45 of whom underwent a straight coloanal anastomosis and 20 of whom underwent a colonic pouch–anal anastomosis with either a 6- or 12-cm J pouch (Fig. 1). They reported a significant decrease in frequency of defecation in the patients with a colonic pouch, and at 1 year, 86% of patients with a colonic pouch had a frequency of fewer than three per day compared with 33% of patients with a straight anastomosis. These results were echoed by Parc et al [64], who reported no urgency or incontinence in the patients with an 8-cm colonic pouch, but 25% of patients required enemas for pouch evacuation. Nicholls et al [65] reported significantly reduced frequency in patients with a colonic pouch, but three of nine videoproctography studies demonstrated incomplete evacuation in patients with a colonic pouch. Kusunoki et al [66] began a randomized study that

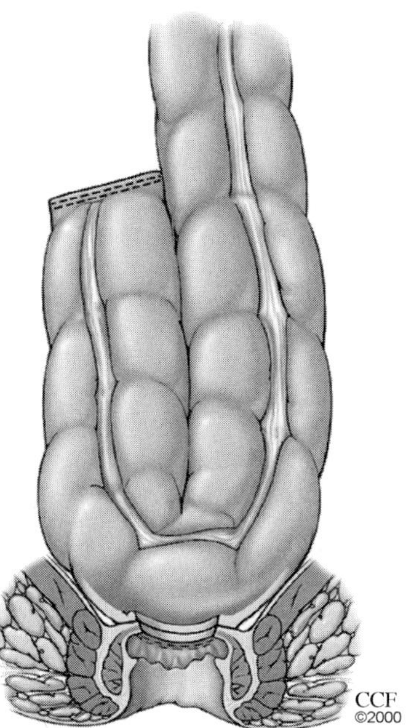

Fig. 1. 8 cm stapled colonic J pouch with double stapled coloanal anastomosis.

compared functional outcome of straight coloanal anastomosis versus colonic pouch–anal anastomosis, but it was stopped because of superior functional results in the colonic pouch group. Several randomized trials that compared straight anastomosis and colonic pouch anastomosis consistently demonstrated reduced frequency at 1 year in patients with a colonic pouch, with a proportion showing decreased urgency and reduced incontinence (Table 2). Functional improvement seems to be preserved over time, although the differences are less dramatic. Dehni et al [67] and Lazorthes et al [68] showed consistent superiority in bowel frequency in patients with a colonic pouch at follow-up of 60 and 24 months, respectively. Joo et al [69], however, reported that by 24 months there was no difference between a straight coloanal and a pouch anal anastomosis in terms of bowel frequency. Any benefits in terms of urgency and incontinence also disappeared by 2 years in all three studies (Table 3) [67–69].

Physiology and pouch size

It seems that the colonic pouch acts as a neorectum in physiologic terms. Maximum tolerated volume and threshold volume are both greater in patients with a colonic pouch compared with a straight anastomosis [65,70,71], although Ho and Seow-Choen [72] failed to demonstrate any difference in a randomized study. Hallbook et al [71] reported improved maximum tolerated volume and compliance in patients with colonic

Table 2
Randomized studies of straight anastomosis versus J pouch after coloanal anastomosis with follow-up at 12 months

Authors	Procedure	No. patient	Functional frequency	*P*	Urgency < 15 min	*P*	Normal continence	*P*	Physiologic resting pressure mm Hg	*P*	Squeeze pressure mm Hg	*P*	Maximum tolerated volume	*P*
Ortiz [101]	Straight	15	1–3/d 10 > 4 11	< 0.05	9	NS	3	NS	42.2 +/− 14.2	NS	135.2 +/− 61.9	NS	148.5 +/− 34.8	< 0.05
	Pouch	15	1–3/d 10 > 4 5		6		6		27.4 +/− 14.2		96.1 +/− 82.0		335 +/− 195.3	
Seow-Chen [102]	Straight	20	2 (0.5–10)	< 0.05	4	NS	14	< 0.01						
	Pouch	19	2 (0.5–4)		2		19							
Hallbook et al [83]	Straight	43	3.5 (2.4–4.5)	< 0.001	45%	< 0.001	2	0.002						
	Pouch	50	2 (1.3–2.3)		7%		5							
Ho [72]	Straight	16	6 (3–7)	0.02	5	NS	16	NS	71.1 (5.8)	0.049	152.7 (14.5)	0.5	174.8 (25.7)	NS
	Pouch	17	3 (2–7)		1		15		55.0 (6.7)		143.5 (18.4)		149.2 (12.2)	

Table 3
Long term functional outcome of straight anastomosis versus J pouch after coloanal anastomosis

Authors	Procedure	No. patient	Follow-up	Frequency	*P*	Urgency < 15 min	*P*	Normal continence	*P*
Lazorthes et al [68]	Straight	16	12 mo	4.5	< 0.01	3		14	NS
	Pouch	15		2.5		2		15	
	Straight	12	24 mo	3.5	< 0.01	0		12	NS
	Pouch	13		2		1		13	
Dehni et al [67]	Straight	34	60 mo	2.8 +/− 1.95	0.001	18		88	NS
	Pouch	47		1.6 +/− 1.1		7		87	
Joo et al [69]	Straight	30	12 mo	4.0 +/− 2.0	< 0.005	11	< 0.05	2.2 +/− 3.7[a]	< 0.05
	Pouch	26		2.4 +/− 1.3		2		0.8 +/− 1.6	
	Straight	27	24 mo	2.5 +/− 1.1	NS	5	NS	1.3 +/− 2.6	NS
	Pouch	15		2.2 +/− 0.9		1		0.8 +/− 1.5	

[a] Incontinence score.

pouches, and Ramirez et al [73] concluded that the colonic pouch acted as a neorectum, because in a comparison between patients who had undergone a high anterior resection and patients who had undergone a coloanal anastomosis with a colonic pouch, there was no difference in terms of manometric or functional outcome.

Pouch size seems to have an impact on function. Berger et al [74] reported that 25% of patients required enemas for evacuation after formation of an 8-cm colonic J pouch. Similar difficulties were reported in other series—in 37% of patients with a 9-cm pouch by Mortensen et al [70] and in 33% of patients with a 10-cm pouch by Nicholls et al [65]. Hida et al [75] randomized patients to either a 5- or 10-cm J pouch. Although the 10-cm pouch had a greater maximum tolerated volume and compliance than the 5-cm pouch, the proportion of patients able to expel a balloon placed in the pouch was significantly less (10 of 20 compared with 18 of 20, respectively). The same group reported that the width of the pouch, assessed by pouchography, was significantly greater in the 10-cm pouch than the 5-cm pouch at 1 and 2 years, with poorer evacuatory function and greater evacuatory difficulty in the 10-cm pouch. They concluded that the 5-cm pouch produced superior function [76]. A mathematical model determined that the optimum pouch size is between 6 and 7 cm [77], although a small study by Lazorthes et al [78] that compared 23 patients with "small" pouches to 24 patients with "large" pouches reported no functional difference between the groups. The consensus is that a pouch size between 5 and 7cm is optimum [79].

Pouch formation, adjuvant therapy, and leak rate

The sigmoid colon and descending colon have been used to form the J pouch. Heah et al [80] compared the two choices and reported no difference, although it was in a population with a low incidence of diverticular disease. With diverticular disease common in Western society and concerns over sigmoid blood supply, the descending colon is preferable for pouch formation, although it requires splenic flexure mobilization [19,79]. Complications related to pouch construction are increased by the use of chemoradiotherapy, which also may have an adverse functional effect [81,82].

Use of a colonic pouch seems to result in a reduction in anastomotic leak rate. Berger et al [74] reported a leak rate of only 3%, which is lower than that reported for most coloanal anastomoses. In a prospective, randomized, controlled trial of straight anastomosis versus colonic pouch, the symptomatic leak rate was 15% in the straight group and only 3% in the pouch-anal group [83]. Researchers reported more than 50 years ago that a colorectal end-to-side anastomosis may have a slightly lower leak rate than a colorectal end-to-end anastomosis [84]. This rate may be caused by perfusion, because Hallbook et al [85] showed that the blood flow of a colonic pouch at the area of anastomosis was superior to that of a straight coloanal pouch using laser Doppler flowmetry.

Coloplasty

There may be problems creating a colonic J pouch–anal anastomosis in some patients, usually men. The narrow male pelvis may make it impossible to bring a bulky colonic pouch down to the anal canal, particularly in patients with fatty mesocolon. If a hand-sewn anastomosis is required, it may be impossible to obtain "reach," with difficulty in bringing down a colonic pouch through the pelvis and through the anal canal, which is usually long and narrow with bulky musculature in men, and generating the risk of tearing the bowel or the blood supply when trying to traverse the canal. An alternative reservoir technique is the coloplasty, which was first described in an animal model by Z'graggen et al [86]. A 4-cm exit conduit is preserved at the distal end of the colon, and an 8-cm longitudinal incision is made through the bowel proximal to this point, which is then closed transversely to form a reservoir [87]. Functional and physiologic results have been found to be comparable to those found with colonic J pouch (Table 4). In a matched study that compared coloplasty with J pouch with straight anastomosis, Mantyh et al [88] reported that reservoir procedures were superior to straight anastomosis with bowel frequency of 2.6 versus 3.1 versus 4.5 bowel movements per day, respectively. These early results—approximately 6 weeks after surgery or ileostomy closures—do seem to persist, however. Ho et al [89] randomized 44 patients to either J pouch or coloplasty. There was a significantly higher leak rate in the coloplasty group (0 versus 15.9%; $P = 0.0121$), but this has not been demonstrated by other studies. The follow-up on the patients was at 4 months and 12 months. Frequency improved over time in the J pouch group (4.5/d to 3/d) and the coloplasty group (4.6/d to 3.4/d). There was no difference between J pouch and coloplasty in resting pressure, squeeze pressure, maximum tolerated volume, or compliance. Furst et al [90] randomized 40 consecutive patients to either J pouch or coloplasty after proctectomy for distal rectal cancer. There was no difference in postoperative complications between the two groups, and they showed no difference in bowel frequency, continence, or urgency. Anorectal physiology testing showed similar results.

Furst et al [90] reported that in 5 of 20 patients randomized to the J pouch group, formation of a pouch was not attempted because of extensive colonic adipose tissue or a narrow male pelvis. Harris et al [91] reviewed reasons for failure to construct a colonic J pouch. Out of 107 patients, it was impossible to construct a colonic J pouch in 28 (26.2%). Seven reasons were identified for failure, either technical (eg, narrow pelvis, bulky anal sphincters, or need for mucosectomy, diverticulosis, insufficient colon length, or pregnancy) or nontechnical (eg, complex surgery or distant metastases present). The coloplasty pouch–anal anastomosis was introduced toward the latter end of the study, and it reduced the incidence of failure to form a reservoir from 27 of 88 (30.7%) to 1 of 19 (5.3%).

A large multicenter, prospective, randomized trial conducted by the Cleveland Clinic that compared coloplasty with colonic J pouch after

Table 4
Functional and physiologic outcome of straight anastomosis versus J pouch versus coloplasty after coloanal anastomosis

Author	Methodology	Reservoir	No. patient	Follow-up	Frequency/24 h	*P*	Maximum volume (mL)	*P*	Compliance mL/mm Hg	*P*
Mantyh et al [88]	Matched	Straight	17	6 wk	4.5 (1–8)	< 0.05[a]	83.3 (34.4)	< 0.05[a]	3.2 (2.1)	< 0.05[a]
		J pouch	16		3.1 (2–6)		150 (56.4)		5.2 (3.1)	
		Coloplasty	20		2.6 (1–5)		116.9 (43.8)		4.9 (2.9)	
Ho et al [89]	Randomized	J pouch	44	52 wk	3 (0.2)	NS	108.3 (13.2)	NS	1.7 (0.4)	NS
		Coloplasty	44		3.4 (0.3)		123.1 (32.4)		3.1 (1.2)	
Furst et al [90]	Randomized	Straight	15[b]	26 wk	2.75 +/− 1	NS	89 +/− 18	NS		
		Coloplasty	20		2 +/− 2		77 +/− 21			

[a] Significant comparing coloplasty and J pouch versus straight anastomosis.
[b] Twenty patients randomized to J pouch but formation impossible because of technical reasons.

proctectomy recently completed recruitment and is awaiting completion of follow-up.

Technical aspects

Selection

Careful selection of patients for coloanal anastomosis is important. Inappropriate selection may result in a compromised oncologic outcome with inadequate tumor clearance or a poor functional outcome, with the patient suffering from intolerable fecal incontinence.

A patient should be assessed with digital rectal examination and rigid proctoscopy to confirm the site and position of the tumor. Local tumor staging should be undertaken using either endoanal ultrasound or MRI [92], with consideration of adjuvant therapy depending on the tumor stage and the management protocols of the institution. At the Cleveland Clinic, low rectal cancers that are staged as T3 or T4 undergo preoperative chemoradiotherapy. Patients who undergo preoperative adjuvant therapy are re-examined after treatment but before surgery to assess tumor response, although the decision over what procedure to undertake is made before adjuvant therapy. All patients should undergo staging to assess for distant disease with an abdominal CT scan, chest radiograph, and a colonoscopy to rule out synchronous neoplasms.

Consideration of whether a coloanal anastomosis is feasible depends on the ability to obtain adequate tumor clearance and assessment of the likely postoperative function. Tumor invasion into the external sphincter necessitates APER, and compromising oncologic outcome for sphincter preservation must be avoided, as commented by Heister more than 200 years ago "...it is surely better to part with one of the conveniences of life than to part with life itself" [93]. The determination of obtaining clearance is made from a combination of clinical assessments, which may include examination under anesthesia and staging investigations. It may be necessary to undertake intersphincteric dissection to obtain adequate clearance from the tumor. If adequate clearance is deemed possible, postoperative function if an anastomosis is undertaken should be considered. Preoperative anorectal physiology, with measurement of resting and squeeze pressures, may predict postoperative function [54]. Endoanal ultrasound to assess for occult sphincter damage may be valuable in female patients [94]. Church et al [95] reported that a comprehensive history and examination by an experienced surgeon are likely to be the best predictors of postoperative function, however.

Mobilization

All patients are given preoperative antibiotics and mechanical bowel preparation. Patients are placed in the modified lithotomy position using

Lloyd-Davies stirrups. A midline incision is performed, and after a full laparostomy, the colon is mobilized from the pelvic brim to the middle colic vessels, including the splenic flexure. The inferior mesenteric artery is divided high near its origin from the aorta, and the inferior mesenteric artery is divided a second time at the lower border of the pancreas to allow adequate length of descending colon to be brought down into the pelvis. The descending colon is divided at its junction with the sigmoid, and the perfusion of the proximal end of colon is assessed by observation of pulsatile flow from the marginal artery and mucosal bleeding. The blood supply of the descending colon depends on the marginal vessel supplied from the middle colic artery. Poor blood supply— such as may result from damage to the arcade of Riolan at the splenic flexure or secondary to atherosclerotic disease—may necessitate resection of the left colon, mobilization of the hepatic flexure, and anastomosis using transverse colon based on ileocolic artery perfusion.

The pelvis is entered using electrocautery in the plane between Waldeyer's fascia and the investing fascia propria of the rectum, with preservation of the hypogastric nerves and ureters. Waldeyer's fascia is divided and dissection continues beyond the tip of the coccyx to the pelvic floor. Dissection is extended laterally and finally anteriorly in a plane in front of Denonvillier's fascia, and a total mesorectal excision is performed. Dissection continues into the infralevator plane beyond the caudal extent of the mesorectum to expose the muscle tube of the most distal rectum, which consists of the circular muscle fibers that continue as the internal anal sphincter and the longitudinal muscle fibers that extend to the anorectal ring. Low pelvic dissection in an obese man with a narrow pelvis may be difficult and may be aided by pushing on the perineum [18].

Rectal division

The surgeon must assess the level of the tumor to determine whether adequate clearance can be obtained by transecting the distal rectum with a stapler or whether intersphincteric dissection with division of the internal anal sphincter in the anal canal is required. This assessment is best done by digital rectal examination. If the surgeon believes that adequate distal margin can be obtained with pelvic division of the rectum with a stapler, the rectum is washed out with cytocidal solution (Turnball 70% alcohol solution in our practice), the rectum is cross-clamped below the tumor, and a transverse stapler of appropriate size (usually a PI-30) is placed across the muscle tube. The level of placement on the muscle tube depends on the assessment of the tumor position, and attainment of adequate clearance from the tumor is vital. It is possible to place the stapler as low as the level of the upper anal canal, particularly in women. Upon release of the stapler, the staple line retreats to within the muscle groups of the levators. In low tumors it may be impossible to place a clamp between the tumor and the transverse stapler, but with copious irrigation of the rectum anally using cytocidal solution during stapler application, oncologic outcome does not seem to be compromised.

If it seems that the transverse stapler will encroach onto the tumor, it may be necessary to divide the internal sphincter within the anal canal, below the tumor, continue the dissection up the intersphincteric plane, and break into the pelvis just above the anorectal ring. Our preference is to place one vicryl effacing anal suture to facilitate exposure of the anal canal. Diathermy is used to divide the mucosa and internal sphincter circumferentially at the appropriate level depending on the tumor height, often just above dentate, and the dissection continues into the pelvis between the internal and external sphincters. Once the pelvis is entered, the specimen is freed and can be removed. If the top of the anal canal has been stapled via the pelvis and the rectum is removed but the surgeon decides to perform a hand-sewn anastomosis, the proximal part of the internal sphincter and the staple line may be excised via the transanal approach.

Reservoir formation

The decision regarding whether to undertake a straight coloanal, pouch–anal, or coloplasty anal anastomosis depends on various factors. There must be adequate length of colon to reach the upper anus, and either the end of the colon or the proposed apex of the pouch should be grasped with a Babcock forceps and placed in the pelvis to ensure adequate reach to enable formation of a tension-free anastomosis. The reach of a straight anastomosis is likely to be slightly longer than either reservoir procedure but is usually only indicated if—after mobilization of the colon—it is impossible to get adequate length for reservoir formation and anastomosis without tension. The surgeon also must assess the shape and size of the pelvis and the size of the colon and mesentery to determine whether a colonic J pouch will fit in the pelvis or whether a coloplasty is more appropriate. It is important in all cases to observe brisk bleeding from the cut distal end of the colon to ensure adequate blood supply.

Colonic J pouch

A linen tape is tied around the proximal colon to minimize fecal spillage. A colonic J pouch of approximately 8 to 10 cm long usually is created (Fig. 2). The apex of the proposed pouch is identified after measurement and grasped with a Babcock forceps and placed in the pelvis to ensure adequate reach. A longitudinal enterotomy is made with diathermy at the proposed apex of the pouch, and a linear staple cutter is inserted along both limbs of the colon. We usually use a singly firing ILA-100 linear stapler, which creates a side-to-side anastomosis between the two colonic limbs. The pouch interior is checked for hemostasis by direct observation of the internal staple

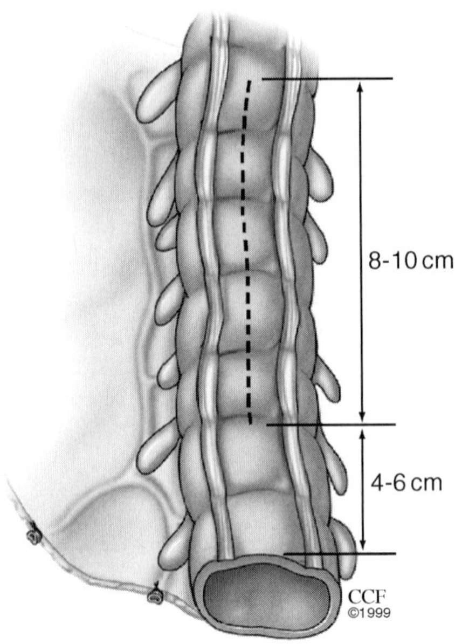

Fig. 2. A longitudinal colotomy is made 4 to 6 cm from the distal end of the colon and around 8 to 10 cm in length.

line by grasping it with a Babcock forceps and everting the staple line as required. Then the open distal end of the colon, which forms the tip of the J pouch, is closed with a transverse stapler, and the staple line is oversewn with 3-0 polyglycolic acid sutures. The pouch is irrigated to confirm absence of leaks, remove any blood from the pouch interior, and assess pouch size. If a stapled anastomosis is planned, a 0 prolene purse string suture is placed in the apex enterotomy.

Coloplasty

After placement of the linen tape, the distal colon is irrigated [87]. A longitudinal colotomy is made 4 to 6 cm from the distal end of the colon and is approximately 8 to 10 cm long. The aim is to create an exit conduit approximately 3 to 4 cm long. If a stapled anastomosis is planned, the colotomy begins 4 cm from the distal end of the colon. If a hand-sewn anastomosis is planned, the colotomy is started 6 cm from the distal end because it may be necessary to excise the most distal tissue, which can be traumatized when delivering the colon transanally. The colotomy is closed transversely, in the fashion of a Heinecke-Mikulicz strictureplasty, with a single layer of interrupted 2-0 polyglycolic acid sutures (Figs. 3A and 3B). The colon is irrigated with saline to assess the integrity and size of the coloplasty. If a stapled anastomosis is planned, a 0 prolene purse string suture is placed in the distal end of the colon (Fig. 4).

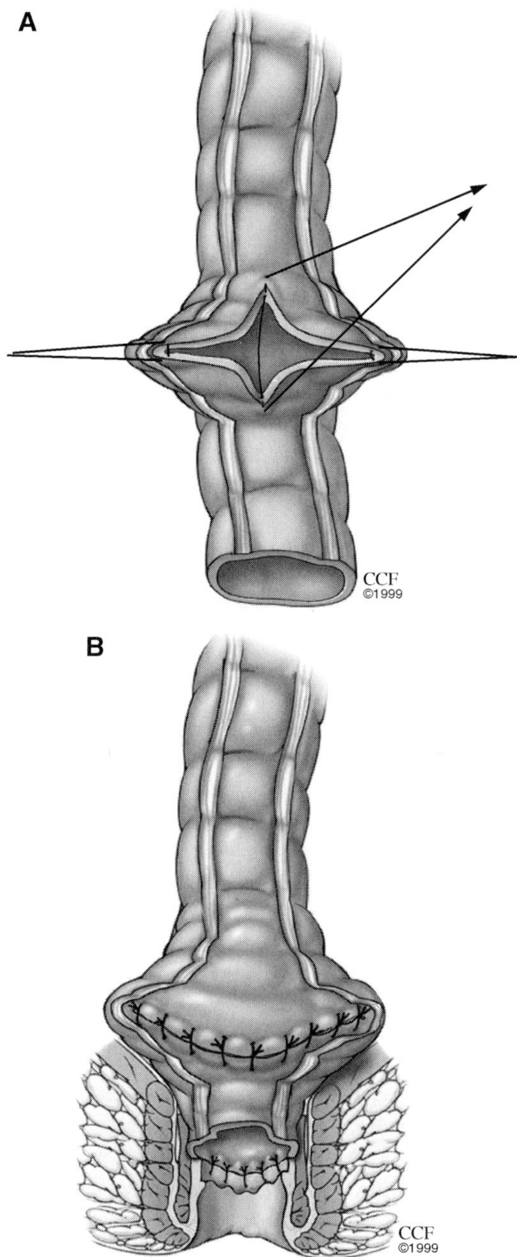

Fig. 3. (*A*) The colotomy is closed transversely, in the fashion of a Heinecke–Mikulicz strictureplasty, (*B*) with a single layer of interrupted 2/0 polyglycolic acid sutures.

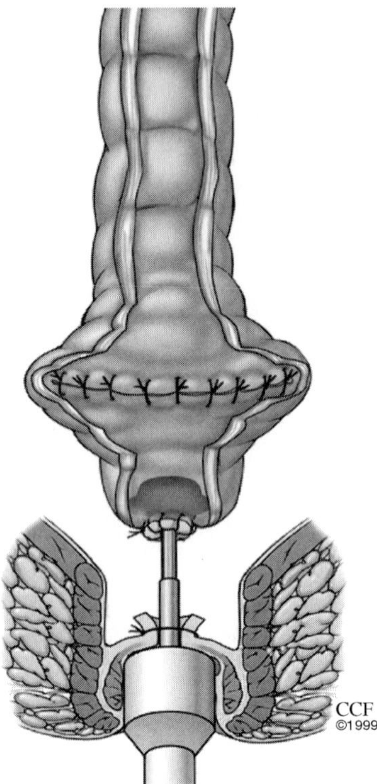

Fig. 4. The colon is anastomosed to the top of the anal canal by either hand-sewn anastomosis of double stapled anastomosis, having placed an 0 prolene purse string suture in the distal end of the colon.

Anastomosis

Stapled anastomosis

If it is possible to staple the distal rectum, a stapled anastomosis usually can be undertaken. A 29-mm EEA circular stapling gun is normally used, the anvil is placed in the distal end of the colon or J pouch, and the purse string is tied. The circular staple gun is inserted gently through the anal sphincters. Inevitably the staple line is low and great care must be taken not to rupture the staple line when inserting the gun. We lubricate the gun well and use large Allis forceps applied to the anal verge to aid insertion of the gun. The operating surgeon may insert the gun bimanually to enable the staple line to be supported with one hand while the gun is inserted and ensure appropriate placement of the circular ring of the cartridge section centered on the staple line. An assistant may open the gun and advance the central pin while the operating surgeon holds the shaft of the gun and confirms that the gun position is such that the central pin penetrates the bowel just posterior to the staple line, particularly in women. In this way, the ultimate anastomosis is far less likely to cause injury to the posterior vaginal wall. The anvil then can be engaged into the central shaft of the gun. As the gun is closed, it is important to ensure that no additional tissue, such as the posterior vaginal wall, is trapped within the gun by using an appropriately placed lighted anterior deep pelvic retractor. After closure of the gun, it then can be fired. The gun is rotated gently and removed while the colon is supported to avoid any damage to it.

The tissue rings contained within the gun are inspected to confirm that they are complete. The pelvis is irrigated with saline and air is insufflated through the anus, with the colon occluded at the pelvic brim. Any air leak is noted.

Hand-sewn anastomosis

If a hand-sewn anastomosis is performed, patient already has sutures placed to efface the anus. Alternative methods of exposure include the Lone Star retractor or intra-anal retractors, such as Parks or Eisenhammer, although they cause some degree of sphincter dilatation. A mucosectomy is performed—if it has not already been done to remove the specimen—to divide the mucosa around the level of the dentate line and divide the internal anal sphincter at some point cranial to this, depending on the resection margin indicated.

A Babcock forceps is passed through the anal canal and the distal end of the colon is grasped. The distal colon is brought down into the pelvis and through the anal canal. A second Babcock forceps may be applied to spread the tension and aid delivery of the colon. It is important that excess force is avoided so that the colon is not damaged. The colon or J pouch should be placed down in the pelvis and "sat" by the pelvic surgeon because it aids delivery through the anal canal, which passes forward and anteriorly from the pelvis. Once the surgeon confirms that the colon will pass through the anal canal without tension, it is removed and the anal canal sutures are placed. Four sutures of 2-0 polyglycolic acid are placed at the four quarters of the clock, with a further suture placed between each, which results in a total of eight sutures. The sutures are placed through mucosa just below the level of mucosal division at the level of the dentate line and passed through the internal sphincter into the anal canal. It is important that a substantial amount of internal sphincter is taken to provide support for the anastomosis. Each suture is held with a hemostat. The colon is then delivered through the anal canal again, and the individual sutures are passed from outside the colon to inside. It is important to take a substantial amount of colon with the sutures at approximately 1 cm. If the distal end of the colon seems traumatized, it is excised and the sutures are tied. The anastomosis is re-assessed, and at any position in which there is a gap in the anastomosis large enough to pass a pair of forceps, a further stitch is placed. The everting anal sutures are removed and the anastomosis "disappears" from view up the anal canal.

Drainage

We routinely drain the pelvis for all low colorectal or coloanal anastomoses with a closed suction drain.

Ileostomy

The decision to perform a diverting loop ileostomy is the same whether the anastomosis is low colorectal, straight coloanal, pouch-anal, or coloplasty-anal. All hand-sewn anastomoses are defunctioned, which is done if there is any concern over factors influencing the integrity of the anastomosis, such as preoperative radiotherapy, incomplete tissue rings, or a leak detected during testing of the anastomosis.

Closure

Patients are reviewed in the office approximately 4 to 6 weeks after discharge, and the anastomosis is assessed by digital rectal examination. Flexible endoscopic examination is performed to inspect any reservoir formed, and a gastrograffin enema is administered to confirm anastomotic and reservoir integrity. If there is no evidence of a leak, the ileostomy is closed approximately 3 months after the original surgery.

If an anastomotic leak is identified, ileostomy closure is deferred. Anastomotic leaks close if there is adequate drainage of any cavity present behind the anastomotic defect. The anastomosis must be examined, which may require administration of anesthesia. It may be necessary to widen the anastomotic defect to ensure adequate drainage, and a mushroom catheter may be inserted through the defect for a period of a few weeks to encourage drainage. The catheter can be removed easily later in the office. It may take a few months for any cavity to close, and the anastomosis can be reassessed by further gastrograffin studies. Once the leak has closed, the ileostomy can be reversed.

Summary

There has been a gradual progression in rectal cancer surgery from the time of Miles, when APER was the procedure of choice, to the current time, with the use of coloanal anastomosis and surgeons striving for sphincter preservation. The incidence of APER can be as low as 10%, although it is still the appropriate procedure for many patients [96]. Technical developments have allowed the use of coloanal anastomosis, which have been shown to be equivalent in terms of local recurrence and survival and have the advantage of avoidance of a permanent stoma. Acknowledgment of the importance of functional outcome for patients has encouraged the use of reservoirs to preserve function. Surgeons should perform sphincter-preserving surgery for most cases of rectal cancer with significant functional preservation.

References

[1] Ruo L, Guillem J. Major 20th-century advances in the management of rectal cancer. Dis Colon Rectum 1999;42:563–78.

[2] Miles E. A method of performing abdominopelvic excision for carcinoma of the rectum and of the terminal portion of the pelvic colon. Lancet 1908;2:1812–3.

[3] Mayo W. The radical operation for cancer of the rectum and rectosigmoid. Trans Am Surg Assoc 1916;34:261–72.
[4] Kraske P. Zur exstirpation hochsitzender mastdarmkrebse. Verhdt Chir 1885;14:464.
[5] Hochenegg J. Mein operation der folge bei rektumkarzinom. Wien Klin Wochenschr 1900; 13:399.
[6] Babcock W. Experience with resection of the colon and the elimination of colostomy. Am J Surg 1939;46:186–95.
[7] Bacon H. Evolution of sphincter muscle preservation and re-establishment of continuity in the operative treatment of rectal and sigmoid cancer. Surg Gynecol Obstet 1945;81: 113–27.
[8] Black B. Combined abdomino-endorectal resection. Arch Surg 1952;65:406–16.
[9] Dixon C. Surgical removal of lesions occurring in the sigmoid rectosigmoid. Am J Surg 1939;46:12–7.
[10] Turnbull RJ, Cuthbertson F. Abdomino rectal pull-through resection for cancer and for Hirschprung's disease. Cleve Clin Q 1961;28:109–15.
[11] Cutait D, Figlioni F. A new method of colorectal anastomosis in abdomino-perineal resection. Dis Colon Rectum 1961;4:335–42.
[12] Parks A. Transanal technique in low rectal anastomoses. Proc R Soc Med 1972;65:975–6.
[13] Localio S, Eng K, Gouge T, et al. Abdomino-sacral resection for carcinoma of the mid-rectum: 10 years' experience. Ann Surg 1978;188:745–8.
[14] Mason A. Trans-sphincteric exposure for low rectal anastomosis. Proc R Soc Med 1972; 65:974.
[15] Parks A, Percy J. Resection and sutured colo-anal anastomosis for rectal carcinoma. Br J Surg 1982;69:301–4.
[16] Knight C, Griffen F. An improved technique for low anterior resection of the rectum using the EEA stapler. Surgery 1980;88:710–4.
[17] Heald RJ, Smedh RK, Kald A, et al. Abdominoperineal excision of the rectum: an endangered operation: Norman Nigro lectureship. Dis Colon Rectum 1997;40(7):747–51.
[18] Read T, Kodner I. Proctectomy and coloanal anastomosis for rectal cancer. Arch Surg 1999;134:670–7.
[19] Tytherleigh M, Mortensen N. Options for sphincter preservation in surgery for low rectal cancer. Br J Surg 2003;90(8):922–33.
[20] Church J, Raudkivi P, Hill G. The surgical anatomy of the rectum: a review with particular relevance to the hazards of rectal mobilization. Int J Colorectal Dis 1987;2(3):158–66.
[21] McMinn R. Last's anatomy. London: Churchill-Livingstone; 1990.
[22] Westhues H. Die pathologisch-anatomischen grundlagen der chirurgie des rektum karzinoms. Leipzig: Georg Thieme; 1934.
[23] Dukes C. The classification of cancer of the rectum. J Pathol Bacteriol 1932;35:323–32.
[24] Grinnell R. Distal intramural spread of carcinoma of the rectum and rectosigmoid. Surg Gynecol Obstet 1954;99:421–9.
[25] Goligher J, Dukes C, Bussey H. Local recurrences after sphincter saving excisions for carcinoma of the rectum and rectosigmoid. Br J Surg 1951;39:199–211.
[26] Pollett WG, Nicholls RJ. The relationship between the extent of distal clearance and survival and local recurrence rates after curative anterior resection for carcinoma of the rectum. Ann Surg 1983;198(2):159–63.
[27] Wolmark N, Fischer B. An analysis of survival and treatment failure following abdominoperineal and sphincter saving resection in Dukes B and C rectal carcinoma. Ann Surg 1986;204:480–7.
[28] Williams NS, Dixon MF, Johnston D. Reappraisal of the 5 centimetre rule of distal excision for carcinoma of the rectum: a study of distal intramural spread and of patients' survival. Br J Surg 1983;70(3):150–4.
[29] Shirouzu K, Isomoto H, Kakegawa T. Distal spread of rectal cancer and optimal distal margin of resection for sphincter preserving surgery. Cancer 1995;76:388–92.

[30] Andreola S, Leo E, Belli F, et al. Distal intramural spread in adenocarcinoma of the lower third of the rectum treated with total rectal resection and coloanal anastomosis. Dis Colon Rectum 1997;40:25–9.
[31] Karanjia ND, Schache DJ, North WR, et al. Close shave in anterior resection. Br J Surg 1990;77(5):510–2.
[32] Phillips RK, Hittinger R, Blesovsky L, et al. Local recurrence following curative surgery for large bowel cancer: II. The rectum and rectosigmoid. Br J Surg 1984;71(1):17–20.
[33] Hermanek P. Onkologische chirurgie/pathologisch-anatomische sicht. Langenbecks Arch Chir 1991;191:277–81.
[34] Schiessel R, Karner-Hanusch J, Herbst F, et al. Intersphincteric resection for low rectal tumours. Br J Surg 1994;81:1376–8.
[35] Teramoto T, Watanabe M, Kitajima M. Per anum intersphincteric rectal dissection with direct coloanal anastomosis for lower rectal cancer: the ultimate sphincter-preserving operation. Dis Colon Rectum 1997;40(Suppl 10):S43–7.
[36] Rullier E, Zerbib F, Laurent C, et al. Intersphincteric resection with excision of the internal anal sphincter for conservative treatment of very low rectal cancer. Dis Colon Rectum 1999; 42:1168–75.
[37] Fucini C, Elbetti C, Petrolo A, et al. Excision of the levator muscles with external sphincter preservation in the treatment of selected low T4 rectal cancers. Dis Colon Rectum 2002;45: 1697–705.
[38] Rouanet P, Fabre JM, Dubois JB, et al. Conservative surgery for low rectal carcinoma after high-dose radiation: functional and oncologic results. Ann Surg 1995;221(1):67–73.
[39] Grann A, Minsky B, Cohen A, et al. Preliminary results of preoperative 5-fluorouracil, low-dose leucovorin, and concurrent radiation therapy for clinically resectable T3 rectal cancer. Dis Colon Rectum 1997;40(5):515–22.
[40] Rullier E, Goffre B, Bonnel C, et al. Preoperative radiochemotherapy and sphincter-saving resection for T3 carcinomas of the lower third of the rectum. Ann Surg 2001;234:633–40.
[41] Williams NS, Johnston D. The quality of life after rectal excision for low rectal cancer. Br J Surg 1983;70(8):460–2.
[42] Frigell A, Ottander M, Stenbeck H, et al. Quality of life of patients treated with abdominoperineal resection or anterior resection for rectal carcinoma. Ann Chir Gynaecol 1990;79:26–30.
[43] Whynes D, Neilson A, Robinson M, et al. Colorectal cancer screening and quality of life. Qual Life Res 1994;3:191–8.
[44] Jess P, Christiansen J, Bech P. Quality of life after anterior resection versus abdominoperineal extirpation for rectal cancer. Scand J Gastroenterol 2002;37:1201–4.
[45] Lane R, Parks A. Function of the anal sphincter following coloanal anastomosis. Br J Surg 1977;64:596–9.
[46] Keighley MR, Matheson D. Functional results of rectal excision and endo-anal anastomosis. Br J Surg 1980;67(10):757–61.
[47] McDonald P, Heald R. A survey of postoperative function after rectal anastomosis with circular stapling devices. Br J Surg 1983;70:727–9.
[48] Lewis W, Holdsworth P, Stephenson B, et al. Role of the rectum in the physiological and clinical results of coloanal and colorectal anastomosis after anterior resection for rectal cancer. Br J Surg 1992;79:1082–6.
[49] Camilleri-Brennan J, Steele R. Quality of life after treatment for rectal cancer. Br J Surg 1998;85:1036–43.
[50] Williams NS, Price R, Johnston D. The long term effect of sphincter preserving operations for rectal carcinoma on function of the anal sphincter in man. Br J Surg 1980;67(3):203–8.
[51] Rao G, Drew P, Lee P, et al. Anterior resection syndrome is secondary to sympathetic denervation. Int J Colorectal Dis 1996;11:250–8.
[52] Matzel K, Stadelmaier U, Muehldorfer S, et al. Continence after colorectal reconstruction following resection: impact of level of anastomosis. Int J Colorectal Dis 1997;12:82–7.

[53] Molloy R, Moran K, Coulter J, et al. Mechanism of sphincter impairment following low anterior resection. Dis Colon Rectum 1992;35:462–4.
[54] Matsushita K, Yamada K, Sameshima T, et al. Prediction of incontinence following low anterior resection for rectal carcinoma. Dis Colon Rectum 1997;40:575–9.
[55] Farouk R, Duthie G, Lee P, et al. Endosonographic evidence of injury to the internal anal sphincter after low anterior resection: long-term follow-up. Dis Colon Rectum 1998;41: 888–91.
[56] Otto I, Ito K, Ye C, et al. Causes of rectal incontinence after sphincter-preserving operations for rectal cancer. Dis Colon Rectum 1996;39:1423–7.
[57] Gamagami R, Istvan G, Cabarrot P, et al. Fecal continence following partial resection of the anal canal in distal rectal cancer: long-term results after coloanal anastomoses. Surgery 2000;127:291–5.
[58] Holzer B, Feil W, Holbling N, et al. Long-term results after intersphincteric resection of very low rectal cancers. Presented at the Meeting of the European Association of Coloproctology. Erlangen, September 12–14, 2002.
[59] Paty P, Enker W, Cohen A, et al. Long-term functional results of coloanal anastomosis for rectal cancer. Am J Surg 1994;167:90–5.
[60] Yamana T, Oya M, Komatsu J, et al. Preoperative anal sphincter high pressure zone, maximum tolerable volume, and anal mucosal electrosensitivity predict early postoperative defecatory function after low anterior resection for rectal cancer. Dis Colon Rectum 1999; 42:1145–51.
[61] Pedersen I, Hint K, Olsen J, et al. Anorectal function after low anterior resection for carcinoma. Ann Surg 1986;204:133–5.
[62] McAnena O, Heald R, Lockhart-Mummery H. Operative and functional results of total mesorectal excision with ultralow anterior resection in the management of carcinoma of the lower one-third of the rectum. Surg Gynecol Obstet 1990;170:517–21.
[63] Lazorthes F, Fages P, Chiotasso P, et al. Resection of the rectum with construction of a colonic reservoir and colo-anal anastomosis for carcinoma of the rectum. Br J Surg 1986; 73:136–8.
[64] Parc R, Tiret E, Frileux P, et al. Resection and colo-anal anastomosis with colonic reservoir for rectal cancer. Br J Surg 1986;73:139–41.
[65] Nicholls RJ, Lubowski DZ, Donaldson DR. Comparison of colonic reservoir and straight colo-anal reconstruction after rectal excision. Br J Surg 1988;75(4):318–20.
[66] Kusunoki M, Shoji Y, Yanagi H, et al. Function after anoabdominal rectal resection and colonic pouch-anal anastomosis. Br J Surg 1991;78(12):1434–8.
[67] Dehni N, Tiret E, Singland J, et al. Long-term functional outcome after low anterior resection: comparison of low colorectal anastomosis and colonic J-pouch-anal anastomosis. Dis Colon Rectum 1998;41:817–23.
[68] Lazorthes F, Chiotasso P, Gamagami R, et al. Late clinical outcome in a randomized prospective comparison of colonic J pouch and straight coloanal anastomosis. Br J Surg 1997;84:1449–51.
[69] Joo J, Latulippe J, Alabaz O, et al. Long-term functional evaluation of straight coloanal anastomosis and colonic J-pouch. Dis Colon Rectum 1998;41:740–6.
[70] Mortensen N, Ramirez J, Takeuchi N, et al. Colonic J pouch-anal anastomosis after rectal excision for carcinoma: functional outcome. Br J Surg 1995;82:611–3.
[71] Hallbook O, Nystrom P, Sjodahl R. Physiologic characteristics of straight and colonic J-pouch anastomoses after rectal excision for cancer. Dis Colon Rectum 1997;40: 322–8.
[72] Ho Y-H, Seow-Choen F. Prospective randomized controlled study of clinical function and anorectal physiology after low anterior resection: comparison of straight and colonic J pouch anastomosis. Br J Surg 1996;83:978–80.
[73] Ramirez J, Mortensen N, Takeuchi N, et al. Colonic J-pouch rectal reconstruction: is it really a neorectum? Dis Colon Rectum 1996;39:1286–8.

[74] Berger A, Tiret E, Parc R, et al. Excision of the rectum with colonic J pouch-anal anastomosis for adenocarcinoma of the low and mid rectum. World J Surg 1992;16:470–7.
[75] Hida J, Yasutomi M, Fujimoto K, et al. Functional outcome after low anterior resection with low anastomosis for rectal cancer using the colonic J-pouch: prospective randomized study for determination of optimum pouch size. Dis Colon Rectum 1996;39:986–91.
[76] Hida J, Yasutomi M, Maruyama T, et al. Enlargement of colonic pouch after proctectomy and coloanal anastomosis: potential cause for evacuatory difficulty. Dis Colon Rectum 1999;42:1181–8.
[77] Banerjee A, Parc R. Prediction of optimum dimensions of colonic pouch reservoir. Dis Colon Rectum 1996;39:1293–5.
[78] Lazorthes F, Gamagami R, Chiotasso P, et al. Prospective, randomized study comparing clinical results between small and large colonic J-pouch following coloanal anastomosis. Dis Colon Rectum 1997;40:1409–13.
[79] Williams N, Seow-Choen F. Physiological and functional outcome following ultra-low anterior resection with colon pouch-anal anastomosis. Br J Surg 1998;85:1029–35.
[80] Heah S, Seow-Choen F, Eu K, et al. Prospective, randomised trial comparing sigmoid vs. descending colonic J-pouch after total rectal excision. Dis Colon Rectum 2002;45:322–8.
[81] Kusunoki M, Yanagi H, Shoji Y, et al. Anoabdominal rectal resection and colonic J pouch-anal anastomosis: 10 years' experience. Br J Surg 1997;84:1277–80.
[82] Gervaz P, Rotholtz N, Wexner S, et al. Colonic J-pouch function in rectal cancer patients: impact of adjuvant chemoradiotherapy. Dis Colon Rectum 2001;44:1667–75.
[83] Hallbook O, Pahlman L, Krog M, et al. Randomized comparison of straight and colonic J pouch anastomosis after low anterior resection. Ann Surg 1996;224(1):58–65.
[84] Baker J. Low end to side rectosigmoid anastomoses: description of technique. Arch Surg 1950;61:143–57.
[85] Hallbook O, Johansson K, Sjodahl R. Laser Doppler blood flow measurement in rectal resection for carcinoma: comparison between the straight and colonic J pouch reconstruction. Br J Surg 1996;83:389–92.
[86] Z'graggen K, Maurer C, Mettler D, et al. A novel colon pouch and its comparison with straight coloanal and colon J-pouch anal anastomosis: preliminary results in pigs. Surgery 1999;125:105–12.
[87] Fazio V, Mantyh C, Hull T. Colonic coloplasty: novel technique to enhance low colorectal or coloanal anastomosis. Dis Colon Rectum 2000;43:1448–50.
[88] Mantyh C, Hull T, Fazio V. Coloplasty in low colorectal anastomosis: manometric and functional comparison with straight and colonic J-pouch anastomosis. Dis Colon Rectum 2001;44:37–42.
[89] Ho Y-H, Brown S, Heah S, et al. Comparison of J-pouch and coloplasty pouch for low rectal cancers. Ann Surg 2002;236(1):49–55.
[90] Furst A, Suttner S, Agha A, et al. Colonic J-pouch vs coloplasty following resection of distal rectal cancer. Dis Colon Rectum 2003;46:1161–6.
[91] Harris G, Lavery I, Fazio V. Reasons for failure to construct the colonic J-pouch: what can be done to improve the size of the neorectal reservoir should it occur? Dis Colon Rectum 2002;45:1304–8.
[92] Heriot A, Grundy A, Kumar D. Preoperative staging of rectal carcinoma. Br J Surg 1999; 86:17–28.
[93] Heister L. A general system of surgery. London: W. Innys; 1743.
[94] Miller A, Lewis W, Williamson M, et al. Factors that influence the functional outcome after coloanal anastomosis for carcinoma of the rectum. Br J Surg 1995;82:1327–30.
[95] Church J, Saad R, Schroeder T, et al. Predicting the functional result of anastomoses to the anus: the paradox of preoperative anal resting pressure. Dis Colon Rectum 1993;36: 895–900.
[96] Dowdall J, Maguire D, McAnena O. Experience of surgery for rectal cancer with total mesorectal excision in a general surgical practice. Br J Surg 2002;89:1014–9.

[97] Hautefeuille P, Valleur P, Pernicini T, et al. Functional and oncological results after coloanal anastomosis for low rectal carcinoma. Ann Surg 1988;207:61–4.

[98] Cavaliere F, Pemberton JH, Cosimelli M, et al. Coloanal anastomosis for rectal cancer. Long-term results at the Mayo and Cleveland Clinics. Diseases of the Colon & Rectum 1995;38:807–12.

[99] Gamagami R, Liagre A, Chiotasso P, et al. Coloanal anastomosis for distal third rectal cancer. Prospective study of oncological results. Dis Colon Rectum 1999;42:1272–5.

[100] Berger A, Tiret E, Cunningham C, et al. Rectal excision and colonic pouch-anal anastomosis for rectal cancer. Dis Colon Rectum 1999;42:1265–71.

[101] Ortiz H, De Miguel M, Armendariz P, et al. Coloanal anastomosis: are functional results better with a pouch? Dis Colon Rectum 1995;38:375–7.

[102] Seow-Choen F, Goh H. Prospective randomized trial comparing J colonic pouch anal anastomosis and straight coloanal anastomosis. Br J Surg 1995;82:608–10.

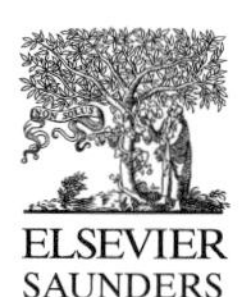
ELSEVIER
SAUNDERS

Surg Oncol Clin N Am
14 (2005) 183–196

SURGICAL
ONCOLOGY CLINICS
OF NORTH AMERICA

Local Excision: Some Reality Testing

Anders Mellgren, MD, PhD[a], Joel Goldberg, MD[a], David A. Rothenberger, MD[a,b,*]

[a]*Division of Colon and Rectal Surgery, Department of Surgery, University of Minnesota Medical School, 393 Dunlap St N #500, St Paul, MN 55104, USA*
[b]*University of Minnesota Cancer Center, MMC 806, 420 Delaware Street SE, Minneapolis, MN 55455, USA*

The role of local therapy for management of rectal cancer has been debated for decades, but its use is generally limited to unusual circumstances and "early-stage" disease. If technically feasible, local therapy may be an appropriate treatment for medically infirm patients with rectal cancer who would not tolerate radical resection or palliation of patients with symptomatic but incurable rectal cancer. More debatable is the use of local therapy for normal risk patients who refuse a recommended radical resection because of a high likelihood that a permanent colostomy will be necessary.

Some physicians argue that it is unethical to compromise the potential for cure because a patient prefers one treatment to another. Their view is that such patient demands should be refused. Other clinicians accept the primacy of a patient's demands and proceed with local therapy after obtaining informed consent of the potential consequences of what they consider to be a compromised form of treatment.

The role of local therapy as the preferred option for curative intent treatment of normal risk patients with favorable rectal cancer is highly controversial. Some surgeons virtually never recommend this approach because of their conviction that local therapy is associated with a higher rate of local recurrence and a lower survival rate than that which can be achieved with radical surgery. Other surgeons aggressively pursue local therapy options in the hope of curing a patient without the risks of mortality and serious morbidity associated with radical resection.

* Corresponding author. University of Minnesota Cancer Center, MMC 806, 420 Delaware Street SE, Minneapolis, MN 55455.

E-mail address: rothe002@umn.edu (D.A. Rothenberger).

doi:10.1016/j.soc.2004.11.007

Rationale for local therapy

The major benefits of local therapy for rectal cancer are negligible mortality, minimal morbidity, rapid postoperative recovery, preservation of genitourinary function, and maintenance of near-normal anal continence with avoidance of a permanent colostomy. Proponents of local therapy also argue that if recurrence develops, salvage radical treatment is often possible with good long-term results [1]. Retrospective reviews have suggested that survival after local therapy for properly selected rectal cancers is equal to that achieved with more radical surgery [2–4]. Conventional management of rectal cancer with radical surgery is far from perfect. The operative mortality rate is 2% to 3% in modern series. Major morbidity is common (30%–46%), and functional results are often suboptimal [5]. In addition to these drawbacks, a significant number of patients with rectal cancer treated by traditional radical therapy are not cured. They may die of disseminated disease that was present but occult at their initial operation, or in 5% to 30% of cases they may develop a fatal local recurrence despite radical extirpation of what seemed to be localized rectal cancer. Other patients may be overtreated if they undergo radical resection for a rectal cancer that on pathologic analysis was a T_1N_0 adenocarcinoma that theoretically could have been cured by local means. For all of these reasons, surgeons remain interested in developing local therapy alternatives to radical surgery.

Terminology and classifications

Terminology of polypoid neoplasms

As screening colonoscopy becomes more commonplace, the diagnosis of cancer arising in a polypoid neoplasm undoubtedly will be made more often. The incidence of invasive cancer in a polyp ranges from 1.5% to 12% in resected adenomas. The probability of cancer arising in a polyp correlates with polyp size and histology and ranges from 0.1% for a tubular adenoma smaller than 6 mm to 40% for a villous adenoma larger than 3 cm.

The terminology used to describe polypoid cancers and cancer that arises in polyps is often confusing. The commonly used but imprecise term "polypoid neoplasms" encompasses a wide spectrum of lesions. If cancer cells are confined to the mucosa of a polyp or a polypoid mass, the lesion may be labeled as high-grade dysplasia, severe dysplasia, carcinoma in situ, or intramucosal carcinoma. These terms are synonyms for a noninvasive adenocarcinoma that is classified as a $TisN_xM_x$ tumor. Such lesions do not have access to lymphatic drainage of the lamina propria and there is no risk of recurrence or metastasis if removed in their entirety. Snare polypectomy and local excision (LE) are appropriate methods of definitive treatment for such lesions.

If an adenocarcinoma penetrates the muscularis mucosa and invades into the submucosa, it has gained access to lymphovascular channels and acquired the potential to recur locally or metastasize distantly. Any such lesion is considered an invasive cancer.

A malignant polyp is a term generally used to describe an adenoma harboring a cancer that has invaded through the muscularis mucosa into—but not beyond—the submucosa. It is classified as $T_1N_xM_x$.

A polypoid carcinoma is a descriptive term usually applied to an adenocarcinoma with the gross morphology of a polyp but without residual benign adenoma on histology. The T stage is variable and is best defined by the pathologist using the TNM system.

TNM system

The TNM system defines four levels of invasive cancer in the bowel wall. T_1 is invasion into the submucosa. T_2 is invasion into muscularis propria. T_3 is invasion through the muscularis propria into the subserosa or into nonperitonealized pericolic or perirectal tissues. T_4 is invasion directly into other organs or structures or perforation into the visceral peritoneum.

Haggitt classification

Haggitt et al [6] classified TIS and T_1 cancers that arise in polyps based on their level of invasiveness. Haggitt level 0 connotes a noninvasive in situ carcinoma confined to the mucosa, whereas levels 1, 2, and 3 define invasive carcinomas that invade into the head, neck, and stalk of a pedunculated polyp, respectively. Haggitt level 4 defines a cancer that invades into submucosa at the base of the stalk of a pedunculated polyp or in any sessile polypoid neoplasm. If invasion is into the muscularis propria, the cancer is T_2, and the Haggitt classification does not apply.

Submucosal invasion

A more precise staging system to predict adverse outcomes for patients with Haggitt level 4 submucosal invasion would be of value, especially for high operative risk patients or patients with distal rectal polyps in which the radical surgery option would require proctectomy and permanent colostomy.

A new classification system based on extent of submucosal invasion has been proposed by Kikuchi et al [7] to assess the risk of T_1 cancers. In this system, Sm_1 is slight submucosal invasion (upper third); Sm_2 is intermediate submucosal invasion (middle third); Sm_3 is invasion near the muscularis propria (lower third). Using this classification scheme, Haggitt level 1, 2, and 3 polyps would all be Sm_1 lesions, whereas Haggitt level 4 polyps, whether sessile or pedunculated, could be Sm_1, Sm_2, or Sm_3, depending on the depth of submucosal invasion.

Local therapy options

Options of local therapy used for management of rectal cancer include endocavitary radiation, fulguration, and LE techniques. This article focuses on the curative intent treatment of rectal cancer by the two most commonly used methods of local therapy: polypectomy and transanal LE. Endocavitary radiation requires special equipment, and expertise and is not widely available. Fulguration is currently used primarily for palliation to control bleeding from an incurable rectal cancer with minimal morbidity. Because of their limited use, these techniques are discussed only briefly.

Excision of a rectal tumor can be performed by polypectomy or surgical excision. Local surgical excision can be performed by transanal or posterior approaches. Transanal approaches include LE of a full-thickness disc of the rectal wall that harbors the rectal cancer or transanal endoscopic microsurgery. Transanal endoscopic microsurgery requires specialized equipment and training and is available in only a few centers. Its primary advantage is providing adequate exposure for proximally based rectal lesions that are difficult to expose for traditional LE. Posterior approaches by a transsacral incision or a transsphincteric dissection are rarely used.

Polypectomy

Snare polypectomy is performed at colonoscopy or rigid proctoscopy. The goal is to remove the polyp in a single piece and orient it for the pathologist so that depth of invasion and margins of excision can be evaluated. For larger polyps and polyps with suspicious clinical findings (eg, ulceration, firmness, and sessile lesions), the distance from the anal verge should be measured with the rigid proctoscope, and the site of the lesion should be marked with a submucosal injection of India ink. It is essential to mark the site of the original lesion in the event that it is necessary to perform an excision of a margin or more formal cancer operation.

Local excision

LE is the technique most frequently used to remove a distal rectal tumor. Several factors contribute to the ease and success of this procedure. Patients usually undergo a complete bowel preparation to decrease the risk of infection, prevent postoperative fecal impaction, and provide a clean surgical field. The prone jack-knife position offers the best exposure for most tumors and facilitates exposure for the assistant. Lithotomy position may be preferred for distal posterior tumors.

After the rectum is effaced as much as possible with a Lone-Star retractor (Lone-Star Medical Products, Inc., Stafford, Texas), exposure of the tumor is achieved with an anoscope, such as a Pratt bivalve retractor. A traction suture may be placed 2 to 3 cm distal to the lesion to facilitate excision for more proximal lesions. The area around and under the lesion may be infiltrated with either saline or local anesthesia with epinephrine to raise the lesion and minimize bleeding.

A full-thickness excision using electrocautery is performed with a 1-cm margin. If the lesion is extraperitoneal, surgeon preference determines whether to close the defect. Many surgeons recommend closing the defect to achieve better hemostasis and prevent postoperative bleeding [8]. If the lesion is at or above the peritoneal reflection, then the defect must be closed. Whenever the defect is closed, a rigid proctoscopy should be performed to ensure that the rectal lumen has not been compromised.

The specimen should be oriented and pinned out for the pathologist, who inks the margins before formalin fixation.

Transanal endoscopic microsurgery

Transanal endoscopic microsurgery is best used for tumors in the more proximal rectum. This complex technique is generally used for lesions that are not amenable to LE because they are too far from the anal verge (upper third of the rectum). The basic principles of transanal endoscopic microsurgery are the same as for LE. Transanal endoscopic microsurgery is performed through a 4-cm operating anoscope with CO_2 insufflation of the rectum. Long, laparoscopic-like instruments are used to facilitate a full-thickness excision and suture closure of the rectal wall. Morbidity and mortality are comparable to LE, and short-term follow-up shows a 5% local recurrence rate [9].

Posterior approaches

Posterior approaches are rarely used currently. The transsacral (Kraske) approach uses a posterior midline incision to remove the coccyx and sacral vertebrae as necessary. The rectum is opened and the lesion is excised, or a segmental resection with an anastomosis can be performed. The trans-sphincteric (York-Mason) approach uses division of the sphincter complex in the posterior midline to facilitate exposure to the rectum. After excision of the tumor, the sphincter complex is reconstructed. Both techniques are associated with a 20% fistula rate [10], and fecal incontinence is common after the York-Mason procedure.

Preoperative evaluation and staging

In theory, $T_{1\text{-}2}N_0M_0$ accessible rectal cancers that do not invade the anal sphincter and are small enough to be totally excised with clear margins should be curable by LE or possibly by snare polypectomy and should result in minimal morbidity, excellent function, and long-term cancer-free survival. Unfortunately, the ability to assess accurately the T and N stage of rectal lesions by current diagnostic tests is less than perfect.

The preoperative assessment should include the same standard evaluation that all patients with rectal cancer undergo. This evaluation includes tumor visualization and biopsy to determine its precise location and confirm the diagnosis of adenocarcinoma, colonoscopy to exclude synchronous lesions or other colonic pathology, evaluation of liver and lungs to exclude distant metastases, and medical assessment to determine operative risk.

Local staging of the rectal tumor is of utmost importance in patients who are considered for treatment with LE. An appropriate LE can remove the entire tumor in the rectal wall, but possible spread to the regional lymph nodes in the mesorectum is not removed with this procedure. It is important to exclude cancers with high risk for spread to the mesorectal lymph nodes.

The literature indicates that the incidence of lymph node metastases correlates most closely with depth of rectal wall invasion [11–15]. This risk is especially high if the cancer extends through the rectal wall, but lymphatic spread also occurs in up to 12% of T_1 cancers and 22% of T_2 cancers [11–15]. Accurate imaging studies are essential to assess the depth of bowel wall penetration of the tumor and distinguish node-negative from node-positive T_1 and T_2 rectal cancers. Preoperative staging with endorectal ultrasound (ERUS) or MRI is usually used in this assessment.

Clinical evaluation

Routine physical examination is performed, and the surgeon should note the presence of liver enlargement, abdominal tenderness or masses, lymphadenopathy, and prior abdominal scars or ventral hernias. Anal sphincter integrity and function are assessed carefully by digital rectal examination. A patient with pre-existing fecal incontinence or sphincter injury sometimes may be better served with an abdominoperineal resection. LE sometimes may impair sphincter function because of dilation of the sphincter complex at the procedure, and sometimes sphincter function is further compromised if adjuvant radiotherapy is used.

Evaluation of the extent of the primary rectal cancer is imperative for planning appropriate therapy. Suitable tumors for local therapy are usually small, mobile, and readily accessible. A distal rectal cancer that directly invades the anal sphincters is usually an indication that abdominoperineal resection is necessary. The presence of a large, fixed cancer that invades adjacent organs, pelvic sidewalls, or sacrum usually mandates neoadjuvant chemoradiation before radical resection or consideration of palliative measures.

The maximal size permitting LE is debated. Some authors report higher local failure rates if lesions are larger than 3 cm [16,17], whereas others suggest 4 cm as an upper limit [18,19].

Accessibility for LE is another important factor that must be determined preoperatively. The upper end of the tumor must be accessible with a transanal approach and usually is not recommended for tumors more than

8 to 10 cm from the anal verge. The location in the circumference also is of importance in selecting patient position at surgery.

Local staging

ERUS and MRI are the two most useful modalities for determining the depth of rectal wall penetration (T stage) and spread to the mesorectal lymph nodes (N stage). Pelvic CT scanning has proved to be less accurate in this assessment.

Endorectal ultrasound

At ERUS, the ultrasound probe covered with a balloon is usually introduced through a proctoscope to the upper rectum. The balloon is then filled with water to achieve optimal contact with the rectal wall and the probe is slowly retracted. The perirectal tissues are visualized, and enlarged lymph nodes may be visualized (N stage). Pathologic lymph nodes are usually defined as circular or slightly oval-shaped structures, often with an irregular border and with an echogenicity similar to the tumor [20]. At the level of the tumor, rectal wall penetration is assessed using a modification of the TNM classification based on a five-layer rectal wall model [21].

In a combined review of a large number of patients evaluated with ERUS, staging accuracy averaged close to 90% [22]. The accuracy for predicting extent of bowel wall involvement was higher (80%–90%) than the accuracy for identifying lymph node metastases (70%–80%).

The authors recently reviewed the University of Minnesota experience in staging rectal tumors with ERUS [23]. Five colorectal surgeons experienced in the technique performed the examinations. The accuracy was lower than previously reported. Overall accuracy was 64%, with 25% of patients overstaged and 11% of patients understaged.

MRI

MRI may be an excellent tool to visualize the extent of tumor growth in the mesorectum and identify patients with a threatened mesorectal margin. The technique is becoming an increasingly important tool in predicting anatomy before radical surgery [24].

For staging of early tumors, MRI has yet not replaced ERUS. Initially the accuracy of this technique was only 40% to 60% [25,26]. More recent high-resolution MR technology does not require insertion of an endorectal coil and is more accurate, however. In a recent study, Brown et al [27] reported an accuracy of 94% using high-resolution MRI in 98 patients who were undergoing radical surgery for rectal cancer. MRI is expensive, but the fast development of this technique holds significant promise as a useful tool in the preoperative assessment of patients with rectal tumors.

Outcome of local excision for early rectal cancer

Studies on the outcome after LE for rectal cancer are frequently heterogeneous, and results vary significantly. Most studies are retrospective and frequently include benign and malignant tumors. Stage and histopathologic assessment of known risk factors are not always mentioned. Preoperative staging with ERUS or MRI usually is not performed.

The combined experience of different centers suggests that the local recurrence rate after LE is less than 15% [28], with a local recurrence rate for T_1 tumors of approximately 10% and a local recurrence rate for T_2 tumors of approximately 25%. As noted in Table 1, however, the range between different studies is wide [2,13,29–31]. Results may be worse if adverse risk factors are present. Potential adverse risk factors include poorly differentiated histology, lymphovascular infiltration, and compromised margins.

The group at Memorial Sloan-Kettering Cancer Center in New York recently reported their long-term results of LE for rectal cancer [15]. One hundred twenty-five patients with T_1 and T_2 adenocarcinomas of the rectum treated by LE as definitive surgery were reviewed. 25% received adjuvant radiation therapy, and half of this latter group received adjuvant chemotherapy. Median follow-up was 6.7 years. The 10-year local recurrence and survival rates were 17% and 74%, respectively, for T_1 rectal cancers and 26% and 72%, respectively, for T_2 cancers. Median time to relapse was 1.4 years for local recurrence and 2.5 years for distant recurrence. In patients who received radiotherapy, local recurrence was delayed. The authors concluded that the long-term risk of recurrence after LE of T_1 and T_2 rectal cancers is substantial. Two thirds of patients with tumor recurrence had local failure, which implicated inadequate resection as the course of treatment failure. Neither adjuvant radiotherapy nor salvage surgery was reliable in preventing or controlling local recurrence.

The group at the Mayo Clinic in Rochester, Minnesota recently evaluated their results in treating T_1 tumors with LE [32]. They compared 70 patients who underwent LE with 74 patients who underwent radical resection for T_1 tumors in the rectum. The 5- and 10-year outcomes were significantly better for overall survival and cancer-free survival in the radical

Table 1
Studies using local excision for the treatment of T_1 and T_2 rectal tumors

Series	Number	Mean follow-up time (mo)	Local recurrence rate T_1 tumors (%)	Local recurrence rate T_2 tumors (%)
Hager et al [2]	59	36	8	17
Taylor et al [29]	24	52	40	50
Varma et al [30]	32	72	5	45
Mellgren et al [13]	108	53	17	46
Chorost et al [31]	16	22	36	60

resection group, but there were no significant differences in local recurrence or distant metastasis. For lesions with invasion into the lower third of the submucosa (Sm_3), the radical resection group had lower rates of distant metastasis and better survival. The authors concluded that LE is associated with a high incidence of local recurrence and distant metastasis.

The group at the Cleveland Clinic in Ohio recently evaluated all 52 patients with T_1 low rectal cancers who underwent LE alone at their institution between 1980 through 1998 [33]. The 5-year recurrence rate was 29%, and the 5-year cancer-specific survival rate was 89%. Fourteen of 15 patients with recurrence underwent salvage treatment, with a 56% 5-year survival rate. The authors conclude that LE of T_1 rectal tumors with low-grade malignancy has a high rate of recurrence.

Outcome of local excision for early rectal cancer at University of Minnesota

At the University of Minnesota and affiliated hospitals, 108 patients with T_1 and T_2 rectal adenocarcinomas were treated by LE without adjuvant chemoradiation between 1987 and 1996 [13]. At a mean follow-up of 4.4 years, the estimated probability of LE at 5 years was 18% for T_1 tumors and 47% for T_2 tumors. These results were compared with a matched group of 153 patients who underwent radical resection during the same time period. In the latter group, the estimated probability of local recurrence at 5 years was 0% for T_1 tumors and 6% for T_2 tumors.

The results in our study [13] are inferior to the results in several other studies [2,3]. Patients underwent treatment with LE at the surgeon's discretion after discussion with the patient. Many patients did not undergo preoperative staging, and there were no set criteria—for size or other parameters—to identify suitable patients for this treatment modality. It is unknown whether more stringent evaluation and selection of patients would have improved the outcome.

Salvage surgery may be possible if a local recurrence is found in time after LE. We reported results of salvage procedures after evaluating the charts of 29 patients who underwent salvage radical surgery for local recurrence after a full-thickness LE for stage I rectal cancer [1]. The resection was considered curative in 23 patients (79%), and the stage of the recurrent tumor was more advanced than the primary tumor in 27 patients (93%). At a mean follow-up of 39 months after radical surgery, 17 patients (59%) remained free of disease. Salvage surgery can be successful but cannot provide results equivalent to those of initial radical treatment. This finding emphasizes the importance of appropriate selection of the initial treatment of early rectal cancers.

Results of local excision combined with adjuvant chemoradiotherapy

The use of adjuvant chemoradiotherapy after LE in an effort to decrease the risk for recurrence is increasingly common. Indications for adjuvant therapy vary between different centers, but it is usually offered to patients with T_2 or T_3 tumors. Most centers give the adjuvant therapy post-operatively [3,29,34,35], but some centers also use preoperative downstaging chemoradiation followed by LE [36–39].

In 2000, Russell et al [35] reported the results of a multicenter trial that used LE for the treatment of selected patients with rectal cancer. The treatment was designed for patients who would have required abdominoperineal resection as conventional surgical therapy. The tumors were 4 cm or smaller in largest clinical diameter and occupied less than 40% of the rectal circumference. High-risk lesions (T_2, T_3, lymphovascular invasion, size >3 cm or elevated carcinoembryonic antigen) were treated with postoperative chemoradiation therapy. Local failure correlated with T-stage, with a local recurrence rate of 4% for T_1 tumors, 16% for T_2 tumors, and 23% for T_3 tumors. The authors concluded that conservative, sphincter-sparing therapy is a feasible alternative treatment for selected patients with limited cancer that involves the middle and lower rectum. Conversely, the Sloan Kettering group did not find that postoperative adjuvant radiotherapy was effective in preventing or controlling local recurrence (see previous discussion) [15].

In 1990, Marks et al [36] reported on 14 high-risk patients with locally advanced rectal cancer. The patients were treated with preoperative radiation followed by LE. The 3-year actuarial rate of local recurrence was 23%. A few years later, the same group reported on their experience using a technique in which LE was combined with partial excision of the underlying mesorectum [37]. In this study, local recurrence rate at 40 months for T_3 tumors was 67% and the 5-year survival was 50%.

Kim et al [39] reported in 2001 about their experience using LE for T_2 and T_3 cancers after downstaging chemoradiation with a complete clinical response or for patients who were either ineligible for or refused to undergo abdominoperineal resection. Twenty-six patients underwent preoperative chemoradiation followed by full-thickness LE and excision of underlying mesorectum. Pretreatment ERUS classified lesions as uT_2N_0 in 5 patients, uT_3N_0 in 13 patients, uT_3N_1 in 7 patients, and 1 not done. Pathologic partial and complete responses were achieved in 35% and 65% of patients, respectively. Two of nine partial responders underwent immediate abdominoperineal resection. The mean follow-up was 24 months, and the only recurrence was in a patient who refused to undergo abdominoperineal resection after a partial response.

Recommendations and future directions

Current recommendations for treatment of early rectal cancer

Based on an analysis of the available literature, together with our own experience [1,13,14], we restrict the use of curative intent LE to only a few, highly selected patients (Box 1).

Box 1. Suggested criteria for curative intent local excision of rectal cancer

Accessible and amenable to complete excision
$\leq$ 3 cm in largest diameter
$\geq$ 2 mm clear margins
T_1 tumor with Sm_1 invasion
T_1 tumor with Sm_2 invasion
  Well or moderately differentiated
  No lymphovascular invasion

Histologic risk factors have been described and are believed by some authors to be more reliable predictors of greater risk of residual malignancy or metastatic disease than depth of invasiveness. These factors include unfavorable histology (eg, poorly differentiated, signet ring, or mucinous adenocarcinoma) and lymphatic or venous invasion. Although the presence of unfavorable histologic features is associated with an increased risk of lymph node metastasis in early colorectal cancers, it remains unclear whether these histologic features have a variable or uniform influence at each level of invasiveness.

Patients who have undergone a polypectomy with a clear margin ($\geq$ 2 mm) for a Haggitt level 1, 2, or 3 adenocarcinoma that is well or moderately differentiated without lymphovascular invasion run a low risk of recurrence [40]. Observation is prudent for such early-stage cancers.

For T_1 Haggitt level 4 tumors, pedunculated or sessile, the risk of residual cancer or nodal metastases is higher and correlates primarily with the degree of invasion into the submucosa (Sm stage) [41]. Sm_1 cancers have a low risk of recurrence, which is equivalent to the operative mortality of radical surgery in good-risk patients [40]. The presence of histologic risk factors in Sm_2 cancers argues for radical resection (or possibly postoperative adjuvant chemoradiation). Sm_3 cancers have a higher recurrence rate, and radical resection is indicated for most of these patients. For T_2 and T_3 cancers, the curative treatment of choice for good-risk patients is radical resection.

Follow-up

If radical surgery is performed, the complete TNM classification is available. The final stage of disease, a patient's risk factors, and a patient's expectations determine appropriate follow-up.

After LE of a rectal tumor, follow-up can include serial ERUS or MRI studies and proctoscopy examinations. We use ERUS and proctoscopy for good-risk patients every 4 months for 3 years and then every 6 months for 2 more years [1]. We recommend that patients undergo a repeat colonoscopy after 1 year and, if results are negative, another one after an additional

3 years. Some physicians and patients also obtain serial carcinoembryonic antigen testing and imaging of the liver and lungs after 6 to 12 months.

Future directions

Without use of appropriate staging tools, LE remains a technique that neglects possible spread to the mesorectum, which is against all modern principles for treatment of rectal cancer [24,42]. The primary issue concerning the appropriate role of LE in the management of rectal cancer remains whether we can predict accurately the stage of a rectal cancer preoperatively. As discussed previously, ERUS can predict T staging rather satisfactorily, whereas prediction of involved lymph nodes remains problematic [23]. High-resolution MRI may be a better tool to predict spread outside the rectal wall [27]. It remains to be demonstrated, however, whether this technique will be able to better identify patients suitable for LE. Using new positron emission tomography techniques may be another way to identify appropriate patients.

The literature on the use of adjuvant chemoradiation therapy combined with LE reveals varied results [18,35–37,43]. It is difficult to decide from the current literature whether this approach will prove beneficial.

LE may be a treatment alternative in patients who gain a complete clinical response after treatment with neoadjuvant chemoradiation for adenocarcinoma of the rectum. Most surgeons recommend that these patients undergo a radical resection. This resection may involve an abdominoperineal resection, and sometimes there is no remaining tumor found in the specimen. Recently, Habr Gama et al [44] reported on following this group of patients without surgical intervention. Two hundred sixty-five patients with rectal cancer received neoadjuvant chemoradiation, and 71 (27%) of these patients had a complete clinical response. These 71 patients were followed without any surgical intervention and were compared with 22 patients who underwent radical resection and in whom there was no remaining tumor in the specimen ($T_0N_0M_0$). Five-year disease-free survival rate was 92% in the observation group and 83% in the resection group.

References

[1] Friel CM, Cromwell JW, Marra C, et al. Salvage radical surgery after failed local excision for early rectal cancer. Dis Colon Rectum 2002;45(7):875–9.

[2] Hager T, Gall FP, Hermanek P. Local excision of cancer of the rectum. Dis Colon Rectum 1983;26(3):149–51.

[3] Bleday R. Local excision of rectal cancer. World J Surg 1997;21(7):706–14.

[4] Minsky BD. Clinical experience with local excision and postoperative radiation therapy for rectal cancer. Dis Colon Rectum 1993;36(4):405–9.

[5] Longo WE, Virgo KS, Johnson FE, et al. Outcome after proctectomy for rectal cancer in Department of Veterans Affairs Hospitals: a report from the National Surgical Quality Improvement Program. Ann Surg 1998;228(1):64–70.

[6] Haggitt RC, Glotzbach RE, Soffer EE, et al. Prognostic factors in colorectal carcinomas arising in adenomas: implications for lesions removed by endoscopic polypectomy. Gastroenterology 1985;89(2):328–36.
[7] Kikuchi R, Takano M, Takagi K, et al. Management of early invasive colorectal cancer: risk of recurrence and clinical guidelines. Dis Colon Rectum 1996;39(7):827–8.
[8] Ramirez JM, Aguilella V, Arribas D, et al. Transanal full-thickness excision of rectal tumours: should the defect be sutured? A randomized controlled trial. Colorectal Dis 2002; 4(1):51–5.
[9] Guerrieri M, Feliciotti F, Baldarelli M, et al. Sphincter-saving surgery in patients with rectal cancer treated by radiotherapy and transanal endoscopic microsurgery: 10 years' experience. Dig Liver Dis 2003;35(12):876–80.
[10] Christiansen J. Excision of mid-rectal lesions by the Kraske sacral approach. Br J Surg 1980; 67(9):651.
[11] Brodsky JT, Richard GK, Cohen AM, et al. Variables correlated with the risk of lymph node metastasis in early rectal cancer. Cancer 1992;69(2):322–6.
[12] Blumberg D, Paty PB, Guillem JG, et al. All patients with small intramural rectal cancers are at risk for lymph node metastasis. Dis Colon Rectum 1999;42(7):881–5.
[13] Mellgren A, Sirivongs P, Rothenberger DA, et al. Is local excision adequate therapy for early rectal cancer? Dis Colon Rectum 2000;43(8):1064–71.
[14] Garcia-Aguilar J, Mellgren A, Sirivongs P, et al. Local excision of rectal cancer without adjuvant therapy: a word of caution. Ann Surg 2000;231(3):345–51.
[15] Paty PB, Nash GM, Baron P, et al. Long-term results of local excision for rectal cancer. Ann Surg 2002;236(4):522–9.
[16] Willett CG, Compton CC, Shellito PC, et al. Selection factors for local excision or abdominoperineal resection of early stage rectal cancer. Cancer 1994;73(11):2716–20.
[17] Frost DB, Wong R, Rao A. A retrospective comparison of transanal surgery and endocavitary radiation for the treatment of early rectal carcinoma. Arch Surg 1993;128(9): 1028–32.
[18] Bleday R, Breen E, Jessup JM, et al. Prospective evaluation of local excision for small rectal cancers. Dis Colon Rectum 1997;40(4):388–92.
[19] Bailey HR, Huval WV, Max E, et al. Local excision of carcinoma of the rectum for cure. Surgery 1992;111(5):555–61.
[20] Beynon J, Roe AM, Foy DM, et al. Preoperative staging of local invasion in rectal cancer using endoluminal ultrasound. J R Soc Med 1987;80(1):23–4.
[21] Hildebrandt U, Feifel G, Schwartz HP, et al. Endorectal ultrasound: instrumentation and clinical aspects. Int J Colorectal Dis 1986;986(4):203–7.
[22] Marohn MR. Endorectal ultrasound: SAGES postgraduate course syllabus. 1997.
[23] Garcia-Aguilar J, Pollack J, Lee SH, et al. Accuracy of endorectal ultrasonography in preoperative staging of rectal tumors. Dis Colon Rectum 2002;45(1):10–5.
[24] Brown G, Kirkham A, Williams GT, et al. High-resolution MRI of the anatomy important in total mesorectal excision of the rectum. AJR Am J Roentgenol 2004;182(2): 431–9.
[25] Thaler W, Watzka S, Martin F, et al. Preoperative staging of rectal cancer by endoluminal ultrasound vs. magnetic resonance imaging: preliminary results of a prospective, comparative study. Dis Colon Rectum 1994;37(12):1189–93.
[26] Meyenberger C, Huch Boni RA, Bertschinger P, et al. Endoscopic ultrasound and endorectal magnetic resonance imaging: a prospective, comparative study for preoperative staging and follow-up of rectal cancer. Endoscopy 1995;27(7):469–79.
[27] Brown G, Davies S, Williams GT, et al. Effectiveness of preoperative staging in rectal cancer: digital rectal examination, endoluminal ultrasound or magnetic resonance imaging? Br J Cancer 2004;91(1):23–9.
[28] Sengupta S, Tjandra JJ. Local excision of rectal cancer: what is the evidence? Dis Colon Rectum 2001;44(9):1345–61.

[29] Taylor RH, Hay JH, Larsson SN. Transanal local excision of selected low rectal cancers. Am J Surg 1998;175(5):360–3.
[30] Varma MG, Rogers SJ, Schrock TR, et al. Local excision of rectal carcinoma. Arch Surg 1999;134(8):863–7.
[31] Chorost MI, Petrelli NJ, McKenna M, et al. Local excision of rectal carcinoma. Am Surg 2001;67(8):774–9.
[32] Nascimbeni R, Nivatvongs S, Larson DR, et al. Long-term survival after local excision for T1 carcinoma of the rectum. Dis Colon Rectum 2004;47(11):1773–9.
[33] Madbouly KM, Remzi FH, Erkek BA, et al. Recurrence after transanal excision of T1 rectal cancer: should we be concerned? Dis Colon Rectum, in press.
[34] Steele GD Jr, Herndon JE, Bleday R, et al. Sphincter-sparing treatment for distal rectal adenocarcinoma. Ann Surg Oncol 1999;6(5):433–41.
[35] Russell AH, Harris J, Rosenberg PJ, et al. Anal sphincter conservation for patients with adenocarcinoma of the distal rectum: long-term results of radiation therapy oncology group protocol 89–02. Int J Radiat Oncol Biol Phys 2000;15(2):313–22.
[36] Marks G, Mohiuddin MM, Masoni L, et al. High-dose preoperative radiation and full-thickness local excision: a new option for patients with select cancers of the rectum. Dis Colon Rectum 1990;33(9):735–9.
[37] Mohiuddin M, Marks G, Bannon J. High-dose preoperative radiation and full thickness local excision: a new option for selected T3 distal rectal cancers. Int J Radiat Oncol Biol Phys 1994;30(4):845–9.
[38] Mohiuddin M, Regine WF, Marks GJ, et al. High-dose preoperative radiation and the challenge of sphincter-preservation surgery for cancer of the distal 2 cm of the rectum. Int J Radiat Oncol Biol Phys 1998;40(3):569–74.
[39] Kim CJ, Yeatman TJ, Coppola D, et al. Local excision of T2 and T3 rectal cancers after downstaging chemoradiation. Ann Surg 2001;234(3):352–8.
[40] Rothenberger DA, Garcia-Aguilar J. Management of cancer in a polyp. In: Saltz LB, editor. Colorectal cancer: multimodality management. New York: Humana Press; 2002. p. 325–35.
[41] Nivatvongs S. Surgical management of early colorectal cancer. World J Surg 2000;24(9): 1052–5.
[42] Heald RJ, Ryall RD. Recurrence and survival after total mesorectal excision for rectal cancer. Lancet 1986;28(8496):1479–82.
[43] Minsky BD, Enker WE, Cohen AM, et al. Local excision and postoperative radiation therapy for rectal cancer. Am J Clin Oncol 1994;17(5):411–6.
[44] Habr-Gama A, Perez RO, Nadalin W, et al. Operative versus nonoperative treatment for stage 0 distal rectal cancer following chemoradiation therapy: long-term results. Ann Surg 2004;240(4):711–7.

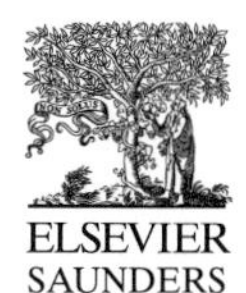
ELSEVIER
SAUNDERS

Surg Oncol Clin N Am
14 (2005) 197–224

SURGICAL
ONCOLOGY CLINICS
OF NORTH AMERICA

Surgical Management of Pelvic Malignancy: Role of Extended Abdominoperineal Resection/Exenteration/Abdominal Sacral Resection

Harold J. Wanebo, MD, FACS[a,b,c,*], Giovanni Begossi, MD[d], Kimberly A. Varker, MD[e]

[a]*Boston University Medical School, 715 Albany Street, Boston, MA 02118, USA*
[b]*Brown University, Providence, RI 02912, USA*
[c]*Department of Surgery, Roger Williams Medical Center, 825 Chalkstone Avenue, Providence, RI 02908, USA*
[d]*The University of Massachusetts Medical Center, 55 Lake Avenue North, Worcester, MA 01655, USA*
[e]*Department of Surgery, The Ohio State University, Columbus, OH 43210, USA*

Locoregional recurrence: incidence and risk factors

Although the incidence of locoregional recurrence of colorectal cancer after primary resection has been reduced by improved surgical techniques and the frequent use of neoadjuvant or adjuvant therapy, local failure remains a significant clinical problem. At diagnosis, 37% of patients with colorectal cancer have localized disease (5-year survival, 91%), 37% have regional disease (5-year survival, 66%), 20% have distant metastases (5-year survival, 8.5%), and 6% are unstaged [1,2]. Stage for stage, the outcome is worse for rectal cancer (5-year survival approximately 20% less) than for colon cancer.

The primary determinants of survival are TNM stage and completeness of resection, with the goal being R0 resection (no gross or microscopic residual disease). Other prognostic factors include histologic type and grade, serum carcinoembryonic antigen (CEA) level, and extramural or submucosal

* Corresponding author. Roger Williams Medical Center, Department of Surgery, 825 Chalkstone Avenue, Providence, RI 02908.
E-mail address: hwanebo@rwmc.org (H.J. Wanebo).

doi:10.1016/j.soc.2004.12.001 *surgonc.theclinics.com*

vascular invasion [3]. Additionally, the presence of bowel obstruction secondary to tumor has been identified as an independent poor prognostic indicator in multivariate analyses [4]. Various potential tumor markers are being studied, including DCC (Deleted in Colon Cancer), p27^{Kip1}, DNA microsatellite instability markers, and thymidylate synthase [5]. Recent data have indicated that loss of the 18q allele in patients with microsatellite-stable Stage III colon cancer confers an inferior prognosis [6]. Other molecular markers of prognosis are likely to be identified in the future.

Natural history data suggest that one third of patients resected for cure will develop recurrence, presumably due to occult micrometastatic disease present at the time of diagnosis [4,7]. Due to the anatomic confines of the pelvis, particularly in males, it is more challenging to achieve complete extirpation with wide margins of rectal cancer than of colon cancer. This may account for the higher risk of locoregional recurrence of rectal cancer.

An older report by Pilipshen et al [2] characterized recurrence patterns after resection of rectal cancer in a group of 412 patients (Table 1). One hundred eighty-two patients (44.2%) developed recurrence, of which 105 (57.6%) were pelvic. Pelvic recurrence involved the predominating site alone (55/103) or extrapelvic sites (50/79). The overall risk of recurrence was similar after low anterior resection (LAR) and abdominoperineal resection (APR), but the incidence of pelvic recurrence with fixation was much higher after APR (89.7% as compared with 27% after LAR).

A series of improvements to standard of care has markedly improved local control rates after primary resection of rectal cancer [8]. Early studies,

Table 1
Recurrence after resection of rectal cancer

Total patients (recurrence rate)	*n* (%)	
Type of recurrence		
Local only	16 (15)	
Distant only	14 (13)	
Local and distant	18 (17)	
Anatomic site of recurrence		
Pelvis	28 (27)	
Liver	19 (18)	
Visceral	22 (21)	
Intra-abdominal	8 (8)	
Recurrence rate	LAR (240 points)	APR (142 points)
	66 (27.5)	38 (27.4)
Anastamotic	9 (14.6)	
Perianastamotic	3 (4.5)	
Pelvic with fixation	19 (27.0)	35 (89.7)
Pelvic without fixation	3 (4.5)	4 (10.3)

Abbreviations: APR, abdominoperineal resection; LAR, low anterior resection.

Data from Pilipshen SJ, Heilweil M, Quan SH, et al. Patterns of pelvic recurrence following definitive resections of rectal cancer. Cancer 1984;53:1354–62.

typified by that of Stearns [9], demonstrated the benefit of adjuvant radiation. The combination of systemic chemotherapy with radiation therapy in the adjuvant setting was shown by the Gastrointestinal Study Group to significantly improve time to recurrence and survival in patients with stages B2 and C rectal carcinoma [10]. Trials by the North Clinical Cancer Study Group and The National Surgical Adjuvant Breast and Bowel Project trials R-01 and R-02 further confirmed decreased local recurrence rates with the combination of adjuvant radiation and chemotherapy as compared with radiation or chemotherapy alone [11].

The technique of total mesorectal excision (TME), introduced by Heald [12] in 1978 and updated in 1998, has greatly improved the results of primary resection. In his series of 519 patients undergoing TME (465 LAR, 37 APR), the overall local failure at 5 years was 3%. The value of a course of high-fraction irradiation was highlighted by the Swedish Rectal Cancer Trail, which demonstrated improved local control and survival with adjuvant radiation [13]. The Dutch Rectal Cancer Study Group combined TME with radiation therapy according to the Swedish Trial protocol, obtaining a low rate of local failure (2.9% for TME plus radiation versus 8.25% for TME alone) [14].

Despite improvements in adjuvant therapy regimens and the virtually universal adoption of TME, recurrent rectal cancer remains a reality. Nonsurgical management options, such as external beam radiation therapy (EBRT) and systemic chemotherapy, are not associated with long-term survival, although they can provide temporary tumor stabilization and palliation of pain and other symptoms [15]. For suitable operable candidates, resection of pelvic recurrence can provide 5-year survival rates of up to 30%, similar to those seen after resection of solitary metastases to the lung, liver, or brain [16]. Thus, aggressive resection of pelvic recurrence in highly selected patients seems to be worth pursuing (Wanebo HJ, Begossi G, unpublished observations).

Routine surveillance after primary resection

The appropriate surveillance regimen to follow after primary resection of colorectal cancer is a matter of some controversy. Early identification and treatment of recurrence may be associated with superior outcomes [17]. Follow-up should include history and physical examination, assessment of serum CEA levels, colonoscopy, and CT of the abdomen and pelvis at regular intervals. In addition, endoanal ultrasound may be a useful adjunct after a sphincter-saving procedure (SSP) to assess potential recurrence at the anastomotic site [5].

The optimal schedule for office visits and imaging studies is somewhat arbitrary. Scheduled follow-up should probably occur at least every 3 to 4 months for the first 2 to 3 years because 50% to 75% of recurrences occur within 2 years of primary resection, and 95% of recurrences occur within

3 years postoperatively [18]. Symptoms of recurrent disease often precede any findings on imaging studies, and a high false-negative rate continues to plague the use of the CEA level as a screening tool for the identification of recurrence [19]. Some studies have concluded that the use of extensive surveillance protocols confers only a minimal improvement in survival over expectant management [20].

Kraemer et al [18] have attempted to delineate an optimal screening regimen based on an individualized stratification of risk. The defined high-risk group included patients with Dukes C stage rectal cancer (any T, N1-N2, M0 by TNM stage), tumor invasion of adjacent organ, tumor fixation, or poorly differentiated histology. This group had a recurrence rate of 25.6%. The low-risk group, defined as Dukes A stage, no tumor invasion or fixation, and well differentiated histology had a recurrence rate of 2.9%. The intermediate-risk group included Dukes B stage, no evidence of extra-rectal tumor invasion or fixation, and moderately differentiated histology and had a recurrence risk of 9.8%. These findings suggest that the most intense follow-up regimen should be used for high-risk patients and that a more moderate regimen may be used for low-risk patients [5].

Workup of identified recurrence

Approximately 50% of patients who experience locoregional recurrence of rectal cancer have concomitant distant metastases [21]. Complete imaging workup to assess the extent of locoregional recurrence and to rule out associated metastatic disease is imperative before embarking upon a major exenterative procedure. CT scan of the chest, abdomen, and pelvis is used to exclude hepatic lesions or other metastatic disease. Historically, plain films and bone scan have been used for the determination of possible bone marrow involvement, which precludes aggressive sacral resection [22]. MRI of the pelvis is helpful in confirming sacral invasion by tumor, assessing the proximal and lateral extent of tumor, and planning the level of sacral resection [15,22,23]. MRI may allow differentiation between recurrent pelvic disease and postoperative fibrotic change due to their different signal intensities on T2-weighted images [24]. Gadolinium-enhanced MRI reportedly has 87% sensitivity and 100% sensitivity for the detection of pelvic recurrence, as compared with 80% and 86%, respectively, for standard MRI [25]. In addition, tissue biopsy is essential. This can be obtained per vagina in the female, transanally after low anterior resection, or by CT-guided fine needle aspiration after APR.

Recent studies suggest that 18-fluorodeoxyglucose positron emission tomography (PET) is more sensitive than CT in detecting metastatic or recurrent colorectal cancer and remains accurate after full-dose radiation [26,27]. The role of 18-fluorodeoxyglucose PET in this setting is currently being defined.

Treatment of resectable abdominal or pelvic recurrence

Treatment of anastomotic recurrence

Truly localized (bowel wall only) anastomotic recurrence is uncommon, representing only 10% to 20% of all rectal cancer [28,29]. Locoregional recurrence, with spread to the peritoneal cavity, pelvis, or perineum, is much more common due to the limited resection margins attainable in the pelvis and to the rich lymphatic networks existing in the mesorectum [28,29].

A common theme in many series is that patients who undergo primary resection by APR for cancer present later with more advanced disease and have correspondingly lower resectability rates than those who initially underwent SSP (Table 2A). Broad infiltration of bone and associated ligaments in the pelvis is typically seen in such patients [23].

Occasionally, true anastomotic recurrence can be seen after low anterior resection performed for a small, early cancer. Isolated anastomotic recurrence is amenable to re-resection by repeat anterior resection or by salvage APR with good results [18,28–37]. Even recurrent disease that is tethered to the posterior pelvic floor may be resectable by salvage APR, especially if preoperative radiation therapy is given. The combination of re-resection with intra-operative radiation is another technique available in certain centers that seems to be associated with improved control (Table 2B) [16,37].

Table 2A
Re-resection for recurrent rectal cancer

Author	No. of points	First procedure	Second procedure	Results (5 yr %) (median)
Segal, 1981 [36]	12	LAR	APR	6 NED (6 mo) 4 DOD (24 mo)
Hojo, 1986 [31]	22	LAR	Resect (APR)	11 NED
Vassilopoulos, 1981 [17a]	30	LAR	15 R0 Resect 10 R1 Resect 5 R2 Resect	(49%) 5 yr, (59 mo) (12%) 56, (17 mo) 8 mo
Pihl, 1981 [18a]	35	AR Anast. Recur	14 R0 20 No Resect	41 mo 8.8 mo
Polk and Spratt, 1979 [34]	21	APR	Resect Perineal Recurr (8) Combined Resect13	21/21/DOD 12 mo Med
Schiessel, 1986 [22a]	53	LAR/ARP	21 APR 9 Sacral Res 8 Abdom Excis 3 Eviscertion 10 Re-resection	16/53 (30%; 3 yr)

Abbreviations: APR, abdominoperineal resection; DOD, dead of disease; LAR, low anterior resection; NED, no evidence disease.

Table 2B
Re-resection for locally recurrent rectal cancer (+IORT)

Author	Local recurrence	Re-resection	Results
Willett, 1991 [24a]	30 pelvic	13 complete resect (R0) +IORT	54%; 5 yr Local control 62%
		17 partial resect (R1) +IORT	6%; 5 yr Local control
Beart, 1988 [43a]	24 pelvic	24 resected +IORT	28%; 4 yr
		R1 min residual	20 mo; 13 (54% NED)
		R2 gross residual	8–33%, NED 3 LR/5 Dist

Pelvic exenteration for recurrent rectal carcinoma

Pelvic recurrence with involvement of anterior structures (bladder and prostate) or posterior visceral structures (vagina) can be resected en bloc by pelvic exenteration. It is essential to first rule out involvement of the sacral bone, which necessitates abdominosacral resection (ABSR). Potential sacral involvement is best assessed by MRI.

Multiple published series reveal results of pelvic exenteration procedures (Table 3). Law et al [38] reported a series of 24 patients who underwent total pelvic exenteration, 15 for primary tumor and nine for recurrent disease. Overall 5-year survival was 44%. Survival was significantly higher in patients resected for primary disease (64%). Only one patient who underwent resection for recurrent disease lived more than 24 months. The overall complication rate was 54%, with no postoperative deaths. Estes et al [39] presented 16 cases of exenteration for recurrent disease (anterior exenteration, $n = 3$; posterior exenteration, $n = 6$; total pelvic exenteration, $n = 4$; total exenteration-sacral resection, $n = 3$). Five-year overall survival was 49%, and mean survival was 31 months. Wiig et al [40] reported 47 patients who underwent exenteration, all of whom received preoperative irradiation to 46 to 50 Gy. Twenty-five procedures were done for advanced primary cancer, and 22 procedures were done for recurrence. Five-year actuarial survival was 28% (36% for those with primary tumors, 18% for those with recurrent tumors, $n = 66$).

Meterissian et al [41] presented a series of 40 patients who underwent pelvic exenteration (primary tumor, $n = 29$; recurrent disease, $n = 11$), resulting in 5-year overall survival of 49% and median survival of 56 months. Rodel [42] reviewed 35 previously nonirradiated patients with pelvic recurrence of rectal cancer. All were treated with concurrent chemoradiation with 5-fluorouracil. Twenty-eight patients underwent curative resection, with 16 requiring adjacent organ resections. At median follow-up of 27 months, three patients (18%) had experienced local re-recurrence.

Friel et al [43] reported on 29 patients who underwent salvage surgical resection after failed local excision for early rectal cancer. At mean follow-up

Table 3
Results of published series of pelvic exenteration procedures

Author	Number of patients	Procedure	Survival
Law [38]	24 (primary = 15; recurrent = 9)	TPE	44% 5-yr
Estes [4]	16	Anterior exenteration = 3 Posterior exenteration = 6 TPE = 4 ASR = 3	49% 5-yr
Wiig [40]	47 (primary = 25; recurrent = 22)	PE	28% 5-yr
Meterissian [41]	40 (primary = 29; recurrent = 11)	PE	49% 5-yr
Rodel [42]	28	PE	18% recurrence at 27 mo
Friel [43]	29 (all salvage)	PE	59% disease-free at 39 mo
Ogunbiyi [44]	14 (all recurrent)	PE	86% disease-free survival at 25 mo
Salo [45]	103	PE	24% 5-yr
Huguier [24]	30	PE	19% 5-yr
Lopez-Kostner [46]	43	PE	32% disease-free at 5 yr
Bozzetti [47]	45	PE	19% 5-yr
Garcia-Aguilar [48]	42	PE	35% 5-yr

Abbreviations: ASR, abdominal sacral resection; PE, pelvic exenteration; TPE, total pelvic exenteration.

of 39 months, 17 patients (59%) were disease free. Ogunbiyi [44] reported on 14 patients who underwent curative resection for pelvic recurrence. Disease-free survival was 86% at a median of 25 months. In a review of 131 patients with recurrent disease who underwent exploration with curative intent (103 of whom underwent resection), Salo et al [45] reported 5-year overall survival rate of 24%. Huguier and Houry [24] reported on 30 patients who underwent curative re-resection of recurrent rectal carcinoma. Actuarial 5-year survival was 19% (28% in asymptomatic and 8% in symptomatic patients). Lopez-Kostner [46] reported 117 patients with locally recurrent rectal cancer, of whom 43 underwent salvage surgery, with a 5-year disease-free survival rate of 32%. Bozzetti et al [47] reported on 45 patients with locally recurrent colorectal cancer, 21 of whom underwent R0 resection, with a 5-year survival rate of 19%. Finally, Garcia-Aguilar et al [48] reviewed 42 patients who underwent curative resection of locally recurrent rectal cancer. Estimated 5-year survival was 35%, as compared with 7% in patients who underwent palliative surgery or nonsurgical management.

ABSR

Recurrent colorectal cancer involving anterior or posterior visceral structures within the pelvis is optimally treated by total pelvic exenteration, but disease involving the sacrum must be resected en bloc with the remainder of the specimen. The possibility of sacral involvement is best evaluated by MRI. We have previously reported our experience with ABSR of recurrent colorectal cancers [22,29,49–54].

A thorough assessment of the patient's physiologic status, in particular the cardiac, pulmonary, and renal reserve, must be made before embarking on a procedure of this magnitude. The intra-operative placement of ureteral stents greatly facilitates identification of the ureters during a difficult pelvic dissection. We accomplish the procedure in two stages, 48 hours apart, to allow for patient stabilization between the stages of the operation. The steps in the procedure have been presented in detail elsewhere [5,9,17,25,29,51, 55–57]. The major operative steps are illustrated in Figs. 1 through 16.

The first stage of the operation begins with laparotomy and a careful search for extrapelvic disease (Fig. 1). The presence of liver metastases, serosal seeding, or para-aortic lymphadenopathy constitutes absolute contraindications to attempts at resection. Similarly, involvement of the

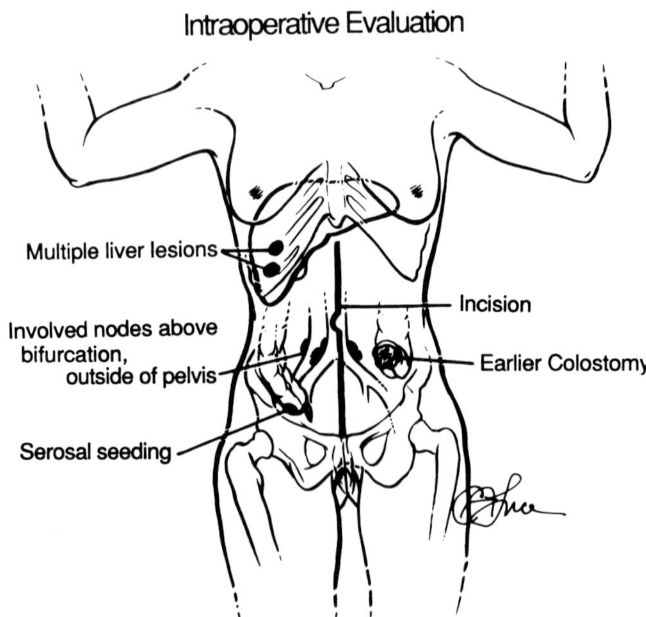

Fig. 1. Intra operative evaluations. Reasons to exclude resection include disease outside of pelvis, multiple liver metastases, serosal seeding, para-aortic nodal metastasis, sacral marrow invasion, and upper side wall invasion at level of common iliac arteries.

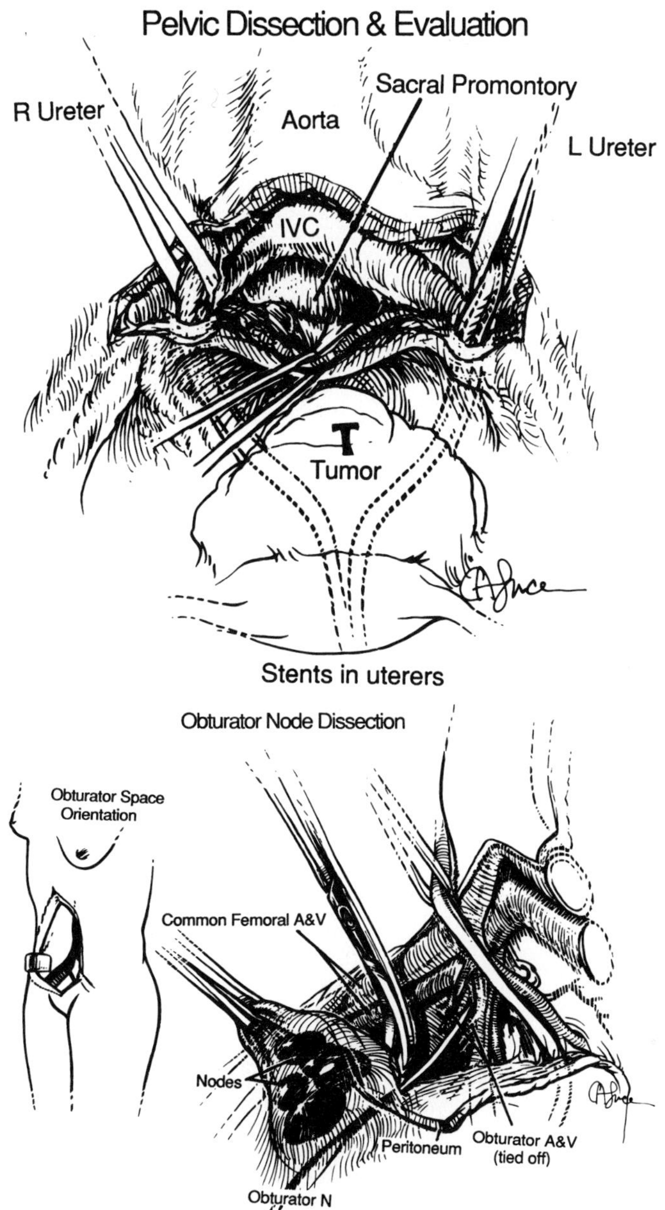

Figs. 2 & 3. The dissection starts at the bifurcation of the aorta. A bilateral aorto-iliac node dissection is done, including internal iliac and obturator node dissection.

pelvic or obturator nodes (assessed by formal node dissection) contraindicates resection. Provided that there are no contraindications to resection, pelvic exenteration with reconstruction as needed (eg, ileal

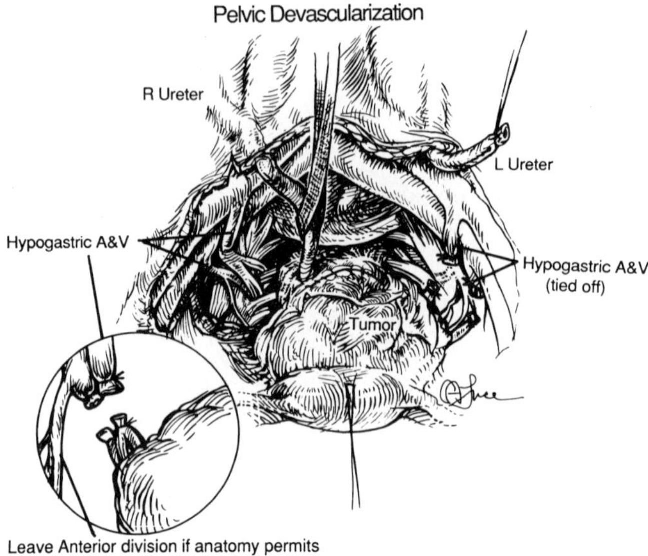

Fig. 4. The internal iliac artery and vein are divided and suture ligated with sutures bilaterally to accomplish devascularization of the pelvis.

conduit) is performed, followed by devascularization of the pelvis. In many cases, previous surgery and radiation leaves a scarred pelvis with dense adhesions and obliterated land marks. The initial dissection is facilitated by beginning the dissection at the aortic bifurcation and continuing along the

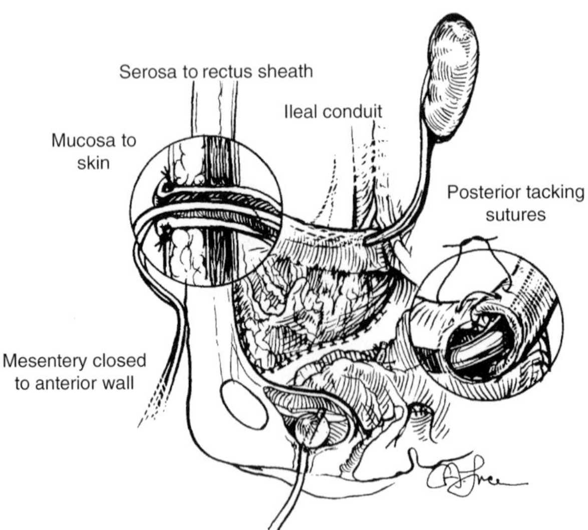

Fig. 5. An ideal conduit is fashioned if bladder resection is required. The boot of the conduit is secured above the aortic bifurcation to prevent its descent into the pelvis.

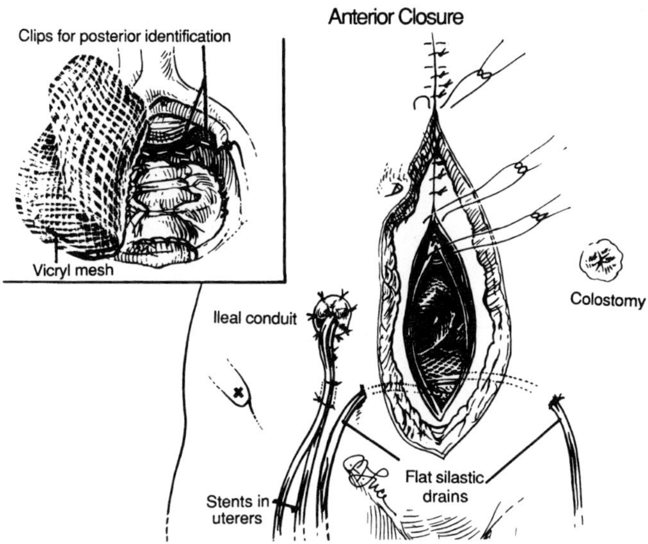

Fig. 6. The abdomen is closed. In some cases mobilization of the rectus abdominus is done to provide additional vascularized tissue for filling the resulting from the pelvic resection. Clips are placed on the pelvic floor to provide a new line of resection.

iliac and internal iliac vessels to mobilize a new posterior pelvic envelope, which is carried into the deeper pelvis until one encounters the upper reaches of the recurrence (Figs. 2, 3). The internal iliac artery is dissected to a comfortable level in posterior pelvis below first or second arterial branches to maintain available vascularity to the posterior pelvis (Fig. 4). The artery is bisected, and sutures are ligated. The internal iliac vein is carefully isolated and divided between vascular clamps (or divided with vascular staples), and the end sutures are ligated. After the internal iliac and obliterator node dissection and isolation and dissection of the distal ureter, a decision is made regarding need for bladder resection and formation of the ileal (or colonic bladder) (Fig. 5). The abdomen is closed. In some cases, a rectus abdominus muscle flap may be developed as bulk filler for the pelvis if a large pelvic space vacuum is envisioned (Fig. 6). Vascular clips are placed along the line of planned posterior resection as a guide. The proximal rectum is bisected and detached from the distal rectum, if present, and an end sigmoid colostomy is performed. If the bladder, prostate, or seminal vesicles are clinically involved by tumor or are determined to be involved by cystoscopy, the ureters are detached, and an ileal conduit is fashioned. The uterus and vagina are resected if clinically involved by tumor; otherwise, they are left in situ. This assists in reconstruction and helps to maintain quality of life. The pelvic organs are left in situ until the second stage of the operation. The laparotomy is closed, and the patient is taken to the intensive care unit.

Forty-eight hours later (assuming clinical stability), the patient is returned to the operating room. The second stage of the operation is

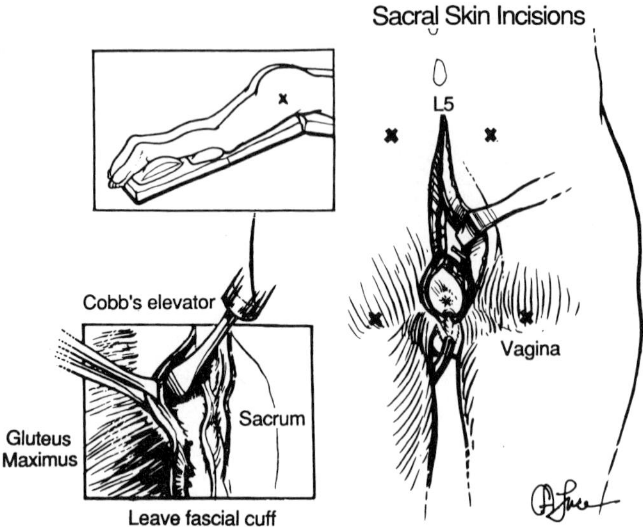

Fig. 7. The patient is repositioned prone. A posterior sacral incision is made from the spinous process of L5 to the perineum, and full-thickness myocutaneous gluteal flaps are raised to the lateral border of the sacrum.

accomplished through a presacral incision, with the patient in the prone position (Fig. 7). This portion of the procedure consists of (1) completion of the perineal dissection; (2) full thickness dissection of the gluteus muscles, including skin, muscle, and fascia from the sacrum (Fig. 8); (3) sacral

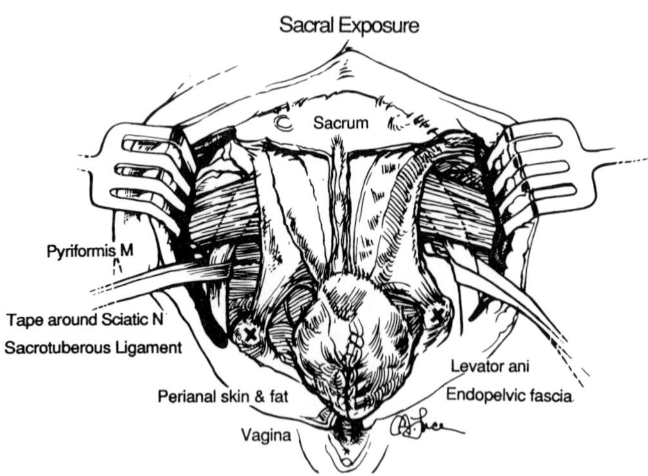

Fig. 8. After dissection of the gluteus maximus and medius muscles from their sacral origins, the sciatic nerve is identified bilaterally and encircled with a vessel loop. The sacrotuberous ligaments and sacro-spinous ligaments (not shown) are isolated and divided. The ischio-rectal fossa is entered and dissected.

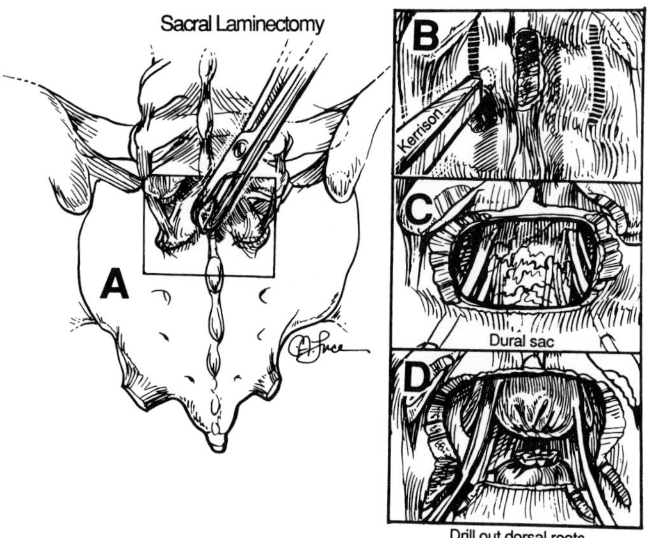

Fig. 9. A sacral laminectomy is done, and generally the L5 and S1 nerve roots are preserved. The S2 and S3 nerve roots may be preserved for tumor confined to lower pelvis. Palpating the previously placed presacral clips may help indicate the level of sacral osteotomy.

laminectomy with preservation of the nerve roots and suture ligation of the dural sac (Fig. 9); and (4) osteotomy of the sacrum at the predetermined level (Figs. 10, 11). Resection of the tumor with contiguous abdominal viscera and involved sacrum is accomplished en bloc (Fig. 12). The large pelvic floor defect may be covered by a Vicryl mesh and a transposed rectus

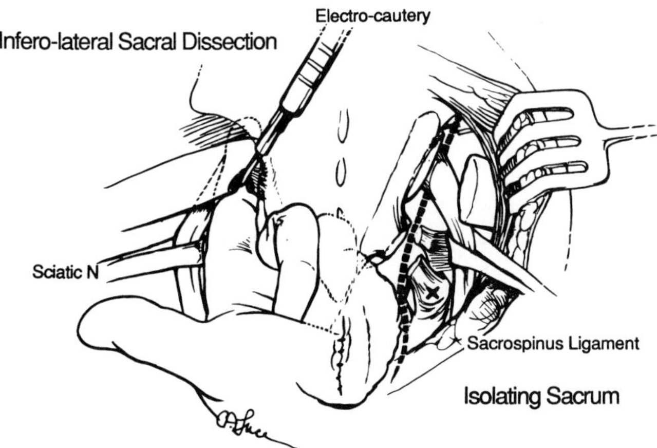

Fig. 10. The surgeon's finger is inserted anteriorly from the medial aspect of the sciatic nerve and advanced deeply beneath the pyriformis muscle through the underlying endopelvic fascia to reach the anterior surface of the sacrum.

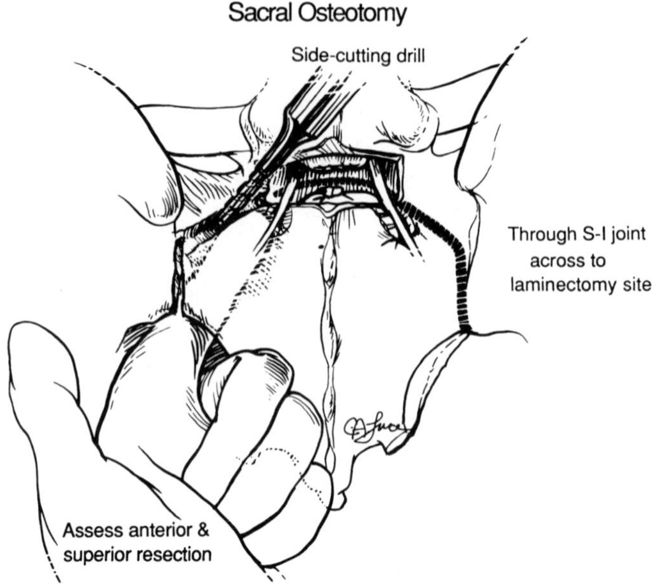

Fig. 11. The sacrum is divided with an osteotome or an oscillating saw; the surgeon's finger is positioned anteriorly to protect the underlying intra-abdominal contents.

abdominus muscle flap to prevent herniation of viscera (Fig. 13). The closure with large musculo-cutaneous gluteus flaps provides a secure posterior closure in most patients but may be supplemented by the addition of the rectus abdominus flap (Figs. 14–16). Our experience has shown that

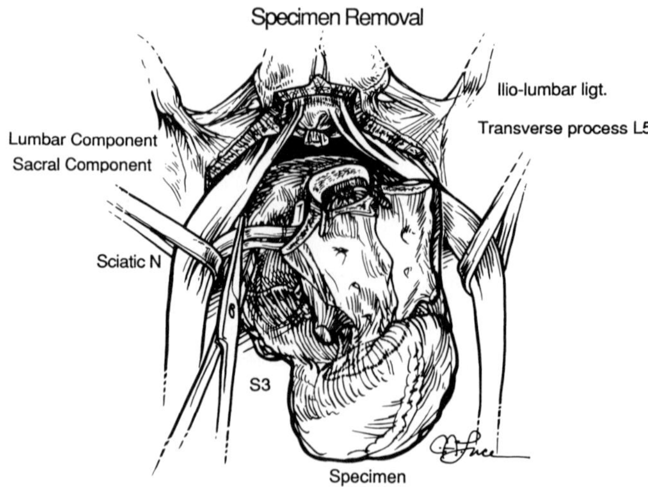

Fig. 12. The sacrum, pelvic side walls, tumor, and attached pelvic structures are removed en bloc.

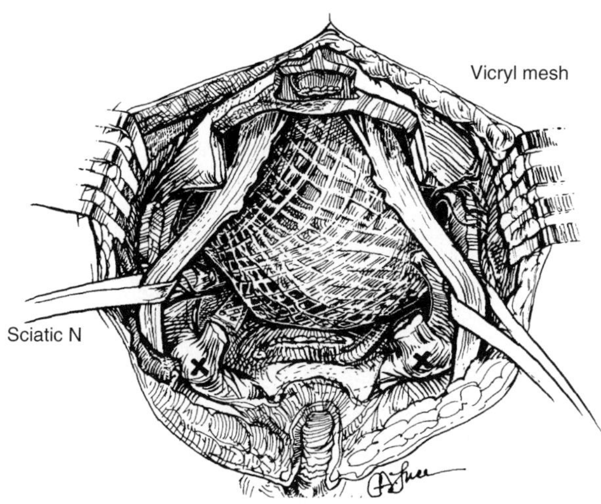

Fig. 13. The pelvic floor has been removed, revealing the internal contents, in this case covered by a Vicryl mesh to prevent early herniation of viscera through the pelvic floor. In some cases, a rectus abdominus muscle may be rotated into the pelvic floor to prevent herniation.

closure of the posterior wound with gluteus muscle flaps is associated with decreased morbidity as compared with primary wound closure [22]. Mean operative time is approximately 20 hours (12 hours for the first stage and 8 hours for the second stage). Total estimated blood loss averages 10,000 mL.

A recent review of our experience as of April 2002 revealed a total of 181 patients who presented or were referred for management of recurrent rectal cancer (Wanebo HJ, Begossi G, unpublished observations). Of these, 80 patients had palliative treatment, including 17 who received systemic supportive care only, 23 who underwent palliative resection, and 40 who underwent pelvic perfusion. A total of 97 patients underwent curative resection: 23 underwent repeat anterior resection or abdominoperineal resection, 63 underwent ABSR, and 15 underwent resection of distant metastases. Seventy-one patients underwent composite ABSR: 63 with curative intent and eight for palliation (Harold J. Wanebo, MD, personal communication, 2004) (Tables 4–12). Six of the eight patients who underwent composite ABSR with palliative intent had known hepatic metastases or extra-pelvic disease. Two patients had extended ABSR (between L5–L1) or extended side wall extension in an effort to control otherwise uncontrolled disease in previously heavily irradiated patients. The median survival in this group was <12 months. We no longer consider such patients appropriate candidates for resection. Of the 63 patients undergoing curative abdominal sacral resection (ASR) (43 male, 20 female, mean age 58 years), the stage of the primary cancer was approximately evenly divided between Stages II and III (Table 4). Likewise, equivalent numbers of

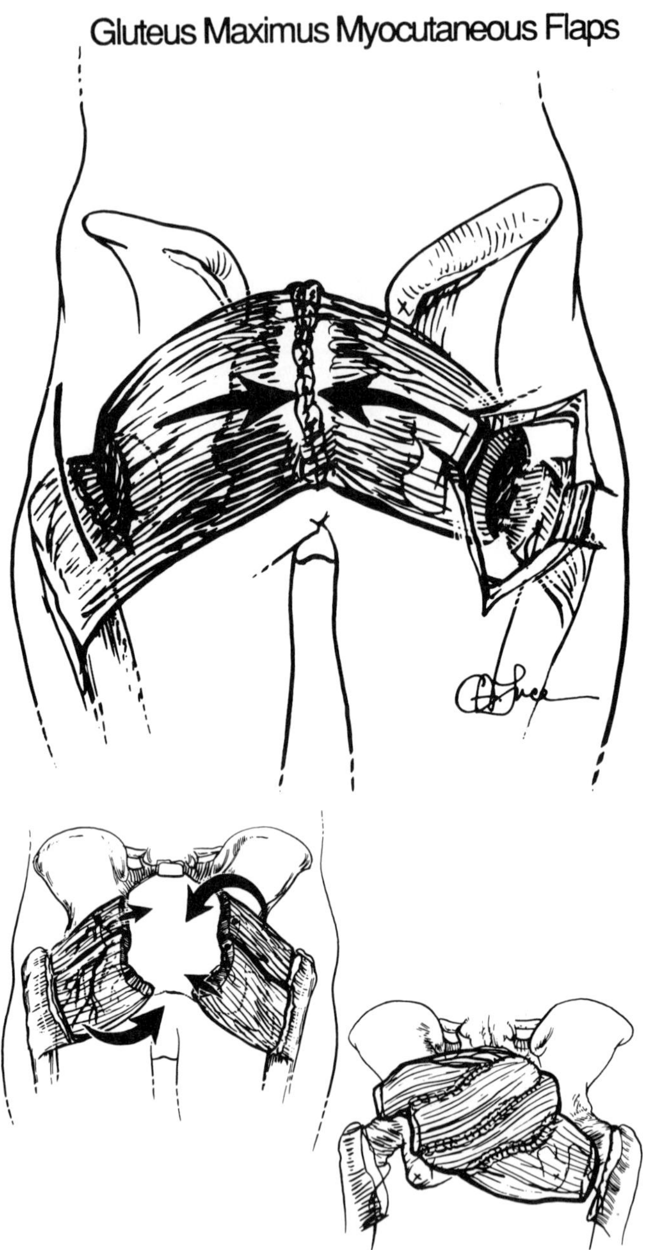

Figs. 14, 15, 16. The gluteus muscles are approximated in the midline. The lateral insertion of the gluteus maximus may have to be incised to allow medial advancement of the muscle. Large gluteus maximus cutaneous flaps are rotated to close the defect.

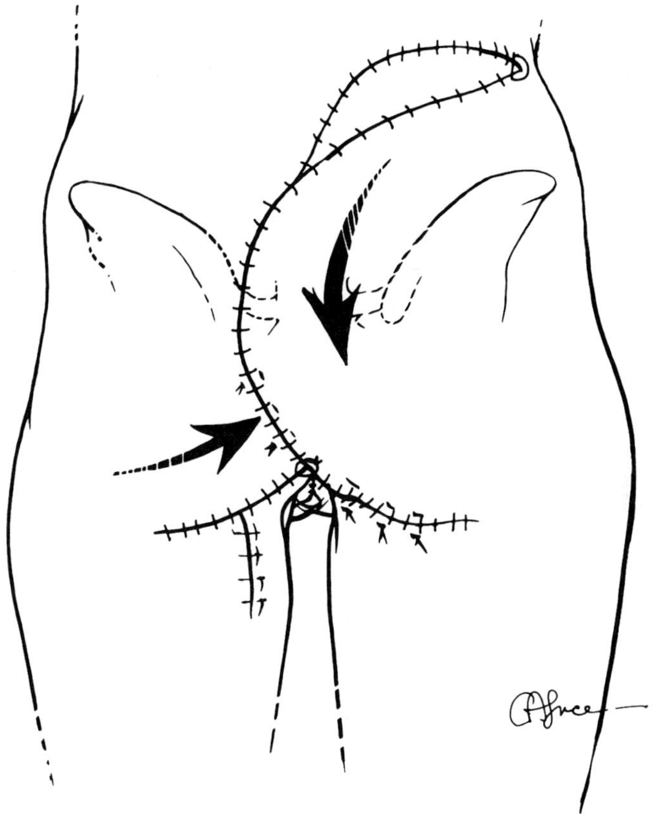

Figs. 14, 15, 16 (*continued*)

Table 4
Abdominal sacral resection: patient characteristics

Variable	n (%)
Gender	
Male	20 (32)
Female	43 (68)
Tumor type	
Advanced rectal cancer	5 (8)
Recurrent rectal cancer	58 (92)
Stage of primary cancer	
Stage I	2 (3.1)
Stage II	29 (46.0)
Stage III	29 (46.0)
Unknown	3 (4.8)

Note: mean age was 57.9 years (range 29–76 years).

Table 5
Abdominal sacral resection: previous treatments

Procedure	n (%)
Primary surgery	
Anterior resection	28 (48.2)
Abdominoperineal resection	30 (51.8)
Resection for second recurrence	
Anterior resection	3 (42.8)
Abdominoperineal resection	3 (42.8)
Hepatic resection	1 (14.4)
Radiation therapy (cGy)	
3000–4500	21 (33.3)
4600–5900	29 (46.0)
>6000	7 (11.1)
No prior radiation	5 (8.0)
Unknown	1 (1.6)

patients had been previously treated with anterior resection and APR. All but 5 of the 63 patients had previously undergone pelvic irradiation (those who had not received radiation therapy before ASR) (Table 5). The preoperative CEA level for the 63 patients was as follows: <5 ng/mL, 30 patients (48%); 5 to 10 ng/mL, five patients (8%); >10 ng/mL, 27 patients (48%); not available, one patient (1.6%).

Of the 63 patients undergoing ASR for cure, 31 (49%) required total cystectomy with ileal conduit, and seven (11%) underwent partial bladder resection; 27 patients (43%) had resection of the prostate or seminal vesicles, 9 (14%) had resection of the vagina, 10 (16%) had hysterectomy, and 12 (9%) had small bowel resection (Table 6). Tumor invasion of the sacral bone or ligaments was observed in 33 patients (52%), of the sacral bone marrow in seven patients (11%), and of the pelvic side walls in 10 patients (16%) (Table 7). Tumor margins were negative in 41 patients (65%), "close" (2-mm margins) in seven patients (11%), and positive in 15 patients (24%) (Table 8). The patients with involvement of the sacral bone marrow or pelvic side walls were included in the positive margin group. Median blood loss (recorded for the first 47 patients in the series) was 9546 mL. Median total operative time was 19.25 hours. Sixty-day operative mortality was 6% (four

Table 6
Abdominal sacral resection: concomitant organ resections

Organ resected	n (%)
Rectum	27 (43)
Cystectomy with ileal conduit	31 (49)
Partial cystectomy	7 (11)
Prostate/seminal vesicles	27 (43)
Vagina	9 (14)
Hysterectomy	10 (16)
Small bowel resection	12 (19)

Table 7
Abdominal sacral resection: tumor invasion and pelvic node status

Tumor location	*n* (%)
Tumor invasion	
Sacral bone or ligaments	33 (52)
Sacral bone marrow	7 (11)
Pelvic side walls	10 (16)
Pelvic nodes	
Negative	61 (96.8)
Positive	2 (3.2)

patients) (Table 9). Complication rates were as follows: wound-related, 70%; cardiopulmonary, 62%; septic, 51%; urologic, 19%; and musculoskeletal, 14% (Table 9). With the routine use of full-thickness myocutaneous flaps for closure of the sacral wound, the rate of wound complications has markedly decreased. Of 58 patients with long-term follow-up as of April 2002, median survival was 32 months, with 5-year survival of 30% (Fig. 17). This compares favorably with a historic control group of patients having recurrent rectal cancer primarily treated with irradiation, rather than resection, in whom median survival was 16 months and 5-year survival was 3% (Fig. 17) [52,53]. The current overall disease-free survival rates are 31% and 20%, respectively (Fig. 18).

In our series, type of primary resection and CEA level (but not age, gender, or stage of primary cancer) were significant prognostic factors (Table 10). Patients whose primary cancer was resected by low anterior resection had a median survival of 53 months and 5-year survival of 35%, whereas patients whose primary cancer was resected by APR had median survival of 22 months and 5-year survival of 20% ($P < 0.05$). Five-year survival was 47% for patients whose CEA was <5 ng/ml and 16% for patients whose CEA was ≥5 ng/ml ($P < 0.05$). We identified a group of very-high-risk patients whose median survival was <12 months. This included patients with bone marrow invasion, positive lateral pelvic nodes, or microscopically positive margins. The former two groups of patients can be identified before completion of the first phase of the procedure. The latter group should undergo re-excision to negative margins, if possible. If the patient has not been previously irradiated, intraoperative radiotherapy (IORT) or postoperative brachytherapy could be added.

Table 8
Abdominal sacral resection: tumor pathology

Surgical margins	*n* (%)
Negative	41 (65)
Close negative (2 mm)	7 (11)
Positive	15 (24)

Table 9
Abdominal sacral resection: mortality and morbidity ($n = 63$)

Event	n (%)
Mortality	
30-d mortality	2 (3.1)
30–60-d mortality	2 (3.1)
Morbidity	
Pulmonary	17 (27)
Cardiovascular	22 (35)
Deep venous thrombosis	8 (13)
Cardiac	5 (8)
Urologic	50 (79)
Acute renal failure	17 (27)
Urinary tract infection	17 (27)
Fistula	7 (10)
Musculoskeletal	
Neurologic	9 (14)
Peroneal nerve	6 (9)
Neuropraxia	1 (1.6)
Sepsis	32 (51)
Wound complication	44 (70)
Infection	10 (16)
Dehiscence	34 (54)

In our series, 76% of patients experienced recurrent disease after ASR, with 52% being distant, 27% being local, and 20% being distant and local recurrence (Table 11). Overall results of our series of 177 patients presenting with recurrent rectal cancer are summarized in Table 12.

Table 10
Abdominal sacral resection: survival statistics

Variable	n	Overall 5-yr survival	Log rank/Cox	Disease-free 5-yr survival	Log rank
CEA level					
<5 ng/mL	25	47%	0.02/0.04	28%	NS
≥5 ng/mL	32	16%		15%	
Primary surgery					
Anterior resection	24	35%	0.02/NS	21%	0.03/NS
APR	29	20%		13%	
Age					
<65 yr	40	31%	NS	20%	NS
≥65 yr	18	29%		22%	
Stage					
I–II	27	34%	NS	13%	NS
III–IV	24	23%		23%	
Gender					
Male	19	35%	NS	28%	NS
Female	39	27%		15%	

Abbreviations: APR, abdominoperineal resection; CEA, carcinoembryonic antigen; NS, not significant.

Table 11
Abdominal sacral resection: recurrence

Event	*n* (%)
Recurrence	44 (76)
5-yr recurrence rate (Kaplan Meier)	80
Recurrence type	
Local	12 (27.3)
Distant	23 (52.3)
Local and distant	9 (20.4)

Published series of abdominal sacral resection

Yamada et al [58] presented a series of 64 patients who had pelvic exenterative procedures, of which 29 incorporated sacral resection. The sacral osteotomy was performed via the anterior lithotomy approach by this group. The 5-year survival for patients undergoing curative resection was 22.9, with a morbidity rate of 56% to 72% (mainly infectious complications). Mannaerts et al [59] reported on 50 patients who underwent ABSR, 13 for locally advanced rectal cancer and 37 for recurrent disease. Three-year overall survival was 41%, with a complication rate of 82%. Zacherl et al [60] reported 12 patients who underwent resection of locally recurrent rectal cancer with sacrectomy. Three-year overall survival was 17%, with a complication rate (mainly wound complications) of 42%. Results are summarized in Table 13. The recent updated series by Moriya is provided elsewhere in this issue.

Treatment of unresectable abdominal or pelvic recurrence

Primary radiation therapy

Treatment of pelvic recurrence of colorectal cancer with primary radiation is rarely curative but can provide excellent short-term (3–6 months)

Table 12
Management of recurrent rectal cancer (personal series)

Procedure	*n*	5-yr overall survival (%)	1-yr survival (%)	2-yr survival (%)	5-yr survival (%)
Curative	97				
Anterior resection or APR	23	28	80	64	24
ASR	63	32	85	55	31
Distant metastases	15	36	76	59	24
No surgical treatment	17	22	60	40	5
Palliative resection	23	21	50	30	5
Pelvic perfusion					
Palliative	30	12	50	20	0
Preoperative	10	29	60	40	10

Abbreviations: APR, abdominoperineal resection; ASR, abdominal sacral resection.

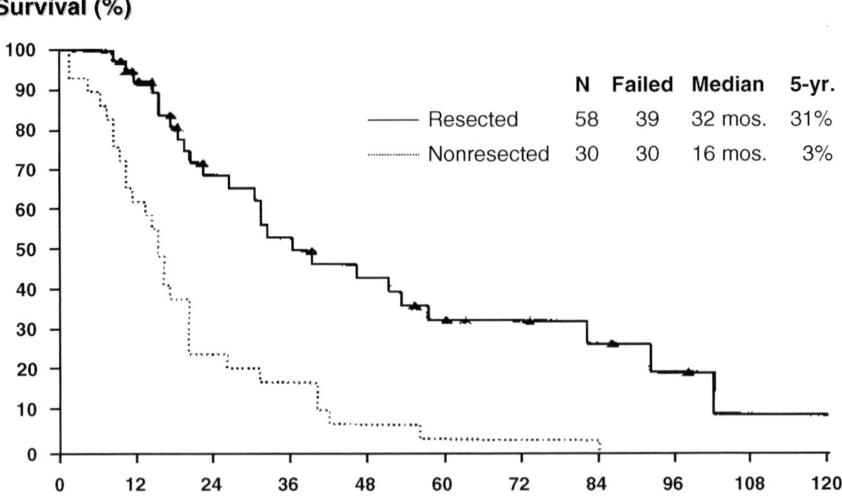

Fig. 17. Overall survival in patients resected for pelvic recurrence of rectal cancer. The median and 5-year survival of 32 months and 31% in the resected group is compared with a median and 5-year survival of 16 months and 3% in a group of patients with locally recurrent rectal cancer who were not resected but were all treated with radiation.

palliation of the boring deep perineal pain in these patients. These patients frequently survive long enough to develop progression of local disease. Many die with uncontrolled local disease and without evidence of systemic metastases [59]. In select patients, irradiation or systemic chemotherapy may provide a bridge to resection of recurrence [32,42].

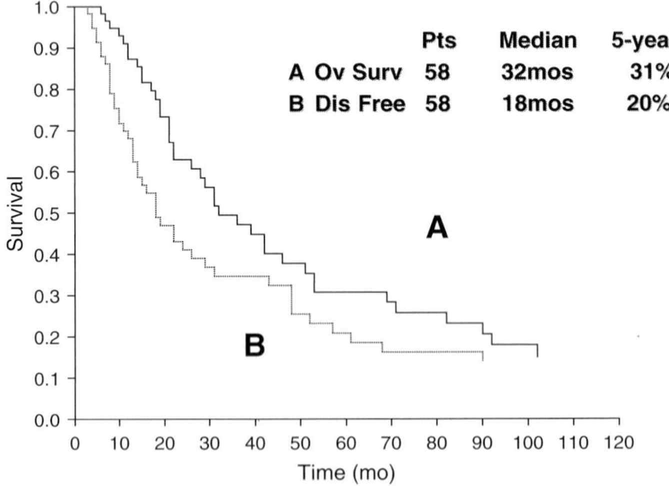

Fig. 18. The overall and disease-free survival after abdominal sacral resection for locally recurrent/advanced rectal cancer. Patient details are listed in Tables 5 through 13.

Table 13
Abdominal sacral resection: results of published series

Author	Number of patients	Mortality/ morbidity (%)	Recurrence rate (%)	Survival
Brunschwig, 1947–1969 [66]	6	33/100	Unknown	25% 5-yr
Sugarbaker, 1982 [67]	6	Unknown	Unknown	66% 3-yr
Takagi, 1979–1983 [65]	7	0/28	Unknown	28% 2-yr
Touran, 1981–1988 [57]	12	0/unknown	100	14% 2-yr
Temple, 1992 [55]	11	9/100	Unknown	20% 5-yr
Maetani, 1978–1996 [68]	59 (43 ASR)	3.3/unknown	76	25% 5-yr
Weber, 1990–1996 [69]	23	0/78	Unknown	30% 5-yr
Zacherl, 1999 [60]	12	Unknown/42	Unknown	17% 3-yr
Mannaerts, 2001 [59]	50	Unknown/82	Unknown	41% 3-yr
Yamada, 2002 [58]	64 (29 ASR)	Unknown/72	Unknown	22.9% 5-yr
Wanebo, (Unpublished data)	63	6.2/unknown	76	31% 5-yr

Surgical palliation

Patients not considered eligible for composite resection due to extent of disease (eg, those having extrapelvic disease, pulmonary or hepatic metastases, or sacral bone marrow invasion) represent a difficult management challenge [61]. Surgery performed for palliation (eg, colostomy proximal to an unresectable obstructing cancer) produces a minimal improvement in survival as compared with expectant management but may provide significant symptom control and improvement in quality of life. Guidelines for patient selection and anticipated results from purely palliative procedures for a variety of malignancies were recently advanced by Miner et al [62]. One group reported 12 patients who underwent palliative procedures for recurrent rectal cancer in whom median survival was 6 months and mean survival was 17 months [24].

Isolated pelvic perfusion

Options are limited for the group of patients who have unresectable pelvic recurrence after primary resection or after resection of recurrent disease. Palliative procedures do not prolong survival. Most of the patients in this group have been heavily pretreated and cannot receive more radiation therapy.

Our group has previously published results with isolated pelvic perfusion [17,63,64]. We and others have shown that isolated pelvic perfusion can provide significant palliation of the often debilitating pain associated with unresectable pelvic recurrence [17,61]. Occasionally, the procedure can function as a bridge to surgical resection [63].

By isolating the circulation to the pelvis, much higher concentrations of the drugs at the target site are achieved, as compared with systemic chemotherapy. In addition, regional perfusion allows for a lower incidence of systemic side effects [17]. Traditionally, we have used sequential infusion of 5-fluorouracil, mitomycin C, and a platinum compound cisplatin or oxaliplatin. The ratio of the level of each drug in the pelvic as compared with the systemic circulation is fairly consistent from patient to patient and ranges from 5:1 to 10:1 [17].

A balloon occlusion catheter (to block proximal flow during the perfusion) and a perfusion cannula are introduced into the distal aorta, and a second set is introduced into the inferior vena cava via the femoral artery and femoral vein, respectively [65]. Distal flow is prevented by tourniquets, inflated to 300 mm Hg, on the patient's thighs. An extracorporeal circuit provides high-flow oxygenated, heated blood containing chemotherapy over 60 minutes [17].

We previously reported on 25 patients (15 palliative, 10 preoperative) in whom a total of 40 isolated pelvic perfusions were performed [63]. Systemic leak ranged from 28% to 38%. Of the 15 patients treated for palliation, there was one objective partial response (by imaging studies). Eight patients experienced partial palliation of pain, ranging form 3 weeks to 3 months. Two patients had complete pain relief. There were 10 patients (five with rectal cancer and five with other pelvic malignancies) who received isolated pelvic perfusion preoperatively. One patient with rectal cancer achieved a complete response, and four patients with other malignancies achieved partial responses [63]. Our most recent update of our experience includes 42 patients with previously irradiated, recurrent cancer of the rectum (Harold J. Wanebo, MD, personal communication, 2004). A complete pathologic response was achieved in two patients, and significant tumor regression occurred in 11 patients, rendering them potentially resectable. Median survival after perfusion was 24 months in the patients rendered resectable, as compared with 8 months for the patients whose disease remained nonresectable. Further follow-up is needed, but these preliminary results suggest potential benefit of isolated pelvic perfusion as a preoperative measure in patients with locally recurrent, previously irradiated rectal cancer.

Summary

Pelvic recurrence of colorectal cancer remains a problem experienced by up to 35% of patients resected for cure. Early diagnosis is often elusive, and pelvic pain or rectal bleeding may be the first indications of recurrence. Factors implicated in a higher risk of recurrence include residual disease after resection, mucinous histologic subtype, poorly differentiated tumor, elevated serum CEA, extramural venous invasion, and bowel obstruction secondary to tumor.

Full staging workup includes physical examination; CT of the chest, abdomen, and pelvis; and serum CEA level. MRI is helpful for suspected sacral involvement. Bone scan or PET scan should be obtained to rule out involvement of the sacral bone marrow, which constitutes an absolute contraindication to surgical resection.

The use of palliative radiation for the treatment of pelvic recurrence of colorectal cancer has been associated with transient or incomplete palliation. For suitable candidates, surgical resection is the ideal treatment for pelvic recurrence. This may consist of salvage APR (for local recurrence after SSP), pelvic exenteration, or ASR, as appropriate for extent of disease. ABSR is a physiologically demanding procedure that should be undertaken only after thorough preoperative evaluation and preparation. Adjuvant radiation should be administered in patients not previously irradiated. Methods vary (eg, EBRT, IORT, or brachytherapy) depending on the extent of disease and previous radiation treatment received by the patient and institutional resources.

For patients with unresectable locoregional recurrence or those who are unfit to undergo a major extirpative procedure, isolated pelvic perfusion may provide partial clinical response and marked palliation.

In conclusion, optimal management of locoregional recurrence of colorectal cancer requires a multidisciplinary approach and a team familiar with the full spectrum of management techniques. Long-term survival rates of 30% can be achieved in carefully selected patients, which is similar to the outcome of resected liver or pulmonary metastases.

References

[1] American Cancer Society. Cancer facts & figures 2004. Available at: www.cancer.org. Accessed February 4, 2004.

[2] Pilipshen SJ, Heilweil M, Quan SH, et al. Patterns of pelvic recurrence following definitive resections of rectal cancer. Cancer 1984;53:1354–62.

[3] American Joint Committee on Cancer. Colon and Rectum. In: Greene FL, Page DL, Fleming ID, Fritz AG, Balch CM, Haller DG, Morrow M, editors. AJCC cancer staging manual. 6th edition. New York: Springer-Verlag; 2002. p. 113–23.

[4] Rousseau DL, Midis GP, Feig BW. Cancer of the colon, rectum, and anus. In: The MD Anderson Surgical Oncology Handbook. 3rd edition. Philadelphia: Lippincott Williams & Wilkins; 2003. p. 213–65.

[5] Varker KA, Wanebo HJ. Colorectal cancer: surgical treatment of abdominal and pelvic recurrences. In: Cancer of the colon, rectum, and anus. Sao Paulo: LemMar, Tezmedd; 2005:435–46.

[6] Watanabe T, Wu TT, Catalano PJ, et al. Molecular predictors of survival after adjuvant chemotherapy for colon cancer. N Engl J Med 2001;344:1196–206.

[7] Gilbertsen VA. The results of the surgical treatment of cancer of the rectum. Surg Gynecol Obstet 1962;114:313–9.

[8] Simmang CL, Gregorcyk SG. Adjuvant therapy for colorectal cancer. In: Cameron JL, editor. Current surgical therapy. 7th edition. St. Louis: Mosby; 2001. p. 246–50.

[9] Stearns MW. Preoperative radiation in carcinoma of the rectum. Proc Natl Cancer Conf 1964;5:489–93.

[10] Gastrointestinal Tumor Study Group. Prolongation of the disease-free interval in surgically treated rectal carcinoma. N Engl J Med 1985;312:1465–72.

[11] Benson AB III. Future directions in adjuvant therapy for rectal cancer. Oncology (Huntington) 2002;16(Suppl 5):45–51.

[12] Heald RJ, Moran BJ, Ryall RD, et al. Rectal cancer: the Basingstoke experience of total mesorectal excision. Arch Surg 1998;133:894–9.

[13] Swedish Rectal Cancer Trial. Improved survival with preoperative radiotherapy in resectable rectal cancer. N Engl J Med 1997;336:980–7.
[14] Kapiteijn E, Marijnen CA, Nagtegaal ID, et al, for the Dutch Colorectal Cancer Group. Preoperative radiotherapy combined with total mesorectal excision for resectable rectal cancer. N Engl J Med 2001;345:638–46.
[15] Wong CS, Cummings BJ, Brierly JD, et al. Treatment of locally recurrent rectal carcinoma: results and prognostic factors. Int J Radiat Oncol Biol Phys 1998;40:427–35.
[16] Beart RW Jr. New success with management of recurrent rectal cancer: a reason to follow patients. Ann Surg Oncol 1999;6:131–2.
[17] Turk PS, Belliveau JF, Darnowski JW, et al. Isolated pelvic perfusion for unresectable cancer using a balloon occlusion technique. Arch Surg 1993;128:533–9.
[17a] Vassilopoulos PP, Yoon JM, Ledesma EJ, et al. Treatment of recurrence of adenocarcinoma of the colon and rectum at the anastomotic site. Surg Gynecol Obstet 1981;152:777.
[18] Kraemer M, Wiratkapun S, Seow-Chen F, et al. Stratifying risk factors for follow-up: a comparison of recurrent and non-recurrent colorectal cancer. Dis Colon Rectum 2001;44:815–21.
[18a] Pihl E, Hughes ES, McDermott FT, et al. Recurrence of carcinoma of the colon and rectum at the anastomotic suture line. Surg Gynecol Obstet 1981;153:495.
[19] Carlsson U, Stewenius J, Ekelund G, et al. Is CEA analysis of value in screening for recurrences after surgery for colorectal carcinoma? Dis Colon Rectum 1983;26:369–73.
[20] Bruinvels DJ, Stiggelbout AM, Kievit J, et al. Follow-up of patients with colorectal cancer: a meta-analysis. Ann Surg 1994;219:174–82.
[21] Sagar PM, Pemberton JH. Surgical management of locally recurrent rectal cancer. Br J Surg 1996;83:293–304.
[22] Wanebo HJ, Antoniuk P, Koness RJ, et al. Pelvic resection of recurrent rectal cancer: technical considerations and outcomes. Dis Colon Rectum 1999;42:1438–48.
[22a] Schiessel R, Wunderlich M, Herbst F. Local recurrence of colorectal cancer: effect of early detection and aggressive surgery. Br J Surg 1986;73:342.
[23] Farouk R, Nelson H, Radice E, et al. Accuracy of computed tomography in determining resectability for locally advanced primary or recurrent colorectal cancers. Am J Surg 1998;175:283–7.
[24] Huguier M, Houry S. Treatment of local recurrence of rectal cancer. Am J Surg 1998;175:288–92.
[24a] Willett CG, Shellito PC, Tepper JE, et al. Intraoperative electron beam radiation therapy for recurrent locally advanced rectal or rectosigmoid carcinoma. Cancer 1991;67:1504.
[25] Torricelli P, Pecchi A, Luppi G, et al. Gadolinium-enhanced MRI with dynamic evaluation in diagnosing the local recurrence of rectal cancer. Abdom Imaging 2003;28:19–27.
[26] Moore HG, Akhurst T, Larson SM, et al. A case-controlled study of 18-fluorodeoxyglucose positron emission tomography in the detection of pelvic recurrence in previously irradiated rectal cancer patients. J Am Coll Surg 2003;197:22–8.
[27] Whiteford MH, Whiteford HM, Yee LF, et al. Usefulness of FDG-PET scan in the assessment of suspected metastatic or recurrent adenocarcinoma of the colon and rectum. Dis Colon Rectum 2000;43:759–67.
[28] Avradopoulos KA, Vezeridis MP, Wanebo HJ. Pelvic exenteration for recurrent rectal cancer. Adv Surg 1996;29:215–33.
[29] Turk PS, Wanebo HJ. Pelvic recurrence: resection and other alternatives. In: Wanebo HJ, editor. Surgery for gastrointestinal cancer: a multidisciplinary approach. Lippincott-Raven Publishers; 1997. p. 745–57.
[30] Cuthbertson AM, Simpson RL. Curative local excision of rectal adenocarcinoma. Aust N Z J Surg 1986;56:229–31.
[31] Hojo K. Anastomotic recurrence after sphincter saving resection for rectal cancer: length of distal clearance of the bowel. Dis Colon Rectum 1986;29:11–4.

[32] Marks G, Mohiuddin MM, Masoni L. High dose preoperative radiation and full-thickness local excision: a new option for patients with select cancer of the rectum. Dis Colon Rectum 1990;33:735–9.
[33] Otmezguine Y, Grimard L, Calitch E. A new combined approach in the conservative management of rectal cancer. Int J Radiat Oncol Biol Phys 1989;17:539–45.
[34] Polk HC Jr, Spratt JS Jr. Results of treatment of perineal recurrence of cancer of the rectum. Cancer 1979;43:952–5.
[35] Sannella NA. Abdominoperineal resection following anterior resection. Cancer 1976;38: 378–81.
[36] Segall MM, Goldberg SM, Nivatvongs S, et al. Abdominoperineal resection for recurrent cancer following anterior resection. Dis Colon Rectum 1981;24:80–4.
[37] Willett CG, Tepper JE, Donnelly S, et al. Patterns of failure following local excision and local excision and postoperative radiation therapy for invasive rectal adenocarcinoma. J Clin Oncol 1989;7:1003–8.
[38] Law WL, Chu KW, Choi HK. Total pelvic exenteration for locally advanced rectal cancer. J Am Coll Surg 2000;190:78–83.
[39] Estes NC, Thomas JH, Jewell WR, et al. Pelvic exenteration: a treatment for failed rectal cancer surgery. Am Surg 1993;59:420–2.
[40] Wiig JN, Poulsen JP, Larsen S, et al. Total pelvic exenteration with preoperative irradiation for advanced primary and recurrent rectal cancer. Eur J Surg 2002;168: 42–8.
[41] Meterissian SH, Skibber JM, Giacco GG, et al. Pelvic exenteration for locally advanced rectal carcinoma: factors predicting improved survival. Surgery 1997;121:479–87.
[42] Rodel C, Grabenbauer GG, Matzel KE, et al. Extensive surgery after high-dose preoperative chemoradiotherapy for locally advanced recurrent rectal cancer. Dis Colon Rectum 2000;43:312–9.
[43] Friel CM, Cromwell JW, Marra C, et al. Salvage radical surgery after failed local excision for early rectal cancer. Dis Colon Rectum 2002;45:875–9.
[43a] Beart RW, Martin JK, Gunderson LL. Management of recurrent rectal cancer. Cancer 1991;67:1504.
[44] Ogunbiyi O, McKenna K, Birnbaum EH, et al. Aggressive surgical management of recurrent rectal cancer: is it worthwhile? Dis Colon Rectum 1997;40:150–5.
[45] Salo JC, Paty PB, Guillem J, et al. Surgical salvage of recurrent rectal carcinoma after curative resection: a 10-year experience. Ann Surg Oncol 1999;6:171–7.
[46] Lopez-Kostner F, Fazio VW, Vignali A, et al. Locally recurrent rectal cancer: predictors and success of salvage surgery. Dis Colon Rectum 2001;44:173–8.
[47] Bozzetti F, Bertario L, Rossetti C, et al. Surgical treatment of locally recurrent rectal carcinoma. Dis Colon Rectum 1997;40:1421–4.
[48] Garcia-Aguilar J, Cromwell JW, Marra C, et al. Treatment of local recurrence of rectal cancer. Dis Colon Rectum 2001;44:1743–8.
[49] Vezeridis MP, Wanebo HJ. Extended radical pelvic surgery including sacral resection. Surg Oncol Clin North Am 1994;3:291–305.
[50] Vezeridis MP, Wanebo HJ. Sacral resection of posterior pelvic malignancy. Cancer Invest 1995;13:375–80.
[51] Wanebo HJ, Marcove RC. Abdominal sacral resection of locally recurrent rectal cancer. Ann Surg 1981;194:458–71.
[52] Wanebo HJ, Gaker DL, Whitehill R, et al. Pelvic recurrence of rectal cancer: options for curative resection. Ann Surg 1987;205:482–94.
[53] Wanebo HJ, Koness RJ, Turk PS, et al. Composite resection of posterior pelvic malignancy. Ann Surg 1992;215:685–93.
[54] Wanebo HJ, Koness RJ, Vezeridis MP, et al. Pelvic resection of recurrent rectal cancer. Ann Surg 1994;220:586–97.

[55] Temple WJ, Ketcham AS. Sacral resection for control of pelvic tumors. Am J Surg 1992; 163:370–4.

[56] Thomas PR, Lindblad AS. Adjuvant postoperative radiotherapy and chemotherapy in rectal carcinoma: a review of the Gastrointestinal Tumor Study Group experience. Radiother Oncol 1988;13:245–52.

[57] Touran T, Frost DB, O'Connell TR. Sacral resection: operative technique and outcome. Arch Surg 1990;125:911–3.

[58] Yamada K, Ishizawa T, Niwa K, et al. Pelvic exenteration and sacral resection for locally advanced primary and recurrent rectal cancer. Dis Colon Rectum 2002;45: 1078–84.

[59] Mannaerts GHH, Rutten HJT, Martijn H, et al. Abdominosacral resection for primary irresectable and locally recurrent rectal cancer. Dis Colon Rectum 2001;44:806–14.

[60] Zacherl J, Schiessel R, Windhager R, et al. Abdominosacral resection of recurrent rectal cancer in the sacrum. Dis Colon Rectum 1999;42:1035–9.

[61] Temple WJ, Saettler EB. Locally recurrent rectal cancer: role of composite resection of extensive pelvic tumors with strategies for minimizing risk of recurrence. J Surg Oncol 2000; 73:47–58.

[62] Miner TJ, Brennan MF, Jaques DP. A prospective, symptom related, outcomes analysis of 1022 palliative procedures for advanced cancer. Ann Surg 2004;240:719–27.

[63] Wanebo HJ, Chung MA, Levy AI, et al. Preoperative therapy for advanced pelvic malignancy by isolated pelvic perfusion with the balloon-occlusion technique. Ann Surg Oncol 1996;3:295–303.

[64] Wanebo HJ, Belliveau JF. A pharmacokinetic model and the clinical pharmacology of cisplatinum, 5-fluorouracil and mitomycin-C in isolated pelvic perfusion. Cancer Chemother Pharmacol 1999;43:427–34.

[65] Takagi H, Morimoto T, Hara S, et al. Seven cases of pelvic exenteration combined with sacral resection for locally recurrent rectal cancer. J Surg Oncol 1986;32:184–8.

[66] Brunschwig A, Barber HR. Pelvic exenteration combined with resection of segments of bony pelvis. Surgery 1969;65:417–20.

[67] Sugarbaker PH. Partial sacrectomy for en bloc excision of rectal cancer with posterior fixation. Dis Colon Rectum 1982;25:708–11.

[68] Maetani S, Onodera H, Nishikawa T, et al. Significance of local recurrence of rectal cancer as a local or disseminated disease. Br J Surg 1998;85:521–5.

[69] Weber KL, Nelson H, Gunderson LL, et al. Sacropelvic resection for recurrent anorectal cancer: a multidisciplinary approach. Clin Orthop 2000;372:231–40.

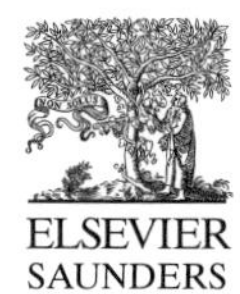

ELSEVIER
SAUNDERS

Surg Oncol Clin N Am
14 (2005) 225–238

SURGICAL
ONCOLOGY CLINICS
OF NORTH AMERICA

Total Pelvic Exenteration with Distal Sacrectomy for Fixed Recurrent Rectal Cancer

Yoshihiro Moriya, MD, PhD*, Takayuki Akasu, MD, Shin Fujita, MD, PhD, Seiichirou Yamamoto, MD

Department of Surgery, National Cancer Center Hospital, 1-1 Tsukiji 5-chome, Chuo-Ku, Tokyo 104-0045, Japan

Four percent to 33% of patients with rectal cancer develop locoregional relapse after undergoing radical surgery with curative intent. Without treatment, the mean survival time for patients with local recurrence is only approximately 8 months, an associated severe symptomatic disease—especially pain—occurs, and their quality of life becomes remarkably deteriorated, probably with a miserable prognosis [1–4].

For cases with locally recurrent rectal cancer (LRRC), external beam radiotherapy, intraoperative radiotherapy, chemotherapies, and surgical treatments have been used singly or as part of a multimodality approach over the last several decades, resulting in certain outcomes that are not yet satisfactory [5–21]. For the purpose of attaining thorough margin-free resection, what we have been performing actively as our standard curative approach for fixed recurrent tumor (FRT) is radical resection with removal of affected neighboring organs and pelvic walls, including the sacrum, as originally reported by Wanebo and Marcove [6]. This article describes the surgical indications, contraindications, surgical techniques, oncologic outcomes, and complications of total pelvic exenteration with distal sacrectomy (TPES).

Patterns of growth in the pelvis

By cause and growth pattern of local recurrence, LRRC can be classified into three main categories.

* Corresponding author.
E-mail address: ymoriya@ncc.go.jp (Y. Moriya).

doi:10.1016/j.soc.2004.11.014

Anastomotic recurrence and perianastomotic recurrence

These suture line recurrences after low anterior resection are caused by implantation of cancer cells into the stump of anastomosis or insufficient resection of the rectal wall or mesorectum (Fig. 1). In the case of extramural invasion, however, it is difficult to distinguish between these two recurrences. When there is no extramural invasion or neighboring organ invasion, the basic surgical procedure is abdominoperineal resection (APR).

Perineal recurrence

Perineal recurrence is a recurrence that occurs after APR near the pelvic floor or perineal wound. From its early stage, perineal recurrence invades the coccyx, gluteal maximus muscle, or pelvic wall. Surgical margin-free resection seldom can be obtained by local excision alone. Many patients need resection of the pelvic wall or intrapelvic organs.

Pelvic recurrence

By occupied site, pelvic recurrence (Fig. 2) can be subdivided into anterior, lateral, and dorsal recurrences. Anterior pelvic recurrence is an LRRC that invades the anterior organs (ie, urogenital organs). For resecting this recurrent tumor, the basic surgical procedure is total pelvic exenteration (TPE). In women, if there is no obvious bladder invasion, it is possible to preserve urinary organs. This recurrence frequently is caused by insufficient resection for T4 rectal cancer. Lateral pelvic recurrence occurs because of lateral lymph node metastasis after total mesorectal excision or insufficient lateral node dissection. It begins to infiltrate the pelvic wall in its early stage. Dorsal pelvic recurrence is presacral extramural recurrence after APR or low

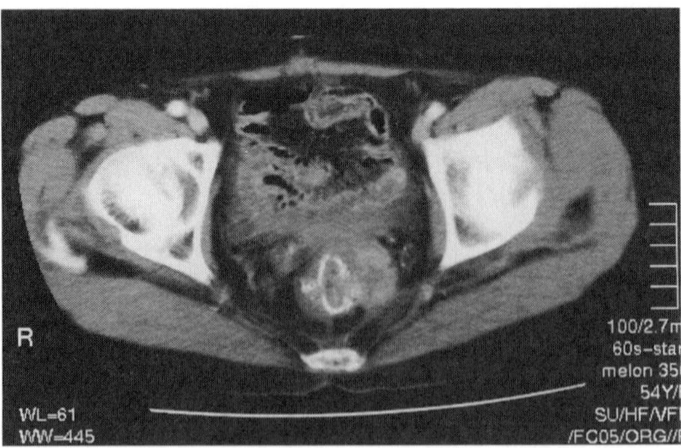

Fig. 1. Perianastomotic recurrence. A 54-year-old female patient underwent TPES for her FRT with 556 mL blood loss and no complication. At initial surgery 4 years ago, she received low anterior resection with D3 lymph node dissection and postoperative 60 Gy radiotherapy.

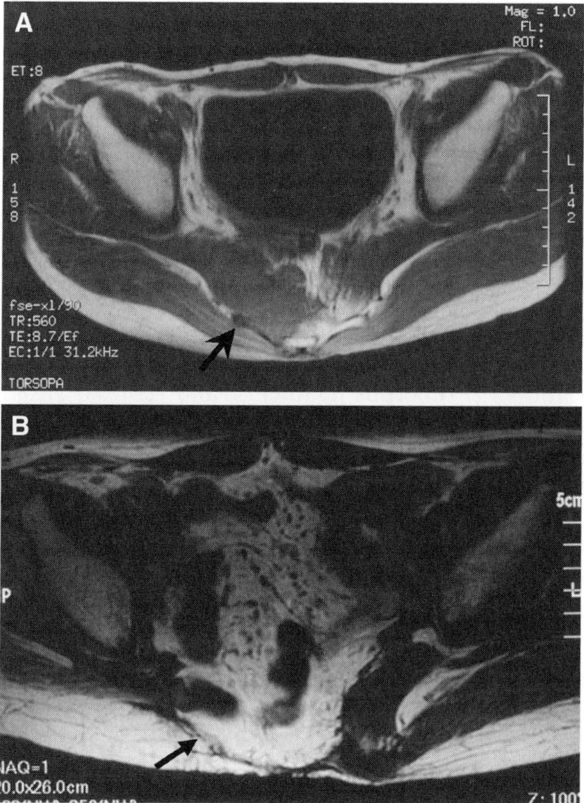

Fig. 2. (*A*) Dorsolateral pelvic recurrence with sacral bone invasion. A 47-year-old male patient underwent TPES for his FRT (*arrow*) with 673 mL blood loss and no complication. At initial surgery 1.5 years ago, he received low anterior resection. (*B*) Postoperative MRI. The patient is alive without re-recurrence 4 years after TPES.

anterior resection that invades the pelvic wall. It forms itself into FRT from its early stage. The cause of this recurrence may be extramesenteric lymphatic spread, insufficient resection of the mesorectum, or a cut into the mesorectum during operation. This pattern of recurrence is common patterns.

Why total pelvic exenteration with distal sacrectomy is the standard surgery for fixed recurrent tumor

Therapeutic policies for LRRC vary remarkably. The probable reasons for this are as follows: (1) there are various LRRCs, ranging from mobile recurrences to huge masses that occupy the pelvis, (2) an inappropriate surgical intervention may cause an iatrogenic cancer spread, leading to impaired quality of life, and (3) although treatments other than complete resection may not bring cure, the invasiveness of surgeries such as TPES is considered excessive. In non-fixed recurrent tumors, complete resection can be achieved more often with limited surgery, such as APR or low anterior resection, and the outcomes are relatively favorable. LRRC grows within the narrow pelvis, and when the tumor size becomes larger to some extent, it can invade the pelvic wall easily and appear in the form of FRT. A challenge for the surgeon is the surgical treatment for FRTs with lateral or dorsal involvement, which comprises a larger percentage.

Such fixation is infrequently confined to one site and is of small range; many of those cases show fixations to the components surrounding the LRRC (eg, bony pelvis, including sacrum and coccyges; non-bony pelvis, including coccygeus muscle, piriform muscle, internal iliac vessels, inferior hypogastric plexus, sacral nerve plexus, obturator internus muscle, and sacrospinous and sacrotuberous ligaments; and residual anterior organs in the pelvis). Their anatomic planes are distorted, and it is difficult to determine and hold uninvolved margins during resection. For FRT cases, composite resection is inevitably required to encompass potentially involved pelvic walls, especially the distal sacrum. Only this strategy enables the R0 extirpation en bloc. Especially after APR, the LRRC grows while being sandwiched between the anterior organs and sacrum. Wanebo and Marcove [6] tackled this difficult problem using the new technique of abdominosacral resection, followed by several surgeons in 1980s [8,9,10,12].

Techniques to preserve the anterior organs and inferior hypogastric plexus for surgical treatment of FRT have been reported [16]. Those approaches, however, are likely to reduce local radicality, because the anatomic pathway around the autonomic nerve plexuses and ureter disappears and is replaced by scar tissue caused by initial surgery, especially after extended surgery. FRT in the deep pelvis also is often fixed more extensively than expected before surgery, which also justifies our experience-based strategy that TPES is positioned as the standard surgery for FRT. This technique is considered to be demanding and formidable because of high rates of mortality and morbidity [6,12,13,19]; consequently, combination of limited resection and intraoperative radiotherapy is likely to become standard in the treatment of FRT [17,22–29]. Whether an emphasis is placed on composite resection or multimodality treatment, surgeons have the same view that the key treatment to obtain local control and survival benefit is R0 surgery [22,28–31]. Is it really possible to carry out R0 resection for FRT by conventional surgery? Having been able to ensure R0 resection for FRT and develop secure surgical techniques, we consider that there are no therapies superior to TPES in treating FRT.

Evaluation by imaging and patient selection

Once the diagnosis of LRRC is made, detailed study should be conducted in terms of surgical indication from two aspects: (1) whether distance metastasis is present and (2) to what extent the tumor spreads within the pelvis. Extrapelvic disease is searched for by the whole body CT scan. MRI and F-18-fluorodeoxy glucose position emission tomography (FDG-PET) are also useful in detecting extrapelvic disease and distinguishing between recurrent disease and scar tissue. CT, MRI, and FDG-PET are useful in distinguishing between solitary and multifocal recurrences in the pelvis and between anterior organ involvement and dorsolateral pelvic wall involvement.

We investigated a total of 196 consecutive patients who underwent laparotomy to remove LRRC between 1983 and 2003. The study excluded patients whose recurrent rectal cancer developed after local excision. We performed a limited surgery, such as APR, in 62 patients, TPE in 41, and TPES in 69. The remaining 24 patients had unresectable LRRC. Clinical and pathologic characteristics of 69 patients are listed in Table 1.

Patients with documented distant metastasis are not candidates for surgical treatment, because the curative potential is low and their life expectancy is not long enough to evaluate treatment outcome. With regard to surgical indication, we conducted TPES for FRT localized in the pelvis. Locally unresectable diseases include tumors that grow into sciatic notch,

Table 1
Clinical and pathologic characteristics of 69 patients

Characteristics	Number
Median age (range) (y)	57 (29–73)
Sex	
Male	55
Female	14
Body mass index (range)	22.9 (15.0–28.7)
Median time to local recurrence (range) (mo)	23 (7–118)
Liver metastasis	
No	65
Yes	5
Initial surgery	
Sphincter-preserving surgery; SPS	33
Abdominoperineal resection; APR	36
Radiotherapy for primary rectal cancer	
Yes	4
No	65
Radiotherapy for local recurrence before re-resection	
Yes	32 (median, 50 Gy; range, 30–80 Gy)
No	37
Dukes classification for primary growth	
A	4
B	18
C	47
Histologic type	
Well-differentiated adenocarcinoma	26
Moderately	34
Poorly	9

encase the external iliac vessels, extend to the sacral promontory, obstruct the bilateral ureters, and cause leg edema secondary to lymphatic or venous obstruction [30,31]. For patients with one or two liver metastases amenable to surgical resection, however, concomitant hepatectomy with surgical treatment of LRRC may be warranted. Lung metastasis and other extrapelvic diseases are excluded from surgical indications.

Surgical technique

TPE for primary pelvic malignancy is performed by first dividing loose connective tissues, such as the Retzius, retrorectal, and obturator spaces, and then dissecting along the parietal pelvic fascia. In recurrent cancer cases, however, those spaces disappear and are replaced by dense scar tissue. Because of this condition, TPES for FRT is a challenging procedure. The operation is performed in the following order.

Abdominal phase

The patient is placed in the lithotomy position. After detaching adhesions caused by initial surgery, the surgeon confirms the localization of the recurrent tumor within the pelvis and the absence of extrapelvic diseases and then makes a final decision to proceed to TPES. First, the Retzius space is opened. The endopelvic fascia and pubo-prostatic ligaments can be identified bilaterally and divided using electric cautery to expose the levator ani muscle. The dorsal vein complex together with the divided endopelvic fascia is bunched with the forceps and doubly tied and divided.

Next, the level of sacral amputation is determined. The anterior area from the aortic bifurcation to the sacral promontory is exposed to enter the anterior surface of the sacrum. The dissection is made using electric cautery down to the distal sacrum, at which point sacral amputation is planned, as is resection of the thickened Waldeyer's fascia with the presacral venous plexuses and scar tissue. During this process, bleeding occurs more or less; however, hemostasis can be obtained using combination of electric cautery and gauze pack. The area from the common iliac artery to the bifurcation between the internal and external iliac arteries is exposed. During dissection of the obturator space while preserving the obturator nerve, components of the sacral nerve plexus, such as the lumbosacral nerve and S1 and S2 sacral nerves, can be identified. Marking the S2 sacral nerve with a rubber loop ensures recognition of sacral nerves during sacrectomy (Fig. 3).

The next step is resection of the internal iliac vessels. The way to manipulate the internal iliac vessels is as follows. First, the trunk of the internal iliac artery is doubly tied and divided at the distal portion of the branching of the superior gluteal artery. Second, several branches that perforate the pelvic wall are divided. Finally, the trunk of the internal iliac vein is doubly tied and divided. Blood loss during TPES mostly occurs from

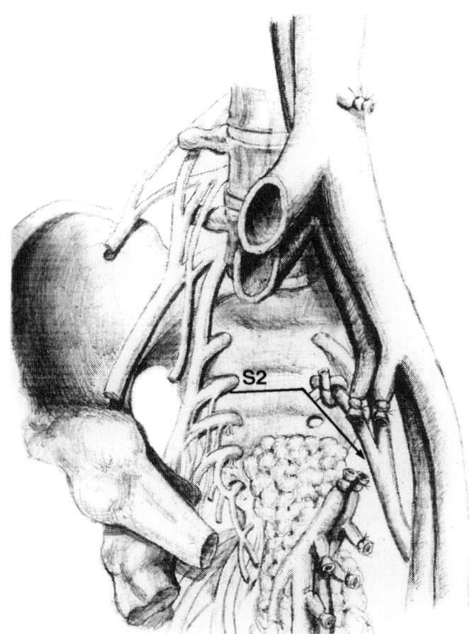

Fig. 3. Line of sacrectomy and marked second sacral nerve.

the venous plexus [31]. By taking the appropriate steps to avoid congestion of the venous plexus at the earliest possible opportunity, the operation can be performed with a minimum amount of blood loss from the venous plexus. Resection of the internal iliac veins is the most important part of this operation, and it requires advanced technical skills and careful maneuvers. FRT extends along the internal iliac vessels more frequently than the primary rectal cancer [32]; bilateral resection of the internal iliac vessels is one of the pivotal steps in TPES. Combined resection of the internal iliac vessels during the abdominal phase greatly contributes to reducing blood loss during sacrectomy.

Perineal phase

Incision of the perineal skin conforms to APR. The levator ani muscle is divided at its attachment and a connection is made through to the pelvic cavity. If the perineal phase is performed after the venous plexus is resected, a considerable amount of blood loss will occur from congested veins around the urogenital diaphragm. The perineal phase should occur before ligation of the trunk of the internal iliac veins so that the phase can be performed with less blood loss.

Sacral phase

The patient is placed in the prone position after temporary closure of abdominal wound. At that point, the padded operating frame for laminectomy is used to prevent an increase in abdominal or vertebral venous pressure. Bleeding caused by the increase of vertebral venous pressure makes sacral amputation complicated. The median incision is made approximately 10 cm longer toward the head from the planned line of sacral amputation. The gluteus maximus muscle is detached from the sacrum so that the posterior surface of the sacrum can be exposed fully. The next step of this phase involves detaching the sacrotuberous and sacrospinous ligaments and piriform muscle that fix the sacrum. After dissecting these structures, the sacral nerve plexus also can be checked.

The surgeon inserts an index finger into the pelvic cavity from the lower edge of the sacroiliac joint and checks the dissected level of the anterior surface of the sacrum to determine the level of sacral amputation. The medial sacral crest is scraped, laminectomy is performed, and the root of the second sacral nerve is identified. The caudal end of the dura usually extends to around the lower edge of the S2. The dura, together with the cauda equine, is tied and divided. The surgeon performs sacral amputation using chisel and hammer at a stretch (Fig. 4). Hemostasis is performed quickly using electric cautery and bone wax. In men, after checking the stump of the urethra, the urethra is closed tightly to prevent transurethral infection. The origins of the gluteus maximus muscle, the subcutis, and the skin are closed tightly.

Urinary diversion, prevention of pelvic sepsis, and wound closure

The patient is placed in the lithotomy position. Reconstruction of the urinary tract using ileal conduit and colostomy is performed. Mobilization of the right colon from the cecum to the hepatic flexure enables construction of a high urostoma. After constructing the ileal conduit, an ileoileostomy

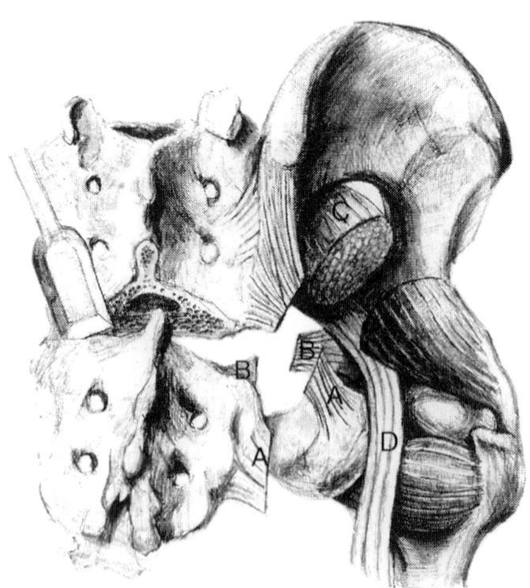

Fig. 4. Sacral amputation in prone position. (*A*) Sacrotuberous ligament. (*B*) Sacrospinous ligament. (*C*) Piriform muscle. (*D*) Sciatic nerve.

should be lifted up above the pelvic brim and fixed to the mesentery so that it will not fall in the pelvic cavity. This procedure is invariably required to prevent anastomotic leakage secondarily caused by pelvic sepsis, especially after radiotherapy. If the greater omentum is long enough with favorable blood flow, omentoplasty into the pelvic cavity should be performed. In patients who have recurrent tumor invading the perineal skin, it is necessary to combine a wide resection of the perineal skin. In such cases, reconstruction should be performed with a musculocutaneous flap [20,30]. It is appropriate that gastrostomy be performed before closing the abdomen, because enteroparalysis continues for a while after TPES. A thick drain is placed in the pelvis, and then the abdomen is closed.

Surgical invasiveness and oncologic outcomes after total pelvic exenteration with distal sacrectomy

Margins were microscopically negative in 57 patients (83%) and positive in 12. A comparison between two periods (1983–1992 and 1993–2003) showed a mean blood loss decrease from 4229 to 2102 mL ($P < 0.001$), with a favorable learning curve (Table 2). There was no difference in operative time and hospital stay. The most common level of sacral amputation was the S3 superior margin in 26 cases, followed by the S3 inferior margin and S2 inferior margin (Table 3). Overall mortality and complication rates were 3% and 58%, respectively. There was no hospital death in the latter period. The most frequent complication was sacral wound dehiscence in 51%, followed by pelvic sepsis in 39%. The incidence of pelvic sepsis in the latter period decreased significantly to 27%, compared with 72% in the former period ($P = 0.038$). Enteroperineal fistulae were observed in four cases.

Survival curves show overall 3- and 5-year disease-specific survival rates of 58% and 40%, respectively. In 57 patients with R0, including 5 patients with hepatic metastasis, 3- and 5-year disease-specific survival rates were 67% and 49%, respectively, whereas there was no 4-year survivor in patients with margin-positive, which showed significantly poor prognosis ($P < 0.001$) (Fig. 5). There was no survival difference between patients with and without radiotherapy before re-resection. Fourteen patients had lateral node metastases around the internal iliac vessels. Of these 14 patients, 6 are alive and 3 were long-term survivors for 64, 71, and 141 months, respectively.

Table 2
Surgical invasiveness and hospital stay

Operative burden	Former period (1983–1992) mean $n = 18$	Latter period (1993–2003) mean $n = 51$	P-value
Operative time (min)	769 (370–990)	702 (480–1100)	NS
Blood loss (mL)	4229 (1800–16,300)	2102 (673–8468)	$P < 0.0001$
Hospital stay (d)	37.5 (23–200)	34 (21–257)	NS

Table 3
Level of distal sacrectomy and complications

Level of sacrectomy	Sepsis in pelvis	Ileus	Fistula[a]
Middle amputation			
S2 inferior margin (n = 12)	6	2	1
S2-3 (n = 26)	9	1	1
Low amputation			
S3 inferior margin (n = 16)	8	1	2
S3-4 (n = 10)	2	1	
S4 inferior margin (n = 5)	2		

[a] Fistula: enteroperineal fistula caused by anastomotic leakage.

Of 57 patients with R0 resection, 34 developed re-recurrence. The most common site was the lung (18 patients) followed by the pelvis (12 patients).

Oncologic outcomes reported in the literature

Factors such as type of surgery, combined therapy, and postoperative follow-up period are diversified, and comparison of reported oncologic outcomes for LRRC is of small significance. For example, a study that includes patients with recurrence after local excision naturally should show favorable outcome, whereas in a study conducted only with cases of FRT, unfavorable outcome can be predicted. Lopez-Kostner et al [33] reported a 5-year survival rate of 32% in 43 patients who underwent surgical treatment, 11 of whom developed recurrence after local excision. On the other hand, Bozzetti et al [18] showed a 5-year survival rate of less than 10% in patients who underwent surgery alone and pointed out a limitation of outcome after surgical treatment alone. Regarding 5-year survival after

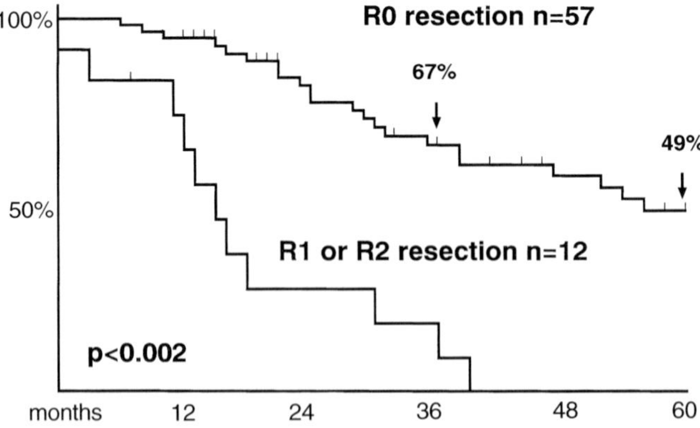

Fig. 5. Disease-specific survival curve. The difference between the two groups was significant ($P < 0.001$).

composite resection, Wanebo et al [19] reported a rate of 31%, Maetani et al [10] reported a rate of 25%, and Yamada et al [21] reported a rate of 18%. Those are not satisfactory outcomes. Incidence of local re-recurrence ranges from 27% to 61% [10,19,31].

As for outcome after multimodality therapy, there are many reports in which the ordinary dosages of radiation used preoperatively were 45 to 50 Gy. Intraoperative dosages of 10 to 15 Gy in R0 cases and 15 to 20 Gy in R-positive cases also were reported [24–29]. Valentini et al [24] reported a 5-year survival rate of 22%, and Mannaerts et al [23] reported a 3-year survival rate of 60%. In the series by Shoup et al [25], who investigated outcomes after resection plus intraoperative radiotherapy, patients with R0 had a median disease-free survival of 31 months and a median disease-specific survival of 66 months.

Lung metastasis and local re-recurrence account for nearly 90% of all re-recurrence patterns [31], and measures to prevent these two types of re-recurrence are important. Compared with 20 years ago, when the only effective antitumor agent was 5-fluorouracil, some effective antitumor agents (eg, CPT-11, UFT, capecitabine, and oxaliplatin) have become available. We think that surgical treatment, combined with composite resection and intraoperative radiotherapy, is indispensable for improving local control rates and that an effective chemotherapy regimen after re-resection is indispensable for inhibiting lung metastasis.

Prognostic factors and staging system

Several factors, such as type of initial surgery, tumor size, presence of symptoms, and serum carcinoembryomic antigen level, have been regarded as significant prognostic indicators, although a consensus has not been reached yet. Willet et al [11] and Wanebo et al [19] found improved resectability in patients who underwent initial low anterior resection compared with patients who had initial APR. If FRT developed after low anterior resection, however, there was no difference in resectability and survival between them [31]. Shoup et al [25] indicated that vascular invasion and R1/R2 resection are factors for poor prognosis. In either report, the most important factor is whether R0 resection was attained [19,24,25,27,31]. Researchers already have shown that in surgical treatment for primary rectal cancer, surgery-related and biologic factors are crucial [34]. Surgical margin status and complications are exclusively determined by a surgeon's technical skills. Complicated surgeries, such as TPES or abdominosacral resection, should be undertaken only in specialized centers with an experienced complex treatment team.

Suzuki et al [14] judged the degree of fixation to surrounding structures according to surgical and pathologic findings and proposed their own staging method. Valentini et al [24] also reported a similar staging system in which they judged from CT scan imaging. They mentioned that degree of fixation is an independent prognostic factor. Wanebo et al [19] proposed a new staging system for stages TR1-2 to TR5, which are determined by extent of invasion. A staging system that uses degree of fixation or other prognostic factors is constructed so that treatment modalities for LRRC, especially surgical treatment, are placed in an appropriate position.

Summary

For primary rectal cancer, there is a difference in therapy between Western countries and Japan. In Western countries, initial surgery is total mesorectal excision or less limited surgery plus radiotherapy. For this reason, fibrosis caused by radiation occurs in the pelvis. On the other hand, in Japan, although preoperative radiotherapy is not given, total mesorectal excision or more extended surgery is performed as initial surgery, and the intrapelvic spaces are covered with postoperative scar tissue. In identifying an anatomic index and doing hemostasis, this scar tissue brings the surgeon more difficulty than the fibrosis caused by radiotherapy. Approximately half of our patients are irradiated preoperatively for recurrence. In those patients, operation is performed under an unfavorable condition because the fibrosis caused by radiation is added to the scar tissue caused by dissection. Composite resection, such as TPES, has been thought to be demanding and formidable because of high mortality and morbidity rates. Improvement of surgical techniques has allowed TPES to be completed with a blood loss of approximately 2000 to 3000 mL, however, which has resulted in a favorable learning curve with low morbidity and mortality rates.

We have excluded tumors that grow into the sacral promontory or sciatic notch from surgical indications. If high sacral amputation is performed, increased surgical invasiveness, more serious complications, and inevitable walking disorders are observed; as a result, a patient may have a remarkably deteriorated quality of life [6,9,12,19]. We have limited the level of sacral amputation in TPES to the S2 lower edge or below to preserve the second sacral nerve. Consequently, patients were able to have favorable quality of life after TPES, except for living with double stomas and temporary pain caused by resection of sacral nerves, and they were able to return to their original occupations [31,35].

If oncologic outcome obtained is superior to that after multimodality treatment, composite resection for FRT also may become an acceptable treatment. Finally, it should be noted that when extended surgeries, such as TPES, are performed for FRT, each of the departments concerned should review surgical indications and the surgeries must be worked on in the form of team medicine. One must realize that only through such process can negative resection margins be obtained as a great boon to patients.

References

[1] Gunderson LL, Sosin H. Area of failure found at reoperation following curative surgery for adenocarcinoma of the rectum. Cancer 1974;34:1278–92.

[2] McDermott FT, Hughes ES, Pihl E, et al. Local recurrence after potentially curative resection for rectal cancer in a series of 1008 patients. Br J Surg 1985;72:34–7.

[3] Pilipshen SJ, Heilweil M, Quan SH, et al. Patterns of pelvic recurrence following definitive resection of rectal cancer. Cancer 1984;53:1354–62.

[4] McCall JL, Cox MR, Wattchow DA. Analysis of local recurrence rates after surgery alone for rectal cancer. Int J Colorectal Dis 1995;10:126–32.

[5] Wong CS, Cumming BJ, Brierly JD, et al. Treatment of locally recurrent rectal carcinoma: results and prognostic factors. Int J Radiat Oncol Biol Phys 1998;40(2):427–35.

[6] Wanebo HJ, Marcove RC. Abdominal sacral resection of locally recurrent rectal cancer. Ann Surg 1981;194(4):458–71.

[7] Pacini P, Cionini L, Pirtoli L, et al. Symptomatic recurrences of carcinoma of the rectum and sigmoid: the influence of radiotherapy on the quality of life. Dis Colon Rectum 1986;29: 865–8.

[8] Takagi H, Morimoto T, Hara S, et al. Seven cases of pelvic exenteration combined with sacral resection for locally rectal cancer. J Surg Oncol 1986;32:184–8.

[9] Maetani S, Nishikawa T, Iijima Y, et al. Extensive en bloc resection of regionally recurrent carcinoma of the rectum. Cancer 1992;69:2876–83.

[10] Maetani S, Onodera H, Nishikawa T, et al. Significance of local recurrence of rectal cancer as a local or disseminated disease. Br J Surg 1998;85:521–5.

[11] Willett CG, Shellito PC, Tepper JE, et al. Intraoperative electron beam radiation therapy for recurrent locally advanced rectal or rectosigmoid carcinoma. Cancer 1991;67:1504–8.

[12] Temple WJ, Ketcham AS. Sacral resection for control of pelvic tumors. Am J Surg 1992;163: 370–4.

[13] Wanebo HJ, Koness J, Vezeridis MP, et al. Pelvic resection of recurrent rectal cancer. Ann Surg 1994;220(4):586–97.

[14] Suzuki K, Gunderson LL, Devine RM, et al. Intraoperative irradiation after palliative surgery for locally recurrent rectal cancer. Cancer 1995;75(4):939–52.

[15] Suzuki K, Dozois RR, Devine RM, et al. Curative reoperation for locally recurrent rectal cancer. Dis Colon Rectum 1996;39(7):730–6.

[16] Wiggers T, de Vries MR, Veeze-Kuypers B. Surgery for local recurrence of rectal carcinoma. Dis Colon Rectum 1996;39(3):323–8.

[17] Goes RN, Beart RW, Simons AJ, et al. Use of brachytherapy in management of locally recurrent rectal cancer. Dis Colon Rectum 1997;40(10):1177–9.

[18] Bozzetti F, Bertario L, Rossetti C, et al. Surgical treatment of locally recurrent rectal carcinoma. Dis Colon Rectum 1997;40(12):1421–4.

[19] Wanebo HJ, Antoniuk P, Koness J, et al. Pelvic resection of recurrent rectal cancer. Dis Colon Rectum 1999;42(11):1438–48.

[20] Mannaerts GHH, Rutten HJT, Martijn H, et al. Abdominosacral resection for primary irresectable and locally recurrent rectal cancer. Dis Colon Rectum 2001;44(6):806–14.

[21] Yamada K, Ishizawa T, Niwa K, et al. Patterns of pelvic invasion are prognostic in the treatment of locally recurrent rectal cancer. Br J Surg 2001;88:988–93.

[22] Magrini S, Nelson H, Gunderson LL. Sacropelvic resection and intraoperative electron irradiation in the management of recurrent anorectal cancer. Dis Colon Rectum 1996;39:1–9.

[23] Mannaerts GHH, Martijn H, Crommelin MA, et al. Intraoperative electron beam radiation therapy for locally recurrent rectal carcinoma. Int J Radiat Oncol Biol Phys 1999;45(2): 297–308.

[24] Valentini V, Morganti A, De Franco A, et al. Chemoradiation with or without intra-operative radiation therapy in patients with locally recurrent rectal carcinoma. Cancer 1999; 86(12):2612–24.

[25] Shoup M, Guillem JG, Alektiar KM, et al. Predictors of survival in recurrent rectal cancer after resection and intraoperative radiotherapy. Dis Colon Rectum 2000;45(5):585–92.
[26] Hahnloser D, Haddock MG, Nelson H. Intraoperative radiotherapy in the multimodality approach to colorectal cancer. Surg Oncol Clin N Am 2003;12:993–1013.
[27] Kuehne J, Kleisli T, Biernacki P, et al. Use of high-dose-rate brachytherapy in the management of locally recurrent rectal cancer. Dis Colon Rectum 2003;46(79):895–9.
[28] Hahnloser D, Nelson H, Gunderson LL, et al. Curative potential of multimodality therapy for locally recurrent rectal cancer. Ann Surg 2003;237(4):502–8.
[29] Rodel C, Grabenbauer GG, Matzel K, et al. Extensive surgery after high-dose preoperative chemoradiotherapy for locally advanced recurrent rectal cancer. Dis Colon Rectum 2000; 43(39):312–9.
[30] Temple WJ, Saettler EB. Locally recurrent rectal cancer: role of composite resection of extensive pelvic tumors with strategies for minimizing risk of recurrence. J Surg Oncol 2000; 73:47–58.
[31] Moriya Y, Akasu T, Fujita S, et al. Total pelvic exenteration with distal sacrectomy for fixed recurrent rectal cancer in the pelvis. Dis Colon Rectum, in press.
[32] Moriya Y, Hojo K, Sawada T, et al. Significance of lateral node dissection for advanced rectal carcinoma at or below the peritoneal reflection. Dis Colon Rectum 1989;32(4):307–15.
[33] Lopez-Kostner F, Fazio VW, Vignali A, et al. Locally recurrent rectal cancer: predictors and success of salvage surgery. Dis Colon Rectum 2001;44(2):173–8.
[34] Porter GA, Soskolne CL, Yakimets WW, et al. Surgeon-related factors and outcome in rectal cancer. Ann Surg 1998;227(2):157–67.
[35] Guren MG, Wiig JN, Dueland S, et al. Quality of life in patients with urinary diversion after operation for locally advanced rectal cancer. Eur J Surg Oncol 2001;27(7):645–51.

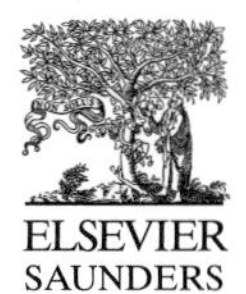

ELSEVIER
SAUNDERS

Surg Oncol Clin N Am
14 (2005) 239–247

SURGICAL
ONCOLOGY CLINICS
OF NORTH AMERICA

New Treatment Concepts for Gynecologic Pelvic Malignancies: Neoadjuvant Therapies

Antonella Restivo, MD[a,b], Mary Gordinier, MD[a,b], Cornelius O. Granai, MD[a,b,*]

[a]*Brown University, Providence, RI*

[b]*The Program in Women's Oncology, Women's and Infant's Hospital of Rhode Island, 101 Dudley Street, Providence, RI 02905, USA*

This article specifically pertains to new ideas and treatments for gynecologic pelvic malignancies, but its underlying substance relates to "change," and the inherent difficulties in changing [1]. Therefore, this vital fundamental process is first considered.

Creating new ideas and re-examining older ideas that lead to improvement—how simple is that? The problem is—it isn't. The truism holds, "Change is hard," and yet it's essential to progress, which benefits all [2]. Even within the "facts rule" domain of science, challenging the status quo is difficult, and not necessarily for reasons that are logical or lofty [3]. Roadblocks to change, often occult, are everywhere, and change-resistant, anachronistic, organizational power structures add to the recalcitrance. Rather than being encouraged, the questioning of current convention can spawn undue costs; and the hallowed halls of academia are not a sanctuary from that counterproductive paradox. These pervasive impediments do not always prevail, however. And, once revealed, the undeniable power of new knowledge slowly transforms even ensconced ideation or, for that matter, the longstanding dogmas of science or medicine.

It is true that not all "seasoned ideas," or their pragmatic representations, should be automatically replaced by something new and shiny (and unproved). Still, no idea, or its embodiment, should be sacrosanct. Instead, if thoughtful consideration suggests an alternative idea that is potentially

* Corresponding author. The Program in Women's Oncology, Women's and Infant's Hospital of Rhode Island, 101 Dudley Street, Providence, RI 02905.

E-mail address: sgranai@wihri.org (C.O. Granai).

doi:10.1016/j.soc.2004.11.004

superior, after validation (eg, clinical trials) the better approach or system should take its (temporary) turn as the new status quo. In the light of day, who could argue with that?

Although this article is not intended to be philosophic, or wander the universe of "macropossibilities," a baseline cognizance of the difficulty of change is relevant. In that context then, when "something" does not occur, it should not be simply presumed it's because the idea was fundamentally bad. This article discusses new ideas that challenge status quo treatments of gynecologic pelvic malignancies. Even in this narrow setting, however, the overarching complex and political influences effecting change and insulating the status quo are likely somewhere at play. A case in point on the history of breast cancer may clarify this concept.

It was only several decades ago that breast cancer was understood as a local or, at most, locoregional disease. Although once believed, this now dated, limited perspective logically led to aggressive locoregional therapies. Radical surgeries were the therapeutic centerpiece, and well-intended general surgeons, with their historically developed cancer operations, led the charge [4]. How naive all this seems now, relatively few years later. Those past perceptions, and their corresponding treatment implications, thankfully have given way to today's more accurate biologic and genetic understandings about the multiple diseases once (simplistically) homogenized as "breast cancer" [5]. Also reflective of the biologic and psychosocial complexity of breast problems are the expert multidisciplinary medical teams, which are now required to advance medical care in this area [6].

Treating neoplasms on their own unique biologic and pathologic terms portends the best outcomes. But, faced with the vastness of expanding information, no individual physician can know but a tiny fraction of today's "data," let alone be sensitive to all the relevant humanism [7]. This is not an indictment of goodness or ability; rather, it's an acknowledgment of the exponential nature of knowledge and human needs.

Based on better understanding, the "radicalness" of surgery is rarely preeminent in breast cancer therapy today. Therapeutic approaches recognizing the true biologic and humanistic scope of the disease are more germane [8]. As implied, concepts such as Hallstedian resections, in the hands and mind of a sole clinician, can no longer a priori dictate or provide what's best. More comprehensive, insightful, and thoughtful approaches are replacing the anecdotal, disjointed, non–patient-centered ways of the past—and the turf-protecting organizational structures that buttressed them. Although surgery and the surgeons still play important roles in the treatment of breast cancer, how different those parts are, and will be, according to unfolding realities and potentials. Hard as this change has been, patients have been the ultimate beneficiaries; after all, this is the ideal that brought physicians here in the first place, and is the quiet inspiration behind challenging the status quo [9].

The treatment of gynecologic pelvic malignancies likely has much to gain from the advances (and political challenges) surrounding breast cancer. By analogy, could less radical pelvic surgery, with its inherently lesser morbidity, result in equal, if not superior, outcomes? Although in many instances, today's status quo treatments for pelvic cancers in women yield great mathematical results, are there nevertheless meaningful ways to improve outcomes if they are more comprehensively defined (eg, sexual function, self-esteem)? In short, are there better treatments and treatment sequences that can result in better quality of life while providing optimal survival, whatever the circumstances?

One concept gaining interest, if not momentum, in the "new management" of gynecologic pelvic cancers is the use of adjuvant chemotherapy or radiation, before contemplated surgery. With the ever-relevant, broader concepts of "change" in mind, this article reviews some of those ideas and current experiences.

Neoadjuvant chemotherapy in the treatment of ovarian cancer

The current standard therapy for advanced-stage epithelial ovarian cancer is primary surgical cytoreduction followed by a combination of platinum- and taxane-based chemotherapy [10]. A favorable long-term outcome can often be achieved when maximal debulking occurs at the time of primary surgery, leaving a residual tumor bulk of less than 2 cm. Optimal cytoreduction can only be achieved in 40% of patients with stage III–IV ovarian cancer, however.

The value of surgical debulking was first documented by Griffiths [11]. His analysis of prognostic factors and size of residual masses in 102 patients found that, in addition to clear cell histology and tumor grade, the size of the largest residual mass was strongly correlated with survival. Improved survival was associated with residual disease of less than 1.5 cm. Similarly, Bolis et al [12] showed that patients who had residual tumor of less than 1 cm following primary debulking had a better 5-year survival rate. A recent meta-analysis by Bristow et al [13] further supported the theory that maximal cytoreduction is a powerful prognostic factor in patients with advanced ovarian cancer. The authors found that with each 10% increase in maximal cytoreduction, there is an associated 5.5% increase in median survival [12].

Maximal cytoreduction is supported by the mathematical model of Goldie and Coldman [14]. This model asserts that chemotherapeutic resistance develops secondary to random spontaneous mutations occurring at a rate proportional to the growth rate and volume of tumor cells present. Thus, a minimal amount of residual tumor decreases the likelihood of developing chemotherapeutic resistance by allowing fewer random spontaneous mutations.

The question is what to do when optimal cytoreduction is not attainable. There are some patients whose imaging studies show widespread disease not amenable to optimal cytoreduction. In addition, there are patients, including those with recent pulmonary emboli, severe malnutrition, uncontrolled respiratory or thyroid disease, and recent myocardial infarctions, who are not good surgical candidates. It is these patients that are prime candidates for neoadjuvant chemotherapy followed by a maximal surgical effort.

Neoadjuvant chemotherapy was first described by Frei, in 1982, for the treatment of head and neck cancer [15,16]. Since that time, neoadjuvant treatment has been recognized as a useful modality for the treatment of advanced-stage cancers. A study by Lawton et al showed that in a cohort of 36 patients treated with neoadjuvant chemotherapy, tumors in 28 patients (89%) were optimally cytoreduced to less than 2 cm [17,18]. Similarly, Onnis et al studied patients with advanced ovarian cancer and found that the percentage of patients whose tumors were optimally debulked was higher in the group who received neoadjuvant chemotherapy as compared with those whose tumors were primarily debulked [15,19].

Some proponents of neoadjuvant chemotherapy propose it as the primary approach in all cases of advanced-stage disease, citing less intraoperative blood loss, decreased ICU stays, decreased number of postoperative hospitalizations, and increased patient comfort. They argue that shrinking the tumor not only makes the surgical procedure more feasible but also increases patient comfort by decreasing the amount of ascites present [18].

Although significant ascites is removed at the time of primary surgery, it often reaccumulates within the immediate postoperative period, causing significant patient discomfort and difficulty breathing. Likewise, pleural effusions may contribute to a difficult postoperative course. Chemotherapy has been documented to hasten the resolution of ascites and effusions within one to two cycles. Vergote et al [20], in a retrospective review of 285 patients, found that neoadjuvant chemotherapy not only helped in avoiding unnecessary morbidity but was also shown to increase patient survival [21].

Although further prospective studies must be completed before the implementation of neoadjuvant therapy as the primary modality for the treatment of stage III and IV ovarian cancers, it is clearly appropriate in a select population and affords patients another avenue to optimal care.

Chemotherapy and radiation in the treatment of vulvar cancer

Among gynecologic malignancies, neoadjuvant chemotherapy and radiation have the most solid indication in the treatment of vulvar cancer. Vulvar cancer constitutes 3% to 5% of all gynecologic malignancies [22]. Although a primary surgical approach is preferred in most situations because of ease of resection and effectiveness of surgical treatment, there are some situations where resection may compromise significant structures or be excessively mutilating or morbid.

In the later stages of disease, local resection often involves midline structures, including the anus, clitoris, urethra, and vagina. Primary surgical resection may be difficult and extensive, necessitating a colostomy or an exenterative procedure to obtain adequate margins. The size of resection is another consideration. Patients whose tumors require a massive perineal resection are plagued with numerous complications, including wound separation, infection, seroma formation, and lower extremity lymphedema [22]. The neoadjuvant approach may spare the patient ultraradical surgery and complications.

The effectiveness of the neoadjuvant approach is well documented. A retrospective review performed at Yale–New Haven Hospital between 1973 and 1998 showed that primary chemoradiation to the vulva followed by surgical excision results in improved relapse-free and overall survival when compared with primary radiation alone [23]. Another study sponsored by the Gynecologic Oncology Group (GOG 101) by Moore et al [24] found that 46.5% of patients with stage III and IV vulvar cancers treated with neoadjuvant chemoradiation had complete regression at time of surgery. The authors recruited 73 patients with stage III and IV vulvar tumors and treated them with a split course of chemoradiation. The regimen included anterior posterior–posterior anterior (AP-PA) radiation to 4760 cGy with concomitant 5-fluorouracil at a dosage of 1000 mg/m^2/day $\times$ 4 days and cisplatin at a dosage of 50 mg/m^2 given on day 1. Definitive surgery was then performed. Of 73 patients evaluated, 34 had a complete clinical response, and 31 underwent surgical resection, with 84.8% having adequate negative margins.

The preservation of sexual function is another potential benefit of primary chemoradiation, particularly among the younger women with vulvar cancer. Periclitoral tumors, treated with primary surgery, require the complete resection of the clitoris. Radiation with concurrent chemotherapy may eradicate disease or decrease it to such an extent that loss of this organ is not necessary, thus allowing for the normal anatomic and physiologic function of the vulva to be retained.

The recurrence rates of vulvar cancer vary with stage and treatment modality but typically decrease in number after complete inguinofemoral lymphadenectomy. Because recurrence in an undissected groin is nearly always fatal, inguinal lymphadenectomy or sentinel node biopsy is advised before commencement of chemoradiation. This technique will allow for a more accurate definition of the radiation fields and affords the patient improved local micrometastatic control.

A final option is to administer neoadjuvant chemotherapy alone, without radiation, to help shrink tumors while avoiding the adverse effects of radiation. This approach alleviates the moist desquamation that is often seen in irradiated vulvas. At present, this treatment option has intellectual appeal but there are no studies documenting its efficacy. Therefore, combined chemoradiation remains the standard of care.

Neoadjuvant radiation in the treatment of endometrial cancer

Endometrial cancer is the fourth most common malignancy in females. It typically occurs in women who are postmenopausal, with approximately 75% of all cases occurring in patients who are 50 years or older [25]. Although surgery is undoubtedly the best primary treatment modality, with a cure rate of 90% and low morbidity, primary radiation therapy has been used in women who are not surgical candidates [26].

Multiple retrospective studies have been performed to evaluate the efficacy of intracavitary radiation combined with external bean radiotherapy in the treatment of stage I and II endometrial cancers [27]. Kucera et al [28] studied 280 patients with stage I endometrial cancer treated with high-dose-rate (HDR) brachytherapy alone and found intracavitary radiotherapy to be an effect treatment option in patients who medically cannot withstand surgery. The authors noted 5-year overall survival rates of 41% to 73% in patients treated with radiotherapy alone compared with 80% to 94% in patients who had undergone primary surgical resection. This study also uncovered a 17.5% rate of local recurrence in the cohort treated with radiation alone, further solidifying the need to maintain surgical resection as the primary treatment modality whenever possible.

Controversy arises when trying to decide between low-dose-rate (LDR) and HDR brachytherapy. Since 1970, HDR brachytherapy has been used increasingly in the treatment of these malignancies because it requires a shorter hospital stay and causes less morbidity [29]. Although large studies have been done in India and Japan, there are no prospective, randomized studies in the United States confirming the equivalency of LDR and HDR. Furthermore, there is a lack of standardization in the delivery of HDR. Patients who receive LDR brachytherapy have a low but not negligible risk of developing complications, most notably pulmonary emboli caused by prolonged immobilization. This possibility combined with a longer hospital stay makes HDR brachytherapy a more attractive choice for those women who cannot endure surgery [30].

In addition to patients who are not surgical candidates because of medical conditions, another subset of patients who benefit from primary radiotherapy includes those whose tumor's origin cannot be defined. Stage IB endocervical adenocarcinoma arising from the upper endocervical canal can be indistinguishable from a primary endometrial carcinoma originating in the lower uterine segment. Often, both histology and physical examination are unrevealing. In this nebulous situation, surgery should be preceded by a 72-hour brachytherapy treatment with intracavitary cesium delivered by means of tandem and ovoid. This approach addresses both tumor histologies. The direct application of radiation dose within the cervix takes advantage of the patient's natural geometry to deliver a dose of radiation to the pelvis in excess of the dose that may be safely delivered with an external beam [31]. Surgery may then be performed with 48 to 72 hours of the treatment, before radiation-related tissue changes occur [31]. The patient thus receives the advantages of surgical staging that ultimately benefit endometrial carcinoma, and radiation to the parametria, which aids with local recurrence in cervical cancer.

Neoadjuvant chemoradiation in the treatment of cervical cancer

The survival of women with locally advanced cervical cancer (stage IB and IIA) has remained somewhat unchanged over the last two decades. The overall 5-year survival rates range from 30% to 50% [32]. Administration of neoadjuvant chemotherapy followed by radical surgery is one approach that has emerged to increase tumor shrinkage, thus allowing for more optimal debulking.

Several randomized trials have been performed to investigate the value of neoadjuvant chemotherapy in this setting. A retrospective review conducted in Italy by Benedetti-Panici et al [32] randomized 409 patients to receive neoadjuvant chemotherapy plus radical hysterectomy or radiation alone. They found that both treatment modalities were well tolerated, but sequential neoadjuvant chemotherapy followed by surgery was more effective than radiation therapy alone. At 5 years, the investigators found a 10% to 15% survival advantage for the patients who received neoadjuvant chemotherapy. The rates of overall survival (58.9% versus 44.5%) and progression-free survival (55.4% versus 41.3%) were higher in the neoadjuvant chemotherapy arm.

Aoki et al [33] evaluated 21 patients with untreated stage IB–IIA cervical cancer who were given two cycles of preoperative chemotherapy (cisplatin [CDDP], vinblastine, and peplomycin). All patients then underwent radical hysterectomy. The authors noted an 86% response rate which compared favorably with the historical controls.

A final study performed by Keys et al [34], in 1999, randomized 374 women with bulky stage IB cervical cancer to receive radiation therapy alone or chemoradiation followed by hysterectomy. They found the rates of progression-free survival and overall survival to be significantly higher at 4 years in the chemoradiation treatment group. Thus, it was concluded that adding weekly infusions of cisplatin to radiotherapy followed by hysterectomy helped to reduce the risk of recurrence in women with bulky stage IB disease.

There is some controversy, however. Many earlier trials have found conflicting data. A French trial randomized 151 patients with stage IIB or III cervical cancer to chemotherapy (cisplatin, methotrexate, chlorambucil, vincristine) followed by radiation versus radiation alone. Although 42% of the patients treated with chemotherapy responded, there was no difference in survival. Likewise, Souhami et al [35], in a similar study, randomized 107 patients with stage IIIB cervical cancer to receive chemotherapy (CDDP, bleomycin, mitomycin, vincristine) followed by radiation versus radiation alone. They found that length of survival was worse in the patients receiving neoadjuvant chemotherapy plus radiation.

The current role of neoadjuvant chemotherapy in the treatment of cervical cancer is therefore still unclear. The approach is promising, but is most appropriate in the setting of a clinical trial. Coming back to the broader perspective, for many reasons change is hard, but its potential is worth it.

References

[1] Johnson S. Who moved my cheese? An amazing way to deal with change in your work and in your life. New York: GP Putnam's Sons; 1998.

[2] Ever wonder why change is sooooo hard. Available at: www.sunrisem.comid66_m.htm. Accessed September 8, 2004.

[3] Davidoff F. Shame: a major reason why most medical doctors don't change their views. Available at: curezone.com.

[4] The cancer breakthrough you've never heard of. Available at: www.texascancercenter.com/unhistory.html.

[5] Legare RD, Strenger R. Adjuvant therapy in breast cancer. Obstet Gynecol Clin North Am 2002;29(1):2798.

[6] Legare RD. Screening and management of hereditary breast cancer. Med Health R I 1999; 82(5):172–5.

[7] Kanbour-Shakir A, Harris KM, Johnson RR, Kanbour AL. Breast care consultation center: role of the pathologist in a multidisciplinary center. Diagn Cytopathol 1997;17(3):191–6.

[8] Scalia JL, Legare RD. The identification and management of hereditary breast and ovarian cancer. Med Health R I 2003;86(2):48–51.

[9] Granai CO. What matters matter? P values, H values, leadership, and us. Obstet Gynecol 2003;102(2):393–6.

[10] Mazzeo F, Berliere M, Kerger J, et al. Neoadjuvant chemotherapy followed by surgery and adjuvant chemotherapy in patients with primarily unresectable advanced-stage ovarian cancer. Gynecol Oncol 2003;90:163–9.

[11] Griffiths CT. Surgical resection of tumor bulk in the primary treatment of ovarian carcinoma [monograph]. National Cancer Institute. 1975;42:101–4.

[12] Bolis G, Villa A, Guarnerio P, et al. Survival of women with advanced ovarian cancer and complete pathologic response at second-look laparotomy. Cancer 1996;77:128–31.

[13] Bristow RE, Tomocruz RS, Armstrong DK, Trimble EL, Montz FJ. Survival effect of maximal cytoreductive surgery for advanced ovarian carcinoma during the platinum era: a meta-analysis. J Clin Oncol 2002;20:1248–59.

[14] Goldie JH, Coldman AJ. A mathematic model for relating the drug sensitivity of tumors to their spontaneous mutation rate. Cancer Treat Rep 1979;63:1727–33.

[15] Shibata K, Kikkawa F, Mika M, et al. Neoadjuvant chemotherapy for FIGO stage III or IV ovarian cancer: survival benefit and prognostic factors. Int J Gynecol Cancer 2003;13: 587–92.

[16] Sardi JE. Neoadjuvant chemotherapy in gynecologic oncology. Surg Clin North Am 2001; 183:274–9.

[17] Surwit E, Childers J, Atlas I, et al. Neoadjuvant chemotherapy for advanced ovarian cancer. Int J Gynecol Cancer 1996;6:356–61.

[18] Lawton FG, Redman CW, Wesley DM, et al. Neoadjuvant (cytoreductive) chemotherapy combined with intervention debulking surgery in advanced, unresected epithelial ovarian cancer. Obstet Gynecol 1989;73:61–5.

[19] Goff BA. Surgical treatment of unusual endometrial cancer. Presented at the 40th annual meeting of the American Society of Clinical Oncology. New Orleans, June 5–8, 2004.

[20] Vergote I, De Wever I, Tjalma W, Van Gramberen M, Decloedt J, Van Dam P. Neoadjuvant chemotherapy or primary debulking surgery in advanced ovarian carcinoma; a retrospective analysis of 285 patients. Gynecol Oncol 1998;71:431–6.
[21] Hoskins WJ, McGuire WP, Brady MF, et al. The effect of diameter of largest residual disease on survival after primary cytoreductive surgery in patients with suboptimal residual epithelial ovarian carcinoma. Am J Obstet Gynecol 1994;170:974–80.
[22] Leiserowitz GS, Russell AH, Kinney WK, et al. Prophylactic chemoradiation of inguinofemoral lymph nodes in patients with locally extensive vulvar cancer. Gynecol Oncol 1997; 66:509–14.
[23] Han SC, Kim DH, Higgins SA, Carcangiu ML, Kacinski BM. Chemoradiation as primary or adjuvant treatment for locally advanced carcinoma of the vulva. Int J Radiat Oncol Biol Phys 2000;47:1235–44.
[24] Moore DH, Thomas GM, Montana GS, Saxer A, Gallup DG, Olt G. Preoperative chemoradiation for advanced vulvar cancer: a phase II study of the Gynecologic Oncology Group. Int J Radiat Oncol Biol Phys 1998;42:79–85.
[25] Hoskins WJ, Perez CA, Young RC, et al. Principles and Practice of Gynecologic Oncology. 4th edition. Philadelphia: Lippincott, Williams, and Wilkins; 2005.
[26] Graham J. The value of preoperative treatment by radium for carcinoma of the uterine body. Surg Gynecol Obstet 1971;132:855–60.
[27] Patel FD, Sharma SC, Negi PS, Ghoshal S, Gupta BD. Low dose rate vs. high dose rate brachytherapy in the treatment of carcinoma of the uterine cervix: a clinical trial. Int J Radiat Oncol Biol Phys 1994;28:335–41.
[28] Kucera H, Knocke TH, Kucera E, Potter R. Treatment of endometrial carcinoma with high-dose-rate brachytherapy alone in medically inoperable stage I patients. Acta Obstet Gynecol Scand 1998;77:1008–12.
[29] Roberts JA, Brunetto VL, Keys HM, et al. A phase III randomized study of surgery vs. surgery plus adjuvant RT in intermediate risk endometrial carcinoma. Gynecol Oncol 1998; 68:135.
[30] Nguyen C, Souchami L, Roman TN, Clark BG. High-dose-rate brachytherapy as the primary treatment of medically inoperable stage I–II endometrial carcinoma. Gynecol Oncol 1995;59:370–5.
[31] Petereit DG, Sarkaria JN, Potter DM, Schink JC. High dose-rate versus low dose-rate brachytherapy in the treatment of cervical cancer: analysis of tumor recurrence. The University of Wisconsin experience. Int J Radiat Oncol Biol Phys 1999;45:1267–74.
[32] Benedetti-Panici P, Greggi S, Colombo A, et al. Neoadjuvant chemotherapy and radical surgery versus exclusive radiotherapy in locally advanced squamous cell cervical cancer: results from the Italian multicenter randomized study. J Clin Oncol 2002;20:179–88.
[33] Aoki Y, Tomita M, Sato T, et al. Neoadjuvant chemotherapy for patients younger than 50 years with high risk squamous cell carcinoma of the cervix. Gynecol Oncol 2001;83:263–7.
[34] Keys HM, Bundy BN, Stehman FB, et al. Cisplatin, radiation, and adjuvant hysterectomy compared with radiation and adjuvant hysterectomy for bulky stage IB cervical carcinoma. N Engl J Med 1999;340:1154–61.
[35] Souhami L, Gil RA, Allan SE, et al. Detrimental effect of neoadjuvant chemotherapy in patients with stage IIIB carcinoma of the cervix: results of a randomized trial. Int J Oncol 1992;1:289–92.

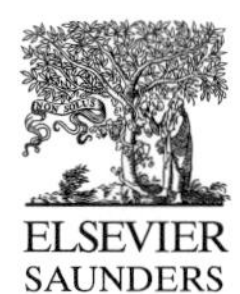
ELSEVIER
SAUNDERS

Surg Oncol Clin N Am
14 (2005) 249–266

SURGICAL
ONCOLOGY CLINICS
OF NORTH AMERICA

Cervical Cancer: Current Management of Early/Late Disease

Wayne A. McCreath, MD[a], Emery Salom, MD[b], Dennis S. Chi, MD[c,*]

[a]*Ob/Gyn Division, Crystal Run Healthcare, 61 Emerald Place, Emerald Corporate Center, Rock Hill, NY 12775, USA*
[b]*Department of Obstetrics and Gynecology, University of Miami, Jackson Memorial Hospital, 1611 NW 12th Avenue, Miami, FL 33136-1094, USA*
[c]*Gynecology Service, Department of Surgery, Memorial Sloan-Kettering Cancer Center, 1275 York Avenue, New York, NY 10021, USA*

Worldwide cervical cancer remains an important public health concern, partially because of the unavailability and underuse of the Pap smear. It is the most frequent cancer among women in Africa, Asia, and South America [1]. In comparison, in the United States, cervical cancer screening is routine, resulting in a lower disease case-to-fatality ratio. Each year in the United States, approximately 12,200 women are diagnosed with cervical cancer and approximately 4000 die of this disease [2]. This comparatively lower mortality rate observed in the United States emphasizes the importance of effective screening.

Screening identifies preinvasive disease and occult cancers, thereby diagnosing disease at earlier stages. The stage represents the extent of invasive disease at diagnosis. Table 1 shows the International Federation of Gynecology and Obstetrics (FIGO) staging for cervical cancer [3]. Stage IA–IIA is considered early disease whereas stage IIB–IVB is deemed advanced disease. This division of cervical cancer into early and late disease is determined by differences in survival, cure rates, and treatment options. Early disease is associated with higher survival and cure rates compared with late disease. Five-year survival rates for stage IA1 to IIA range from 95% for stage IA1 to 76% for stage IIA, whereas 5-year survival rates for stage IIB–IVB decrease from 73% for stage IIB to 22% for stage IVB [4].

* Corresponding author.
E-mail address: chid@mskcc.org (D.S. Chi).

doi:10.1016/j.soc.2004.11.006 ***surgonc.theclinics.com***

Table 1
Staging of carcinoma of the cervix uteri

TNM classification		
Primary tumor (T)	FIGO classification	Definition
TX	C	Primary tumor cannot be assessed
T0	C	No evidence of primary tumor
Tis	0	Carcinoma in situ, intraepithelial carcinoma
T1	I	Cervical carcinoma confined to cervix (extension to the corpus should be disregarded)
T1a	IA	Invasive carcinoma, diagnosed microscopically only. All gross lesions even with superficial invasion are stage IB cancers. Invasion is limited to measured stromal invasion with maximum depth of 5 mm and maximum width of 7 mm.[a]
T1a1	IA1	Minimal microscopically evident stromal invasion. Measured stromal invasion with maximum depth of 3 mm and maximum width of 7 mm.
T1a2	IA2	Measured stromal invasion with depth from 3–5 mm and maximum width of 7 mm
T1b	IB	Clinical lesions confined to the cervix or preclinical lesions larger than stage IA
	IB1	Clinical lesions no larger than 4 cm
	IB2	Clinical lesions larger than 4 cm
T2	II	Cervical carcinoma invades beyond the uterus but not to the pelvic wall or to the lower third of the vagina
T2a	IIA	No obvious parametrial invasion
T2b	IIB	Obvious parametrial invasion
T3	III	Extends to the pelvic wall or involves lower third of the vagina or causes hydronephrosis or nonfunctioning kidney
T3a	IIIA	Tumor involves the lower third of the vagina. No extension to the pelvic wall.
T3b	IIIB	Tumor extends to the pelvic wall or causes hydronephrosis or nonfunctioning kidney
T4	IV	Carcinoma extends beyond the true pelvis or has clinically involved the mucosa of the bladder or rectum. A bullous edema as such does not permit a case to be allotted to stage IV.
T4a	IVA	Spread of the growth to adjacent organs
T4b	IVB	Spread to distant organs

Abbreviation: TNM, tumor-node-metastasis.

[a] The depth of invasion should not be more than 5 mm taken from the base of the epithelium, either surface or glandular, from which it originates. Vascular space involvement, either venous or lymphatic, should not alter the staging.

Data from International Federation of Gynecology and Obstetrics, 1995.

Historically, early-stage disease has been treated with radical hysterectomy and pelvic lymph node dissection. Over time, the following other surgical options have become available: cone biopsy, simple hysterectomy, modified radical hysterectomy, laparoscopic surgery, and vaginal trachelectomy. These operations are used in special circumstances and must meet specific treatment requirements, which will be described later.

Traditionally, late-stage disease has been treated with radiation therapy in the form of whole pelvic external beam irradiation and brachytherapy. To deliver effective brachytherapy, the uterus is used as a conduit. Removing the uterus surgically in late disease places the patient at a disadvantage because brachytherapy cannot be effectively administered. Surgery, therefore, plays a minor role in the treatment of advanced disease.

In recent years, multiple randomized trials have shown that the concurrent administration of low-dose chemotherapy with radiation improves survival compared with radiation therapy alone in the treatment of cervical cancer [5–9]. Concurrent chemoradiation therapy therefore has become the standard whenever radiation is administered in early and late disease [10]. This newly established approach is believed to represent the most significant contribution in cervical cancer treatment since the advent of mega-voltage irradiation in the 1950s [11].

This article discusses the current management of cervical cancer, including the history of surgical management, technical aspects of surgical procedures, and current standards used for treating early and late disease states.

Evolutionary milestones

The initial treatment for cervical cancer was surgery; this approach dates back to 1889 when the disease was first treated with a simple vaginal hysterectomy. During this early period, mortality was high (approaching 75%), whereas survival was low (approaching 5%). Because of these unfavorable outcomes, only 15% of patients diagnosed with the disease underwent surgery [12].

Schuchardt later reported survival rates of 14% by increasing the margins of the simple hysterectomy, thereby creating the first "radical" hysterectomy. Subsequently, Schauta reported survival rates of 38%, with decreased mortality to 18%, and Americh emphasized the importance of anatomic support [12–16]. These contributions of Schauta and Americh significantly improved the morbidity and mortality of vaginal surgery. Thus, the radical vaginal hysterectomy is known today as the Schauta-Americh operation. The approach was used extensively for cancer of the uterus and cervix but was contraindicated when parametrial infiltration caused fixation, a practice that still exists today.

In 1885, Emil Reis [17] introduced the abdominal surgical approach on animals. John Clark, a surgeon at Johns Hopkins, later used the abdominal approach and successfully completed the first radical abdominal hysterectomy on humans [18]. Although the contributions of Clark and Reis have been recognized, it was Ernst Wertheim (a student of Schauta) in 1898 who perfected the surgical technique for the abdominal approach. His surgical modifications significantly decreased morbidity and mortality, especially in relation to sepsis-, bladder-, and ureteral-related injury.

In his monograph published in 1912, Wertheim [19] reported on 1096 patients with cervical cancer, more than 500 of whom were treated surgically. Wertheim reported a 5-year survival rate of 42.9% for those patients managed by surgery. In 1898, 30% of the patients underwent the Wertheim operation, but by 1911, 62% of patients with cervical cancer were treated with the Wertheim abdominal radical hysterectomy.

During these early years, radiation therapy also began to make its entry into the evolutionary timeline for cervical cancer management. Radiochemistry began in 1898 when Madam Curie discovered radium [12]. Around the time of the publication of Wertheim's monograph, Wichman and Degras applied the principles of radiochemistry to effectively treat cervical cancer [20]. These results led to two possible treatment approaches and great debate over the superiority of one over the other during that time. To some degree, that debate still exists today.

Wertheim's influence

Wertheim influenced many surgeons, such as Victor Bonney, Fred Taussig, and Joe Meigs. After Wertheim's death in 1920, Bonney [21] continued to perform Wertheim's operation, and in 1935, reported 5- and 10-year survival rates of 40% and 30%, respectively, in 385 patients undergoing the procedure. He emphasized the importance of surgery at a time when radiation therapy was another choice of management. Taussig [22] believed that lymph nodes infiltrated with cancer were resistant to radiation therapy, and he hypothesized that lymphadenectomy before administering radiation therapy provided a survival advantage. He observed a 3.5-year survival rate of 61% in 26 patients who underwent lymphadenectomy before primary radiation therapy. Taussig's results showed the impact of nodal metastasis on survival, and this observation led Meigs to combine Taussig's lymphadenectomy with Wertheim's hysterectomy to achieve a mortality rate of 0% and a 5-year survival rate of 43%. Meigs [23] showed that the operation could be performed safely with acceptable results, and with Wertheim, established a standard abdominal approach for treating cervical cancer. Today, the Wertheim-Meigs operation is the standard approach used for treating cervical cancer using the abdominal approach.

Cervical cancer surgery

Types and technical aspects

The possible surgical procedures used to treat early cervical cancer are as follows: cervical conization; simple, modified radical, and radical hysterectomies; and radical trachelectomy. Conization and radical trachelectomy are fertility-preserving procedures. Table 2 provides a comparison between these types of surgical procedures.

In 1973, Piver et al [24] characterized five classes of abdominal hysterectomies, which are outlined in Table 3. The purpose of the classification system was to use the appropriate operation for treating the patient without significantly increasing her morbidity or decreasing survival. The differences in the classes vary depending on the management of the ureters, superior vesical arteries, cardinal ligaments, uterosacral ligaments, and vagina.

The class I hysterectomy is also known as an extrafascial hysterectomy. It ensures removal of all cervical tissue without removal of the parametria or significant dissection of the ureter, which are procedures that can lead to partial denervation of the bladder. Class II and III hysterectomies involve partial and complete resection of the parametria, respectively. The class I hysterectomy is reserved for treating benign disease and the earliest stage of cervical cancer, stage IA1 disease, when there is no evidence of lymph-vascular space invasion (LVSI). The class II and III hysterectomies are indicated for patients with the diagnosis of stage IA1 with LVSI and stages IA2 to IIA disease.

Knowledge of the six spaces within the pelvic floor is paramount before commencing a class II or III hysterectomy. The six spaces of the pelvic floor are as follows: the retropubic, vesicovaginal, rectovaginal, presacral, paravesical, and pararectal spaces. The parametrial tissue or cardinal ligament to be removed lies between the paravesical and pararectal spaces (Fig. 1). The tissue extends from the uterus and cervix to the pelvic sidewalls. The uterine arteries and ureters run within the parametrial tissues. As the uterine artery courses from its origin on the hypogastric artery along the pelvic sidewall to the uterus it crosses under the ureter. The point at which the crossing occurs defines the lateral border of the class II hysterectomy. In a class II radical hysterectomy, also known as a modified radical hysterectomy, the paracervical tissue and its portion of the uterine artery are ligated medial to the ureters as shown in Fig. 1. In the class III hysterectomy, also known as a radical hysterectomy, ligation of the uterine artery occurs at its origin from the hypogastric artery, thus removing the entire parametrium (Fig. 2).

The posterior margin of a class II hysterectomy is formed by partially resecting the uterosacral ligaments at a midpoint between the uterus and the sacrum (see Fig. 2). In a class III hysterectomy, complete resection of the

Table 2
Comparison of extent of resection for surgical procedures to treat early-stage cervical cancer

Tissue	Cervical conization	Total abdominal/ vaginal hysterectomy	Modified radical hysterectomy	Radical abdominal hysterectomy	Radical vaginal trachelectomy	Radical vaginal hysterectomy
Cervix uteri	Partially removed	Completely removed	Completely removed	Completely removed	Majority removed	Completely removed
Corpus uteri	Preserved	Completely removed	Completely removed	Completely removed	Preserved	Completely removed
Ovaries and tubes	Preserved	Preserved	Preserved	Preserved	Preserved	Preserved
Parametria and paracolpos	Preserved	Preserved	Removed at level of ureter	Removed lateral to ureter	Partially removed	Removed at level of ureter
Uterine vessels	Preserved	Ligated at level of cervical internal os	Ligated at level of ureter	Ligated at origin from hypogastric vessels	Descending cervicovaginal branch ligated	Ligated at level of ureter
Uterosacral ligaments	Preserved	Ligated at uterus	Divided midway to rectum	Divided near rectum	Partially removed	Partially removed
Vaginal cuff	Preserved	None removed	1–2 cm removed	≥2 cm removed	1–2 cm removed	≥2 cm removed

From Chi DS, Abu-Rustum NR, Hoskins WJ. Cancer of the cervix. In: Rock JA, Jones HW, editors. Te Linde's operative gynecology. 9th edition. Philadelphia: Lippincott, Williams & Wilkins; 2003; with permission.

Table 3
Piver's five classes of abdominal hysterectomies

Class	Type of hysterectomy	Indications	Surgical margins
I	Extrafascial	FIGO stage IA1 without LVSI	No vagina or parametrial tissue excised, no ureteral mobilization
II	Modified radical	FIGO stage IA1 with LVSI, IA2	1-cm margin of vagina and midportion of ureterosacral ligament, parametria margin to the level of the ureter
III	Radical	FIGO stage IA1 with LVSI, IA2–IIA	One third of vagina and all the uterosacral ligament, parametrial margin to the origin of the uterine artery on the anterior division of the hypogastric artery
IV	Radical	Recurrent disease	Three fourths of the vagina, superior vesicle artery is sacrificed, ureter completely dissected from pubovesicle ligament
V	Radical	Recurrent disease	Resection includes portion of the distal ureter or bladder

From Piver SM, Rotledge F, Smith JP. Five classes of extended hysterectomy for women with cervical cancer. Obstet Gynecol 1974;44(2):265–72.

uterosacral ligaments occurs at their sacral origin (see Fig. 1). For both types of hysterectomies, the upper one third of the vagina serves as the inferior surgical margin.

The amount of parametrial tissue removed therefore determines the "radical" nature of the hysterectomy. Surgeons who offer patients a modified radical hysterectomy do so because more extensive lateral and posterior resection can be associated with decreased vascularity and innervation to the bladder, bladder atony, urinary retention, and vesicovaginal and ureterovaginal fistula formation. Not all authorities agree that a class II hysterectomy is an equally efficacious alternative to a class III hysterectomy in the treatment of cervical cancer, however.

In 1996, Massi et al [13] described a class division for vaginal hysterectomies in a similar fashion to Piver's classification of abdominal hysterectomies. Although the surgical techniques between the vaginal and abdominal approach differ, the anatomic landmarks, which define the boundaries between each class, are the same for both approaches. Massi et al [13] only described three classes, which represent the vaginal equivalent to Piver classes I–III. Unlike Piver, the authors did not describe classes of hysterectomy for recurrent disease [13].

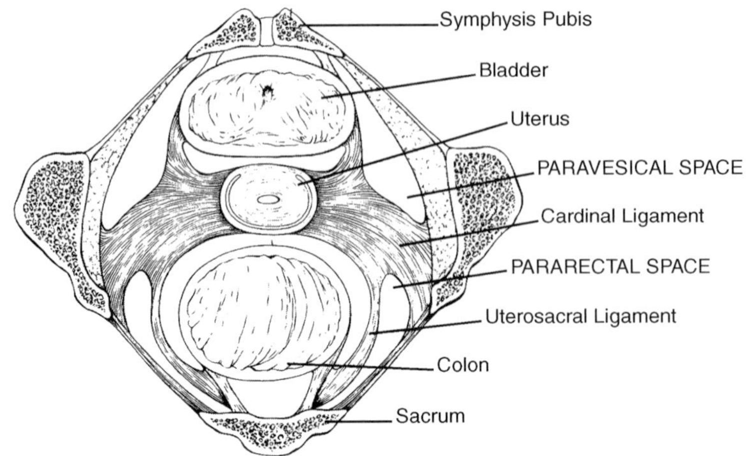

Fig. 1. Cross-section of pelvis showing paravesical and pararectal space. The base of the broad ligament (cardinal ligament) extends to the lateral pelvic wall and contains the major lymphatics draining the cervix. (*From* Chi DS, Abu-Rustum NR, Hoskins WJ. Cancer of the cervix. In: Rock JA, Jones HW, editors. Te Linde's operative gynecology. 9th edition. Philadelphia: Lippincott, Williams & Wilkins; 2003. p. 1403; with permission.)

Oophorectomy at the time of the class II and III hysterectomies is not necessary in early reproductive women because of the low incidence of ovarian metastasis. An incidence of 0.5% for squamous cell carcinoma and 1.7% for adenocarcinoma of the cervix has been reported [25]. This fairly low incidence of metastasis offers young premenopausal patients the opportunity to preserve ovarian function and maintain the benefits of endogenous estrogen. Class IV and V hysterectomies are reserved for patients with recurrent disease, which is not the focus of this article (see Table 3).

Laparoscopy

The current use of laparoscopy in the management of cervical cancer includes the following: staging lymphadenectomy for advanced cervical cancer, total laparoscopic radical hysterectomy, laparoscopically assisted radical vaginal hysterectomy (LARVH), and laparoscopically assisted radical vaginal trachelectomy. Laparoscopically staging lymphadenectomy has been used to determine the status of the para-aortic nodes before the initiation of pelvic radiation therapy in patients with advanced cervical cancer [26]. The radiation therapy can then be more individualized and tailored to the patient by giving standard pelvic radiation therapy to those patients with negative para-aortic nodes while extending the radiation field to include the para-aortic nodes in those patients with documented metastasis.

Class III abdominal hysterectomies with bilateral pelvic lymphadenectomy can be performed completely laparoscopically [27,28]. In an LARVH,

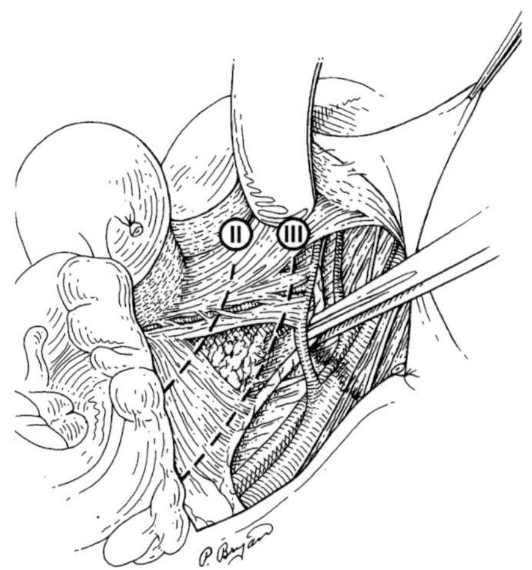

Fig. 2. The cardinal ligament is excised medially in women with microscopic lesions (class II operation) or laterally in those with larger volume lesions (class III operation). (*From* Chi DS, Abu-Rustum NR, Hoskins WJ. Cancer of the cervix. In: Rock JA, Jones HW, editors. Te Linde's operative gynecology. 9th edition. Philadelphia: Lippincott, Williams & Wilkins; 2003. p. 1388; with permission.)

the pelvic lymphadenectomy and division of the upper uterine attachments are performed laparoscopically, with resection of the upper vagina, parametria, uterosacral ligaments, and uterine arteries performed vaginally [4]. The main benefit of the LARVH is to give the operator experience in performing radical vaginal surgery so that fertility-sparing, laparoscopically assisted radical vaginal trachelectomy can be safely performed [29,30].

Fertility-sparing surgery

Approximately 10% to 15% of patients with cervical cancer are diagnosed during their reproductive years. Radical surgery, including hysterectomy, has significant emotional and psychosocial implications for women, especially for their future fertility. Over the last two decades, several surgical techniques have been described to afford young women the opportunity to maintain their reproductive potential without compromising their overall survival and chance of cure.

Aburel was the first to perform a radical abdominal trachelectomy, a procedure that removes the cervix, parametria, and upper vagina while preserving the uterus and its vascularity [30]. Today, the procedure is most commonly performed vaginally, with a laparoscopic procedure for nodal retrieval. The concept of a trachelectomy is similar to a hysterectomy except at the level of the uterine artery. To maintain a viable uterus, the uterine artery must be preserved and not transected. Uterine artery collaterals going to the lateral vaginal fornix and to the cervix are divided, and the cervix is amputated and divided 5 mm below the isthmus. Frozen sections are sent to ensure negative superior margins.

Once, negative margins are obtained, the pouch of Douglas is closed, the uterus is sutured to the remaining upper vagina, and a prophylactic uterine isthmus cerclage is placed to decrease the possibility of miscarriage in the event of subsequent pregnancy.

The reported pregnancy rates with this approach are encouraging. Dargent et al reported on 71 patients who underwent radical vaginal trachelectomy for cervical cancer. Three recurrences and one death were observed. Thirty-one patients attempted to get pregnant, and 28 (90%) were successful. Eighteen of these 28 (64%) patients successfully delivered at least one healthy infant.

Overall, the initial data involving laparoscopically assisted radical vaginal trachelectomy in the management of early cervical cancer are promising. In one study, the actuarial 5-year survival (median follow-up, 52 mo) when using this fertility-sparing approach was 100% for tumors smaller than 2 cm, 79.2% for tumors between 2 and 4 cm, and 50.5% for tumors larger than 4 cm [29]. Larger studies with long-term follow-up are needed before any definitive recommendations regarding overall safety and efficacy can be made.

Current management of early disease

Stage IA

The FIGO staging system for cervical cancer is shown in Table 1. In stage IA1, the cancer has a depth of cervical invasion not exceeding 3 mm and a horizontal spread not exceeding 7 mm. Standard therapy consists of a simple hysterectomy, which can be performed abdominally or vaginally. These operations carry a lower morbidity compared with radical abdominal or vaginal hysterectomy. The incidence of lymph node metastasis is less than 1% in patients with stage IA1 disease; therefore, pelvic lymphadenectomy is not necessary [31,32].

Patients with stage IA1 disease are also candidates for conservative management, provided that certain criteria are met. Because the diagnosis of invasive microscopic cervical cancer is generally made on a cervical conization specimen, this conization can serve as conservative treatment with avoidance of any type of hysterectomy if the following criteria are met: the depth and width of invasion are consistent with stage IA1 disease, the surgical margins are negative for both cancer and dysplasia, there is no lymphatic or vascular space invasion, and the patient desires maintaining future childbearing capability. The 5-year survival rate of more than 95% for patients treated conservatively is similar to that of patients treated with simple or radical hysterectomy. The choice of conservative management should be guided by the patient's preference and desire to preserve fertility. Patients undergoing this management must be carefully selected and adequately counseled.

Patients with stage IA1 disease who have LVSI have a reported incidence of lymph node metastasis as high as 6.2% [31,32]. Therefore, these patients would not be adequately treated with a simple hysterectomy or cone biopsy. The standard treatment for these patients is radical hysterectomy and bilateral pelvic lymphadenectomy. The conservative treatment option for these patients is radical trachelectomy (abdominal or vaginal) with bilateral pelvic lymphadenectomy (using laparotomy or laparoscopy).

Stage IB

Patients with stage IB disease have lesions confined to the cervix ranging from 6 mm of microscopic stromal invasion to grossly visible cervical masses of any size, even larger than 10 cm. This broad classification delineated a wide spectrum of disease, recurrence rates, and treatment outcomes. Thus, in 1994, FIGO modified the staging system for stage IB cervical cancer, dividing it into two subgroups: stages IB1 and IB2 (see Table 1). The subdivision was based on cervical tumor size, which numerous studies had shown to be an important prognostic factor in lymph node metastasis, recurrent disease, and overall survival.

Surgery versus radiation therapy

Studies comparing the outcome between patients with stage IB cervical cancer treated with surgery versus radiation therapy have shown similar survival outcomes [25,33–35]. Although reported survival rates of patients with stage IB disease is approximately 85%, survival data for the specific subdivisions of IB1 and IB2 have not been clearly established, because most of the studies evaluating patients with stage IB tumors were performed without the FIGO substaging. In a typical study, Morley and Seski [34] retrospectively evaluated 401 patients with stage IB cervical cancer and found a 5-year survival rate of 87% for patients treated with radiation and 91% for patients treated with surgery.

Previous reports comparing radiation and surgery have limitations. Most of these studies were retrospective with a nonrandomized design using nonstandard treatment regimens while failing to use an intent-to-treat analysis. The use of an intent-to-treat analysis is important because in some studies the patients who had their surgery abandoned at the time of radical hysterectomy were excluded from the analysis, thus skewing the data in favor of surgery. The Gynecologic Oncology Group (GOG) protocol 49 revealed that 8.7% of all patients explored with the intent to perform a radical hysterectomy had the procedure abandoned because of unexpected findings at the time of laparotomy. The authors recommended that survival rates after radical hysterectomy be adjusted to reflect the outcomes of patients in whom the planned procedure was abandoned [36].

Brewster et al [37] incorporated an intent-to-treat analysis into their evaluation of survival outcomes of patients with cervical cancer treated with radiation versus surgery. The 5-year survival rate for patients with bulky (>4 cm) tumors treated with radiation therapy was 72% versus 68% for those treated surgically. Patients with lesions smaller than 4 cm derived greater benefit from surgery, however, with a 5-year survival rate of 86% for those who were treated surgically compared with 71% for those treated with radiation therapy ($P = 0.001$).

Currently, the standard treatment options for a patient with stage IB1 cervical cancer are radical hysterectomy with bilateral pelvic lymphadenectomy and definitive radiation therapy. The conservative fertility-sparing treatment option for these patients is radical trachelectomy (abdominal or vaginal) with bilateral pelvic lymphadenectomy (using laparotomy or laparoscopy). The benefits of surgical treatment include rapid treatment and preservation of normal ovarian and vaginal function. Several studies have shown that patients older than 65 years can tolerate a radical hysterectomy, so age alone should not be considered a contraindication to the surgical approach.

Because of the worse prognosis of patients with bulky (>4 cm) cervical tumors, patients who have undergone radical hysterectomy and pelvic lymphadenectomy for stage IB2 disease have traditionally received postoperative adjuvant pelvic radiation therapy. In a randomized trial, however, Landoni et al [33] showed that radical hysterectomy plus radiotherapy does not improve overall or disease-free survival in patients with stage IB2 tumors as compared with radiation therapy alone. The combined surgical and radiation treatment significantly increased morbidity, however. Furthermore, another randomized trial performed by the GOG showed a significant survival benefit with the addition of cisplatin chemotherapy to pelvic radiation for patients with stage IB2 cervical cancer [5]. Therefore, many authorities believe that chemoradiation should be the standard treatment for patients with stage IB2 cervical cancer. Primary chemoradiation has not yet been compared with primary radical hysterectomy in this patient population; therefore, the optimal primary treatment in this group of patients has not been definitively determined. The GOG protocol 201, which opened in September 2002, is currently addressing this issue by randomizing patients with stage IB2 cervical cancer to primary concurrent chemoradiation versus radical hysterectomy and bilateral pelvic lymphadenectomy. It is hoped that the results of this trial will answer many of the questions regarding the optimal management of patients with stage IB2 cervical cancer.

Adjuvant therapy after radical hysterectomy

Adverse risk factors for recurrence after radical hysterectomy include the following: deep cervical stromal invasion, LVSI, tumor mass larger than 4 cm, parametrial involvement, positive surgical margins, and positive margins. Patients without these risk factors who receive surgery alone to treat their disease have a 5-year survival rate of 82% to 92% [38–40].

After identifying these risk factors in a prospective trial of radical hysterectomy and pelvic lymphadenectomy in patients with cervical cancer, the GOG designed two separate randomized trials of adjuvant therapy. Patients with none of the previously noted risk factors were deemed low risk and did not qualify for the adjuvant trials. Patients with deep stromal invasion, LVSI, or tumors larger than 4 cm were considered at intermediate risk for recurrence and were candidates for a randomized trial of no further therapy versus adjuvant pelvic radiotherapy. In the published report, there was a significant (47%) reduction in the risk of recurrence among patients who received adjuvant radiotherapy, with a 2-year recurrence-free rate of 88% with radiation versus 79% without this therapy [41]. With longer follow-up periods, however, this difference was not sustained. Therefore, the benefit of pelvic radiation therapy in this intermediate risk group remains controversial.

For patients with high-risk factors, such as positive surgical margins, parametrial involvement, or lymph node metastasis, pelvic radiotherapy was traditionally used and decreased the pelvic relapse rate from 50% to 25% but did not affect overall survival because of distant metastasis. In the other adjuvant GOG trial, patients with any of the three previously described high-risk factors after radical hysterectomy and pelvic lymphadenectomy were randomized to receive either pelvic radiation therapy or pelvic radiation therapy plus concurrent 5-fluorouracil (5-FU) and cisplatin chemotherapy [7]. A significant improvement in progression-free and overall survival was seen for the chemoradiation arm compared with the radiation-alone arm (4-y survival rates of 81% and 71%, respectively). These results have helped establish chemoradiation as the standard therapy for patients with high-risk factors after radical hysterectomy and pelvic lymphadenectomy for cervical cancer.

Stage IIA

Stage IIA cervical cancer extends to the vagina but does not involve the lower one third of the vagina or the parametria. Patients with stage IIA tumors are treated similarly to those with stage IB lesions. Generally, patients with tumors of 4 cm or smaller are treated with radical hysterectomy (which includes an upper vaginectomy) and bilateral pelvic lymph node dissection, whereas those with tumors larger than 4 cm are treated primarily with surgery or concurrent chemotherapy and radiation therapy. The 5-year survival rate of patients with stage IIA disease is approximately 76% [4].

Current management of late disease

Stage IIB–IVA

The most important prognostic factor associated with pelvic tumor control and survival in advanced stages is the bulk of pelvic disease within each stage. The treatment of patients with disease stage IIB–IVA traditionally has been radiotherapy using external beam radiation and brachytherapy. External irradiation treats the whole pelvis and parametria, including the iliac and obturator lymph nodes. Central disease in the vagina, cervix, and adjacent parametria is primarily treated with intracavitary sources. Improvement in radiation techniques has improved tumor control and survival over the past few decades, with 5-year survival rates by stage of disease as follows: stage IIB, 73%; stage IIIA, 51%; stage IIIB, 46%; and stage IVA, 30% [4]. An increased risk of treatment failure occurs if patients have large-volume primary tumors, bilateral parametrial disease, nodal metastases, poor performance status, low hemoglobin values, and a smoking history. The amount of radiation required to treat bulky tumors is limited because these levels are toxic to normal tissues. To overcome this problem, novel applications have been introduced, which include the following: large particle radiotherapy, differences in radiation-fractionation schedules, and the concurrent use of hypothermia or chemotherapy. Multiple recent randomized trials have documented a significant survival benefit with the addition of concurrent cisplatin-based chemotherapy to radiation therapy in the treatment of cervical cancer, and currently, weekly cisplatin or cisplatin plus 5-FU given every 3 weeks with irradiation is standard therapy for patients with stages IIB–IVA [6,8,9]. Surgery plays little role, if any, in the management of late disease. Surgical treatment may be an option for the patient with advanced stage IVA disease who develops either a vesicovaginal or rectovaginal fistula. A patient with locally advanced disease and a fistula could be treated with an exenterative procedure, which is discussed elsewhere in this issue.

Stage IVB

Cytotoxic chemotherapy has been used to treat patients with advanced stage IVB persistent and recurrent disease. This treatment is generally considered palliative and given to patients who can no longer be managed by surgery or radiation therapy. Various factors complicate the use of chemotherapy in these patients. Prior radiation treatment can affect the vascular supply to the involved field, which can result in decreased drug delivery to the tumor site. Pelvic irradiation also reduces bone marrow reserve, thus limiting the tolerable doses of most chemotherapeutic agents. A significant number of patients with stage IVB disease may also have impaired renal function, further limiting the use of certain chemotherapeutic agents.

Among the chemotherapeutic agents used for cervical cancer, cisplatin has shown the most consistent activity, with response rates ranging from 18% to 31% [10]. The GOG recently reported the results of a randomized phase 3 trial of cisplatin versus cisplatin plus topotecan versus methotrexate, vinblastine, actinomycin, and cisplatin (MVAC) in the treatment of stage

IVB, recurrent, or persistent cervical cancer. The MVAC arm was closed prematurely because of excessive toxicity. The combination of cisplatin plus topotecan was superior to cisplatin with respect to response, progression-free survival, and overall survival. The cisplatin plus topotecan regimen is the first regimen to show a significant survival advantage over single-agent cisplatin in this patient population. Because of these results, many feel that the combination of cisplatin and topotecan should be the new standard of care. In this trial, however, the difference in median progression-free survival was less than 2 months between the two arms, and the improvement in median overall survival was only 2.2 months (7 mo for the cisplatin arm versus 9.2 mo for the cisplatin/topotecan arm) [42]. These small improvements and the significantly increased toxicity associated with the combination regimen have caused many to question whether these results justify the use of cisplatin and topotecan over single-agent cisplatin in this setting.

Summary

The evolution in the surgical management of cervical cancer dates back to the late nineteenth century. Many improvements have been made in the operative technique of the radical hysterectomy and pelvic lymphadenectomy since their original description. The incidence of complications after this procedure has decreased during the past three quarters of a century, and the survival rates have increased. The operation has achieved its peak of clinical usefulness during this period and is now considered to be the principal method of treatment of early invasive carcinoma of the cervix. When performed by well-trained gynecologic oncologists, the meticulous execution of this operative procedure has reduced the incidence of complications to an acceptable and infrequent occurrence. The operation affords little additional surgical risk to the patient than a hysterectomy performed for benign disease. Newer laparoscopic approaches are promising, with comparable cure rates and the potential to retain fertility in carefully selected patients.

Comparative studies with primary radiotherapy have shown an equal cure rate with primary radical surgery in the treatment of early-stage disease. The complications of irradiation are far more difficult to manage than are those of primary surgery, however. In young women, when preservation of ovarian function is important, primary surgery is a preferable choice of treatment.

The major limiting factor in the long-term surgical cure of cervical cancer is related to the spread of the disease at the time of initiation of treatment. Historically, in patients in whom pelvic lymph nodes were positive for metastatic tumor, the 5-year cure rate was reduced to approximately 60%. Numerous recently reported prospective, randomized trials have shown the benefit of concurrent chemotherapy and radiation therapy in various settings. In the management of high-risk patients after radical hysterectomy and pelvic lymphadenectomy, including those with positive nodes, the reported 4-year disease-free survival rate is 81%.

It is important to understand that it is the individual surgical expertise that offers the highest cure rate and lowest incidence of complications to the patient with invasive carcinoma of the cervix. One of the greatest errors in clinical judgment is made by gynecologists who attempt a radical hysterectomy and pelvic lymph node dissection without adequate surgical training and experience. Unless the pelvic surgeon is performing this type of surgery regularly in a well-staffed medical center with trained assistants, he or she would be well advised to refer the patient to an established gynecologic oncologist. From the patient's point of view, the initial treatment, whether primary surgery or irradiation, provides the best chance for long-term cure of this disease. It would be to her advantage to have the treatment conducted in the most expert hands because secondary treatment for recurrent disease offers only limited potential long-term cure.

Gynecologic surgeons who become thoroughly familiar with the pathology and natural history of cervical cancer, who appreciate the history of the development of radical hysterectomy and pelvic lymphadenectomy as primary treatment of the disease, and who then thoroughly master the technical details of performing the operation can feel enormous pride in their achievement because there is no greater challenge in gynecologic surgery and no greater personal satisfaction than that which comes to those who are able to perform the operation correctly and save a woman from the intense suffering and undignified death that cervical cancer can cause [4].

References

[1] Parkin DM, Pisani P, Ferlay J. Estimates of the worldwide incidence of eighteen major cancers in 1985. Int J Cancer 1993;54:594–606.

[2] Jemal A, Murray T, Samuels A, et al. Cancer statistics, 2003. Cancer J Clin 2003;53:5–26.

[3] Benedet J, Odicino F, Maisonneuve P, et al. Carcinoma of the cervix uteri. J Epidemiol Biostat 1998;3(1):5–34.

[4] Chi DS, Abu-Rustum NR, Hoskins WJ. Cancer of the cervix. In: Rock JA, Jones HW, editors. TeLinde's operative gynecology. 9th edition. Philadelphia: Lippincott, Williams & Wilkins; 2003. p. 1373–444.

[5] Keys H, Bundy B, Stehman FB, et al. Cisplatin, radiation, and adjuvant hysterectomy compared with radiation and adjuvant hysterectomy for bulky stage IB cervical carcinoma. N Engl J Med 1999;340(15):1154–61.

[6] Morris M, Eifel PJ, Lu J, et al. Pelvic radiation with concurrent chemotherapy compared with pelvic and para-aortic radiation for high-risk cervical cancer. N Engl J Med 1999; 340:1137–43.

[7] Peters WA III, Lui PY, Barrett RJ II, et al. Concurrent chemotherapy and pelvic radiation therapy compared with pelvic radiation therapy alone as adjuvant therapy after radical surgery in high-risk early-stage cancer of the cervix. J Clin Oncol 2000;18(8):1606–13.

[8] Rose PG, Bundy BN, Watkins EB, et al. Concurrent-based radiotherapy and chemotherapy for locally advance cervical cancer. N Engl J Med 1999;340:1144–53.

[9] Whitney CW, Sause W, Bundy BN, et al. Randomized comparison of fluorouracil plus cisplatin versus hydroxyurea as an adjunct to radiation therapy in stages IIB-IVA carcinoma of the cervix with negative papa-aortic lymph nodes: a Gynecologic Oncology Group and Southwest Gynecology Group study. J Clin Oncol 1999;17(5):1339–48.
[10] National Cancer Institute. Concurrent chemo-radiation for cervical cancer. Clinical announcement, February 22 1999. Washington, DC: National Cancer Institute; 1999.
[11] Thomas GM. Improved treatment of cervical cancer-concurrent chemotherapy and radiotherapy. N Engl J Med 1999;340:1198–200.
[12] Ballon SC. The Wertheim hysterectomy. Surg Gynecol Obstet 1976;142(6):920–4.
[13] Massi G, Savino L, Susini T. Three classes of radical vaginal hysterectomy for the treatment of endometrial and cervical cancer. Am J Obstet Gynecol 1996;175(6):1576–85.
[14] Schuchardt K. Eine neue Methode der Gebarmutterexstirpation. Zentralbl Chir 1893;20: 1121–38.
[15] Schauta F. Die operation des Gebarmutterkrebses mittels des Schuchardtschen Paravaginalschnittes. Mschr Geburtshilfe Gynakol 1902;15:133–52.
[16] Americh I. Zur Anatomie und Technik der erweiterten vaginalen carcinomoperation. ArchGynakol 1924;122:497–553.
[17] Reis E. Eine neue Operation Methode des Uterus-carcinomas. Z Geburtshilfe Gynak 1895; 32:266.
[18] Clark JG. A more radical method of performing hysterectomy for cancer of the uterus. Bull Johns Hopk Hosp 6, 1896.
[19] Wertheim E. The extended abdominal operation for carcinoma uteri (based on 500 operative cases). Am J Obstet Dis Women Child 1912;64(2):169–232.
[20] Leonardo RA. History of gynecology. York, UK: Froben Press; 1944.
[21] Bonney V. The treatment of carcinoma of the cervix by Wertheims operation. Am J Obstet Gynecol 1935;30:815–30.
[22] Taussig FJ. Iliac lymphadenectomy with irradiation in the treatment of cancer of the cervix. Am J Obstet Gynecol 1934;28:650–67.
[23] Meigs JV. The carcinoma of the cervix: the Wertheim operation. Surg Gynecol Obstet 1944; 78:195–9.
[24] Piver SM, Rutledge F, Smith JP. Five classes of extended hysterectomy for women with cervical cancer. Obstet Gynecol 1974;44(2):265–72.
[25] Piver MS, Marchetti DL, Patton T, et al. Radical hysterectomy and pelvic lymphadenectomy versus radiation therapy for small (<3 cm) stage 1B cervical carcinoma. Am J Clin Oncol 1998;11:21–4.
[26] Sonoda Y, Leblanc E, Querleu, et al. Prospective evaluation of surgical staging of advanced cervical cancer via a laparoscopic extraperitoneal approach. Gynecol Oncol 2003;91(2): 326–31.
[27] Spirtos NM, Eisenkop SM, Schlaerth JB, et al. Laparoscopic radical hysterectomy (type III) with aortic and pelvic lymphadenectomy in patients with stage I cervical cancer: surgical morbidity and intermediate follow-up. Am J Obstet Gynecol 2002;187:340–8.
[28] Abu-Rustum NR, Gemignani M, Moore K, et al. Total laparoscopic radical hysterectomy with pelvic lymphadenectomy using the argon beam coagulator: pilot data and comparison to laparotomy. Gynecol Oncol 2003;91(2):402–9.
[29] Dargent D. Laparoscopic surgery in gynecologic oncology. Surg Clin North Am 2001;8(4): 949–64.
[30] Dargent DF, Plante M. Laparoscopic surgery in gynecologic cancer. In: Hoskins WJ, Perez CA, Young RC, editors. Principles and practices of gynecologic oncology. 3rd edition. Philadelphia: Lippincott, Williams & Wilkins; 2000. p. 265–95.
[31] Creasman WT, Parker RT. Microinvasive carcinoma of the cervix. Clin Obstet Gynecol 1973;16:261–75.
[32] Ostor AG, Rome RM. Microinvasive squamous cell carcinoma of the cervix: a clinicopathologic study of 200 cases with long-term follow-up. Int J Gynecol Cancer 1995;4(4):257–64.

[33] Landoni F, Maneo A, Colombo A, et al. Randomized study of radical versus radiotherapy for stage IB-IIA cervical cancer. Lancet 1997;350(9077):535–40.

[34] Morley GW, Seski JC. Radical pelvic surgery versus radiation therapy for stage I carcinoma of the cervix (exclusive microinvasion). Am J Obstet Gynecol 1976;126(7):785–98.

[35] Hoskins MP, Morley GW. Radical hysterectomy versus radiation therapy for stage 1B squamous cell cancer of the cervix. Cancer 1991;98:272–7.

[36] Charles WW, Federick BS. The abandoned radical hysterectomy: a Gynecologic Oncology Group study. Gynecol Oncol 1999;79:350–6.

[37] Brewster WR, Monk BJ, Zioga A, et al. Intent-to-treat analysis of stage 1B and IIA cervical cancer in the United States: radiotherapy or surgery 1988–1995. Obstet Gynecol 2002;97: 248–54.

[38] Delgado G, Bundy BN, Fowler WC, et al. A prospective surgical pathological study of stage I squamous carcinoma of the cervix: a Gynecologic Oncology Group study. Gynecol Oncol 1989;35:314–20.

[39] Delgado G. Stage IB squamous cancer of the cervix: the choice of treatment. Obstet Gynecol Surv 1978;33:174–83.

[40] Finan MA, DeCasare S, Fiorica JV, et al. Radical hysterectomy for stage IB1 vs IB2 carcinoma of the cervix: does the new staging system predict morbidity and survival? Gynecol Oncol 1996;62:139–47.

[41] Sedlis A, Bundy BN, Rotman MZ, et al. A randomized trial of pelvic radiation therapy versus no further therapy in selected patients with stage 1B carcinoma of the cervix after radical hysterectomy and pelvic lymphadenectomy: a Gynecologic Oncology Group study. Gynecol Oncol 1999;73(2):177–83.

[42] Long HJ, Bundy BN, Grendys EC, et al. Randomized phase III trial of cisplatin (P) vs. cisplatin plus topotecan (T) vs. MVAC in stage IVB, recurrent or persistent carcinoma of the uterine cervix: a Gynecologic Oncology Group study [abstract]. Gynecol Oncol 2004;92:397.

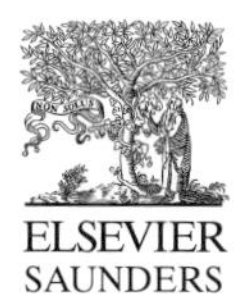

ELSEVIER
SAUNDERS

Surg Oncol Clin N Am
14 (2005) 267–288

SURGICAL
ONCOLOGY CLINICS
OF NORTH AMERICA

Surgical Staging of Gynecologic Malignancies: The Role of Laparoscopy and Sentinel Node Technology

Robert Kim, MD[a], Peter G. Rose, MD[a,b,*]

[a]*Division of Gynecologic Oncology, Department of Obstetrics and Gynecology, Cleveland Clinic Foundation, 9500 Euclid Avenue, A-81, Cleveland, OH 44195, USA*
[b]*Reproductive Biology, Surgery and Gynecology, Case Western Reserve University, Cleveland, OH 44106, USA*

In 1807, Bozzini described the first use of a "vase-like" instrument using candles for illumination to peer into the body of a human being. Jacobaeus coined the modern term "laparoscopy," using the direct insertion of a cystoscope. The first gynecologic procedure was performed by Hope, who used a peritoneoscope to diagnose tubal pregnancies. In 1941, Power and Barnes described the first tubal ligation by coagulating the isthmic portions of a patient's fallopian tubes [1]. For many years laparoscopy was almost completely confined to female sterilization. Advances in light sources, smaller endoscopes, video image resolution, and instruments expanded the use of laparoscopy beyond female sterilization to the management of endometriosis, pelvic floor incontinence, and malignancy.

Hald and Rasmussen, two Danish urologists, were the first to use endoscopy in the management of pelvic tumors. Using a Carlens mediastinoscope in patients with bladder and prostate cancer, they obtained iliac lymph node biopsies through small inguinal incisions [2]. In 1989, Dargent and Salvat [3] reported the first report of pelvic lymphadenectomy for cervical cancer. It was not, however, until Querleu et al [4] presented their series of patients undergoing pelvic lymphadenectomy using a transumbilical transperitoneal approach that laparoscopy was widely accepted as an alternative surgical approach to gynecologic malignancies.

* Corresponding author. Division of Gynecologic Oncology, Department of Obstetrics and Gynecology, Cleveland Clinic Foundation, 9500 Euclid Avenue, A-81, Cleveland, OH 44195.

E-mail address: rosep@ccf.org (P.G. Rose).

doi:10.1016/j.soc.2004.11.012 ***surgonc.theclinics.com***

The use of surgery in the management of gynecologic tumors serves three purposes: staging of disease, tumor resection with curative intent, and tumor debulking. Surgical staging assesses the extent of tumor growth and spread. Radical surgery is a definitive attempt to remove the cancer completely. Finally, cytoreductive surgery involves tumor debulking to as small a residual disease as possible to achieve a better response rate to adjuvant therapies. Although staging often uses clinical examination and noninvasive tests such as radiologic imaging, surgical staging attempts to discern which tumors have metastasized versus those that may be more localized and amenable to complete resection. Traditional surgical methods (ie, exploratory laparotomy) provide more accurate results than noninvasive testing but often require larger, more painful incisions, long recoveries, and may result in greater morbidity. Minimally invasive surgical approaches, as in laparoscopic staging, reduce the invasive component without compromising on diagnostic accuracy.

Laparoscopy offers many potential benefits over traditional laparotomy through its use of magnification and ability to overcome obstructive angles. Proposed benefits include less blood loss during surgery, smaller, less painful incisions, shorter hospital stays, and quicker return to preoperative activities resulting in improved patient quality of life. All of this may occur with less morbidity than laparotomy and result in fewer treatment delays. Given these advantages, many pelvic surgeons have embraced this new technology without much data to support its feasibility in the management of gynecologic malignancies. One must keep in mind that laparoscopy requires a new skill set beyond that of traditional surgical training. The loss of depth perception and tactile sensation from the two-dimensional video screens and use of long instruments, respectively, can disorient even seasoned surgeons unskilled in laparoscopic techniques. As a result, laparoscopy has its own set of complications, and minimally invasive procedures can result in not-so-minimal complications.

Despite these drawbacks, laparoscopy holds considerable promise and utility in the staging of cervical, endometrial, and ovarian cancers. Improvements in instrumentation and equipment and two decades of experience have increased the number of staging procedures performed using these techniques. Ongoing studies are accruing data to address issues of feasibility, adequacy, operative times, economic costs, surgical complications, and, most importantly, impact on disease recurrences and long-term patient survival.

Cervical cancer

Cervical cancer affects more than 400,000 women worldwide, with the most cases and deaths occurring in underdeveloped regions. As a result, sophisticated imaging has not been incorporated into the staging system, and staging for this cancer remains based on clinical findings. In the United States and developed countries, however, oncologists have attempted to assess disease spread more accurately using sophisticated tools, such as CT, MRI, lymphangiography, and positron emission tomography. Each technique has its limitations, especially in its ability to detect small, involved lymph nodes. Considerable benefit could be gained with better detection of disease spread in treatment planning, especially when mapping radiation therapy fields. Pathologic review of actual specimens remains the gold standard for detecting metastases. Laparoscopy has provided a new modality for surgical staging.

Early-stage disease

Laparoscopy has been well described in the treatment of early-stage cervical cancer. There are essentially five different operations used: (1) a total laparoscopic hysterectomy or laparoscopic-assisted vaginal hysterectomy for carcinoma in situ or stage Ia1 disease, (2) laparoscopic-assisted radical vaginal hysterectomy, (3) modifications based on the Schauta technique, (4) laparoscopic radical hysterectomy, and (5) laparoscopic radical vaginal trachelectomy for preservation of fertility. Each of these operations is often combined as part of the staging procedure with pelvic and para-aortic lymphadenectomy.

Laparoscopic pelvic lymphadenectomy

Laparoscopic pelvic lymphadenectomy is the first and necessary step in enabling laparoscopic treatment of gynecologic malignancies. The procedure was first described by Querleu at the Second World Congress of Gynecologic Endoscopy in Clermont-Ferrand, France in June, 1989. He and his colleagues later published in 1991 a series of 39 patients with stage IB-IIB cervical cancer who underwent the procedure [4]. The mean operating time was 80 minutes, an average of only 8.7 lymph nodes (range, 3–22) were removed, and conversion to laparotomy was not required in any of the patients. Five patients in this series had positive lymph nodes.

Childers et al [5] subsequently reported their series of 18 patients. The operating time ranged from 75 to 175 minutes, and the average number of nodes removed was higher at 31.4. Among five patients who underwent immediate laparotomy, an average additional 2.8 lymph nodes were removed. There were no reported complications. Among eight patients with cervical cancer who were candidates for abdominal radical hysterectomy, three were found to have positive lymph nodes. Nine of 13 patients who underwent laparoscopy alone were sent home on postoperative day 1.

Laparoscopic pelvic lymphadenectomy seems to be feasible and adequate. The average number of lymph nodes removed from the pelvic basin is approximately 25 [6]. Fowler et al [7] reported on 12 patients who underwent immediate laparotomy after laparoscopic dissection. A total of 377 lymph nodes were removed, only 75% of which were removed by laparoscopy. None of the patients with negative lymph nodes on laparoscopy, however, had positive lymph nodes on laparotomy. In a review of 594 pelvic sidewall dissections, Nijman et al [8] reported that the mean number of lymph nodes identified was 11.3 (range, 0–42). Using a cutoff value of either the first or tenth percentile, this would give a lower limit of 3 to 6 lymph nodes as an adequate sampling. They found that the laparoscopic approach produced a significantly higher yield of lymph nodes compared with laparotomy (11.9 versus 10.6).

In the largest prospective study to date, the Gynecologic Oncology Group (GOG) reported on 67 patients with stage IA-IIA cervical cancer in whom immediate abdominal radical hysterectomy was planned after laparoscopic pelvic lymphadenectomy [9]. Seventeen patients did not undergo laparotomy because of metastases or complications, and another 10 patients could not be evaluated. Of the remaining 40 patients, the median operating time was 170 minutes, and mean lymph nodes removed numbered 31.1. Seven (10.4%) of all laparoscopy patients sustained vascular injuries, three of which required laparotomy. It was deemed that 6 (15%) of the 40 patients assessed by laparotomy had residual lymph nodes remaining but were all negative for metastases. These results have led some proponents of laparoscopic staging to conclude that laparoscopy samples the significant lymph nodes that are affected by disease. As a result, surgical staging in this setting may provide a minimally invasive approach to deciding whether a woman with presumptive early stage disease might be a candidate for radical hysterectomy.

Advanced-stage disease

Likewise for women with advanced-stage disease, surgical staging may identify areas of spread and assist radiation treatment planning. The standard treatment for stages IIB-IV is chemo-irradiation, and many patients with stage IB_2 are also treated in this manner. Approximately 30% to 50% of women with advanced disease are understaged by clinical methods [10]. Para-aortic lymph nodes are positive in stages IB, II, and III in approximately 6%, 12%, and 30%, respectively [11]. Of women with affected pelvic lymph nodes, one fourth of them have spread to the higher chain para-aortic region.

If the para-aortic lymph nodes are positive, radiation therapy would include an extended field to encompass that area. Without staging, patients with poor risk factors and possible evidence of para-aortic lymph node spread on imaging studies might be administered prophylactic extended field radiation therapy. The risk, however, of grade 4 or 5 radiation toxicity to the gastrointestinal and genitourinary system is approximately 4% [12,13]. Given the inaccuracies of imaging studies, surgery to determine whether para-aortic nodal disease exists can influence treatment decisions and possibly prognosis greatly.

If the para-aortic dissection is carried through to the level of the left renal vein, approximately 20 lymph nodes are sampled [14]. In patients with cervical cancer with para-aortic disease spread, the left side and supra-mesenteric areas are involved approximately 72% and 25% of the time, respectively [15]. The para-aortic dissection should be extended to the left renal vein. The difficulty of the dissection is in the lower portion of the inferior vena cava below the inferior mesenteric artery. Venous tributaries are encountered anterior to the vena cava around 58% at the bifurcation of the inferior vena cava, 19.6% between the inferior mesenteric artery and bifurcation, and only 0.9% above the inferior mesenteric artery to the right ovarian vein [16].

Laparoscopic para-aortic lymphadenectomy

Two laparoscopic approaches toward para-aortic lymphadenectomy have been described. The first technique, using a transumbilical transperitoneal approach similar to that performed for most gynecologic procedures including the pelvic lymphadenectomy, was first described in 1992 by Childers et al [5]. As part of the larger group of 18 patients described above, six patients with stage IIB or greater without evidence of lymphadenopathy on CT scan, underwent laparoscopic pelvic lymphadenectomy. Two patients had disease spread to the pelvic lymph nodes, and one patient had microscopic involvement of the para-aortic lymph nodes. An average of 31.4 lymph nodes were removed without any short-term complications. In the largest study of 28 patients with stage IIB-IIIB disease conducted to assess para-aortic lymphadenectomy, Chu et al [6] performed bilateral lymph node dissection with an average yield of eight lymph nodes and mean operating time of more than 95 minutes. Ten (36%) patients had positive para-aortic lymph nodes and subsequently were treated with either extended field radiation therapy or systemic chemotherapy and whole pelvic radiotherapy. Those without evidence of para-aortic spread received whole pelvic radiotherapy only.

Vasilev and McGonigle [17] were the first to describe a second technique using an extraperitoneal approach through a left incision. In their small series of four patients, they removed an average of five lymph nodes because their dissection was limited to the inframesenteric region. Querleu et al [18] series of 53 patients with bulky early-stage, advanced stage IIB or higher, or recurrent disease is one of the largest series to look at this approach. Two procedures failed, and 9 patients had macroscopically positive lymph nodes. The remaining 42 patients underwent laparoscopic para-aortic lymphadenectomy with an average operating time of 125.9 minutes and lymph node yield of 20.7. An additional 8 patients had microscopic nodal disease. One intraoperative injury to the ureter was managed by stenting. All the patients except one received radiation fields according to their para-aortic lymph node status. With a mean follow-up of 18.9 months, no patient had a recurrence in the para-aortic or common iliac area.

The extraperitoneal approach is considered a more difficult approach because the anatomy is not as familiar, lymphocysts or hematomas may form, and developing the retroperitoneal spaces generally is time consuming. By avoiding entering the peritoneal cavity, however, there is less risk of bowel injury by trocar insertion or traction and dissection and less hernia formation. Operating time may be decreased by avoiding any lysis of adhesions of bowel and omentum. For patients predetermined to undergo radiation therapy, postsurgical adhesions may cause more bowel injuries [19].

Dargent et al [20] conducted a retrospective review of 44 patients who underwent para-aortic lymphadenectomy via three different methods. Success rates for the transperitoneal transumbilical approach were 20% but increased to 32% and 48% for the bilateral extraperitoneal and left extraperitoneal approaches, respectively. The bilateral extraperitoneal and left extraperitoneal approaches resulted in 21.4% (3/14) and 14.3% (3/21) conversions to transperitoneal because of breach of peritoneum during dissection, respectively. Each approach yielded approximately the same number of lymph nodes (transperitoneal: 19 nodes; bilateral extraperitoneal: 16 ± 2 nodes; left extraperitoneal: 15 ± 3 nodes), but the operating time was significantly shorter for the left extraperitoneal approach (119 ± 14 minutes versus 153 ± 22 minutes bilateral extraperitoneal). By omitting the low-yield supramesenteric portion of the dissection, Vergote et al [21] were able to decrease the operating time by approximately one half (120–150 minutes to 70 minutes).

Within the previously mentioned GOG study, adequacy of para-aortic lymphadenectomy was performed by independent review of photographs taken during laparoscopy and inspection of the para-aortic regions at time of laparotomy. All 40 cases of para-aortic lymph node sampling were judged adequate. A mean of 12.1 lymph nodes was removed [9]. This study remains the only one to assess adequacy of laparoscopic pelvic and para-aortic lymphadenectomy. No study to date, however, has been conducted on the adequacy of traditional staging by laparotomy.

Although laparoscopic staging seems feasible and adequate, the question of whether it should be performed exists. In patients who undergo traditional staging, radical para-aortic lymph node dissection has not been shown to improve cure rates [22]. The ability to change treatment fields based on para-aortic disease is reasonable, however, and seems to have a favorable impact on survival. In their study of 274 cases of advanced cervical cancer, Holcomb et al [23] found that the 89 women who underwent pretreatment staging laparotomy and subsequently received extended field radiation therapy or chemotherapy based on those results had a statistically significant longer median survival (29 versus 19 months).

If bulky lymph nodes are encountered during surgical exploration, it is recommended to cease laparoscopic dissection because of the possibility of fragmentation of diseased lymph tissue, dissemination of malignant cells, or promotion of surgical complication [20]. A pathologic specimen may be obtained either by fine-needle aspiration or conversion to laparotomy. The benefit of laparoscopy in the evaluation of lymph nodes lies not only in its minimally invasive approach to obtaining actual tissue specimens but also in its ability to limit further potentially harmful treatment with the goal of local control or enrollment into clinical trials.

It is difficult to assess accurately the impact of laparoscopic pelvic lymphadenectomy on operating duration, hospital stays, and costs because it is often paired with other surgical procedures such as radical hysterectomy. Complications rates vary depending on the series and are likely related to the experience of the surgeon. In the original report by Querleu et al, only 1 of 14 patients could not complete the pelvic lymphadenectomy because of an anesthetic problem, and 1 patient suffered an intraoperative hemorrhage controlled by laparoscopy [4]. All patients except one were discharged home on the same day of surgery. The 5-year survival rate was similar to that of his own experience with laparotomy. In their larger series of 42 patients, 1 patient suffered a lateral injury to the ureter, which was stented [18]. Postoperative complications were recorded in an additional 4 patients. Of Chu et al's 28 patients to undergo para-aortic lymphadenectomy, 1 patient (3.6%) suffered an inferior vena cava injury that required conversion to laparotomy [6]. Possover et al [16] reported ten major vessel injuries in their series of 150 cases. Four of the ten injuries required a laparotomy to control the hemorrhage. For the 26 patients who underwent laparoscopic pelvic and para-aortic lymphadenectomy only, however, mean hospital stay was 3.2 days.

Sentinel node technology

In early-stage cervical cancer, researchers estimate that 10% of lymph nodes contain metastases [24]. Unfortunately, lymph node involvement is not well correlated with clinical stage. Although surgical staging would be a useful adjunct to clinical staging, a large number of patients would undergo surgery, but only a few might benefit from the findings. Although laparoscopic assessment is less invasive than laparotomy and seems adequate, methods to limit the amount of dissection have been sought. Sentinel node mapping is one such emerging technology.

First used in penile cancers in 1977 [25], sentinel node mapping has been used successfully in melanoma and breast cancer. This method involves peritumoral injection of either patent blue dye or a colloidal radioisotope to identify the primary lymph node draining that particular tissue. Application of this technology has extended to gynecologic malignancies in the staging of vulvar [26] and cervical cancers. Use of sentinel node mapping in vulvar cancer is discussed in detail later.

In an early report initially presented at the First International Congress on the Sentinel Node in Diagnosis and Treatment of Cancer in Amsterdam in 1999, Dargent et al [27] injected patent blue violet dye into 35 patients and found 59 sentinel nodes among 69 pelvic sidewall dissections. They identified 11 positive sentinel nodes and concluded that failure to identify sentinel nodes was inversely related to the amount of injected dye into the cervix. Although the negative predictive value was 100%, an additional 170 patients would need to be enrolled to have enough power to confirm those results. At that time, endoscopic probes to detect radioactivity did not exist. More than 15 series have been reported since this initial experience.

Malur et al [28] described the use of dye and radiolabeled albumin in 11 patients. Using both methods to identify sentinel nodes had a detection rate of 90%—far more than the 55% for dye only. Four patients with negative sentinel nodes had a positive pelvic lymph node. Overall, they calculated a false-negative rate of 16.6%, sensitivity of only 83.3%, and negative predictive value of 97%. Levenback et al [29] found a similar false-negative rate of 12%, sensitivity of 87.5%, and 97% negative predictive value. Of their 39 patients, 80% of the sentinel nodes were located in the iliac, obturator, and parametrial node basins. An average of 3.2 sentinel nodes was identified, with an average time lapse between isosulfan blue injection and identification of 7 minutes. Eight sentinel nodes had cancer.

For patients with early cervical disease, the finding of a positive sentinel node is an immediate indication to halt further pelvic lymph node dissection and consider para-aortic lymphadenectomy to determine if an extended field of radiation should be added to their chemoirradiation. If the sentinel node is negative, however, pelvic lymphadenectomy is indicated. In Lambaudie et al's report of 12 patients, 35 sentinel nodes were identified using a combination of patent blue dye and technetium 99m rhenium sulfur colloid injection [30]. One micrometastasis was found in a non–sentinel node on permanent section despite negative sentinel nodes by dye and radioisotope. These early experiences with sentinel node technology are encouraging. It seems that the use of dye and radiocolloid increase the sentinel lymph node detection rate. Although all patients in the series by Levenback et al [29] received a preoperative lymphoscintogram, it made no impact on decision-making.

Until the negative predictive value is near 100%, sentinel node mapping will not be an indication to halt pelvic and para-aortic lymphadenectomy. Intraoperative pathologic assessment of the sentinel node does not seem to be accurate. Barranger et al [31] reported on the inaccuracy of imprint cytology of sentinel nodes to detect metastasis. Marchiole et al [32] reported a high false-negative rate of the sentinel lymph node biopsy. Among five patients with nodal metastasis detected by multilevel sectioning and immunohistochemistry, three had negative sentinel nodes. Possible causes for false-negative results on sentinel nodes may be that lymphatic channels to lymph nodes may be blocked by more advanced cancers, which prevents the uptake of markers. It is possible that inframorphologic metastases may be present in what are negative lymph nodes by current pathologic review [33].

Further study

The GOG has embarked on several trials, such as Protocol 9207, to evaluate laparoscopic lymph node dissection with the current standard of laparotomy in patients with early-stage cervical cancer (stages IA2–IIA) with planned abdominal radical hysterectomy and pelvic lymphadenectomy. To date, 72 patients have been enrolled. Comparison between pelvic and para-aortic lymphadenectomy with newer imaging positron emission tomography and CT scans for diagnostic accuracy and the risks of surgical staging versus prophylactic extended field radiation therapy are areas for future investigation. Since its inception in 1989, many more oncologists are being trained in laparoscopic techniques. With further acceptance, studies with larger patient enrollments and long-term follow-up should become easier to perform. These studies must be conducted before laparoscopy is widely used to stage patients surgically.

Endometrial cancer

In 1987, Creasman et al [34] reported that 11% of endometrial cancer patients entered on a prospective study of surgical staging had nodal metastases. In 1988, the International Federation of Gynecologic Oncology changed the staging of endometrial cancer from one based on clinical evaluation to a surgical-based staging system. Although most oncologists would agree that the staging procedure includes pelvic washings for cytology, an extensive exploration of the abdomen and pelvis, and total hysterectomy, bilateral salpingo-oophorectomy, there is no consensus as to the indications for or degree of lymph node sampling. Currently, no randomized clinical trials have established a standard for pelvic or para-aortic lymphadenectomy. The decision regarding the indication for lymphadenectomy is left to the surgeon, who may use variables such as patient performance status, tumor grade, histology, depth of myoinvasion, and presence of lymphovascular space invasion to determine whether any or all lymph nodes will be removed.

Laparoscopic staging

In 1992, Childers and Surwit [35] were the first to describe their two cases of laparoscopic pelvic and para-aortic lymphadenectomy for endometrial cancer. The following year, they published their series of 59 patients with clinical stage I disease [36]. Fifty-two patients underwent a laparoscopic-assisted vaginal hysterectomy, of whom 29 were candidates for lymph node sampling. Although 93% of patients underwent successful staging, bilateral para-aortic lymphadenectomy was not performed in all of the cases. They found metastatic disease in 14% of patients for all grades and 36% for patients limited to grade 2 or 3 tumors. Comparing 13 patients who underwent pelvic lymph node sampling by laparoscopy to 16 patients by laparotomy, Spirtos et al [37] found similar removal rates with a median of 20 pelvic and eight para-aortic to 22 pelvic and seven para-aortic lymph nodes, respectively. Five years later, Childers team reported on an even larger series of 125 patients [38]. Over that time period, they recorded a decrease in operating time from 196 to 128 minutes, conversion to laparotomy from 8% (2/25) to none (0/100), and hospital stay from 3.2 to 1.8 days. The complication rate remained the same throughout.

Although studies have examined the feasibility and adequacy of laparoscopy in cervical cancer, fewer studies have looked at the role of laparoscopic lymphadenectomy in endometrial cancer. The surgical techniques are similar, except that there is less concern for entering the peritoneal cavity with the risk of adhesion formation because postoperative pelvic radiation therapy is less commonly used.

Only three prospective trials have compared laparoscopic-assisted surgical staging to laparotomy [39–41]. The mean number of pelvic and para-aortic lymph nodes removed by laparoscopy was 10.8 to 21.3 and 2.7 to 9.6, respectively, compared with 4.9 to 21.9 and 4.2 to 8.4 for laparotomy. In only one study was the number statistically significant, and it favored laparoscopy [40]. Two studies showed significant advantages of laparoscopy in terms of mean blood loss (145.5–229.2 mL versus 501.6–594.2 mL) [39,41] and hospitalization (2.3–2.5 days versus 5.2–5.5 days) [40,41]. The mean operating time was generally longer for laparoscopy and significantly different in one study (136.2 minutes versus 101.9 minutes) [41].

Laparoscopy has shown an advantage in terms of blood loss and hospitalizations. Some authors have suggested a better quality of life [37,42]. An average of 1 hour longer operating time is seen in retrospective and prospective studies. As a result, costs have not favored consistently either the laparoscopic or laparotomy approach. Gemignani et al [42] compared clinical outcomes and hospital charges for 320 patients and found that laparoscopy was associated with shorter hospitalizations and lower costs. With a follow-up of 12.4 months, the recurrence rate for the laparoscopic procedure was 4.5% compared with 13.9% at 24 months for laparotomy.

Major and minor complication rates are equivalent. In the original series by Childers et al [36], 3 of 29 intraoperative complications occurred, including a pneumothorax, ureter transection, and bladder cystotomy. In the three prospective studies, the major and minor complication rates for laparoscopy were 0 to 11.6% and 10.3% to 27%, respectively, compared with 2.9% to 8.8% and 12.5% to 36.4% for laparotomy [39–41].

Incompletely staged disease

Gynecologic oncologists have not formulated a standard approach to staging procedures for endometrial cancer. Most endometrial cancer cases in the United States also continue to be managed by nonspecialists in gynecologic oncology. Even in the hands of a skilled surgeon and pathologist, a diagnosis of endometrial cancer may be made in cases of benign polyps, endometrial hyperplasia, endometriosis, or adenomyosis. Poor prognostic factors, such as grade, histology, and myoinvasion, may be upgraded from frozen section analysis on final review. As a result, some patients with high-risk endometrial cancer may be incompletely staged. In these cases, the oncologist must consider whether to perform a surgical staging procedure or empirically treat the patient based on presumed risk factors.

Childers et al [43] examined this dilemma in a review of 13 incompletely staged patients who were subjected to further surgical staging by laparoscopic pelvic and para-aortic lymphadenectomy. The mean number of lymph nodes removed was 17.5, blood loss was 50 mL, and hospitalization lasted 1.5 days. No complications were incurred. Three patients (23%) had evidence of extrauterine disease spread, and four patients received further treatment based on this staging procedure.

Further study

Although many retrospective studies have continued to favor laparoscopy in terms of less blood loss, shorter hospitalizations, and similar lymph node yields and complication rates, large studies and long-term follow-up are not available. Concurrent with cervical cancer studies, the GOG has embarked on several trials to compare laparoscopy to laparotomy. The LAP-2 study is a Phase III, multi-institutional, prospective, randomized, controlled trial designed to compare staging adequacy, operating times, hospitalizations, complication rates, and costs in patients with clinical stage I or IIA disease who undergo either laparoscopic-assisted vaginal hysterectomy or total abdominal hysterectomy. More importantly, it will examine longer term data related to patient quality-of-life indices, and 5-year recurrence and survival rates. To date, 2,085 patients have been entered. Unfortunately, another GOG protocol (Protocol 9402) designed to evaluate the feasibility and adverse effects of laparoscopy in the use of incompletely staged disease within ten weeks of laparotomy was closed because of poor accrual.

Use of sentinel node technology in endometrial cancer is technically more difficult than cervical cancer because the endometrium is not accessible on speculum examination. Hysteroscopic isotope and blue dye injection has been studied for endometrial cancer [44]. In general, the use of sentinel node technology in endometrial cancer has been limited, with reported detection rates of up to 83.3% [45–47]. Endometrial cancers also can involve the endometrium focally or more extensively. The lymphatic network that drains the different anatomic portions of the uterus also varies, which limits the use of sentinel node mapping.

Ovarian cancer

Laparoscopy was first used to evaluate and remove benign adnexal masses. Before progress was made in the areas of cervical and endometrial cancer, laparoscopy was used to evaluate early stage ovarian cancers. In 1973, Bagley et al [48] reported the use of peritoneoscopy four weeks after laparotomy to evaluate diaphragmatic involvement before administering chemotherapy. In 1993, the first adequate staging of an early stage ovarian cancer was reported [49]. One year later, Querleu and LeBlanc [50] published their experience with eight patients who underwent laparoscopic staging after an initial, unsatisfactory laparotomy. All patients underwent a para-aortic lymphadenectomy to the level of the renal veins, with removal of 6 to 17 lymph nodes. The mean hospitalization was 2.8 days. In women with suspected or confirmed ovarian cancer, laparoscopy is used in three distinct roles: the evaluation of a suspicious adnexal mass, staging of apparent early-stage disease, and second-look laparoscopy to evaluate response to chemotherapy.

Evaluation of suspicious adnexal mass

Patients are often evaluated for adnexal masses, and based on physical examination, imaging characteristics, and tumor marker assays, an estimation of the likelihood of benign versus malignant disease can be made fairly accurately. Unfortunately, a comprehensive history, physical examination, imaging study (eg, transvaginal ultrasound, CT scan, MRI), and serum tests, such as CA-125, cannot discern a malignant process from a benign one with 100% accuracy. As a result, ovarian cancer may not be diagnosed until after a woman has undergone surgery to remove the mass for pathologic examination. Because of its minimally invasive approach and the development of instruments such as endobags, laparoscopy has been used to perform the initial surgical assessment. As in laparotomy, a thorough inspection of adnexa, abdomen and pelvis, peritoneal surfaces of the bowel and diaphragm, and omentum is recommended.

For masses that appear benign by imaging, the probability of encountering a malignancy is only 4 to 6 per 1000 [51]. It is estimated, however, that 1% to 15% of suspicious-appearing adnexal masses managed by laparoscopy are found to be malignant [52]. In a retrospective analysis of 819 masses that were laparoscopically managed in 757 patients, 6% were estimated to be malignant [53]. Of these masses, 41% were found to be either borderline (low malignant potential) or cancerous tumors. Although no malignant tumors were missed, almost one half (7 of 15 malignant masses) were punctured at the time of surgery. In a similar study, Canis et al [54] operated on 230 masses judged suspicious based on ultrasound findings. Sixty-two were believed to be malignant at the time of laparoscopic evaluation. Of these 62, 25 were borderline or malignant. A matter of concern was the fact that 5 of 10 borderline and 3 of 15 malignant masses were punctured during the operation.

Three malignant masses also were believed to be benign on initial frozen section analysis.

Dottino et al [55] reported on successful laparoscopic management of 141 of 160 patients with suspicious adnexal masses. Patients with masses that protruded beyond the umbilicus or gross metastases were excluded. There were eight (5%) borderline and nine (6%) malignant tumors. Four malignant tumors were staged laparoscopically. Two borderline tumor cases were converted to laparotomy because of trocar-associated injuries. Although there was no delay in adjuvant treatment, five (3%) of the frozen section analyses were falsely reported as benign.

Complication rates are similar to laparotomy. In the series by Dottino et al [55], three vascular, one small bowel, and one hemorrhage complications were incurred. In the report by Childers et al [56] regarding the management of 138 patients, three major complications were encountered, including a colon enterotomy, inferior vena cava injury, and port site herniation. Of concern in all these studies is the incidental rupture of borderline or malignant tumors, especially in early-stage disease. A rupture of a confined tumor to one ovary could be the difference between a patient being cured by surgery alone and a patient requiring adjuvant chemotherapy. In examining masses ruptured during laparotomy, Dembo et al [57] reviewed 519 patients with apparent stage I disease and found that recurrence risk seemed to correlate with grade, dense adhesions, and large volume ascites. Cyst rupture was not an independent risk factor for recurrence; however, not all patients were fully staged. Although some authors have noted no difference in survival between patients with early-stage tumors with intraoperative rupture [58], there are minimal data specific to rupture at the time of laparoscopy. Some case reports have documented recurrent tumors, but for every patient subjected to adjuvant chemotherapy solely based on intraoperative rupture, it is calculated that 110 to 140 patients could be spared a laparotomy [59]. To avoid rupture, the use of an endobag is recommended. For masses larger than 10 cm or those that adhere densely to surrounding structures or in patients who desire ovarian conservation, laparotomy is advocated [56]. Should a rupture occur, generous irrigation of the abdomen and pelvis is recommended.

Delayed staging

When a malignant tumor is encountered, the surgeon must be prepared to make a decision as to whether to proceed with a complete staging procedure either by laparotomy or laparoscopy or to stop and reschedule the procedure. Although this may not pertain to specialists trained in gynecologic oncology, most laparoscopic evaluation of adnexal masses is performed by nonspecialists. In two classic surveys of oncologists who were referred cases of incompletely staged malignant tumors, most cases were either inappropriately managed or staging was delayed by an interval that ranged from 4.8 to 6.5 weeks [60,61].

Lehner et al [62] reviewed 48 cases later staged by laparotomy after an interval of 17 days. Although 46 tumors were deemed confined to the ovary at the time of laparoscopy, 27 were upstaged to stages IIB–IV by laparotomy. Of 35 cases of malignant masses restaged by laparoscopy, LeBlanc et al [63] upstaged eight cases. Three of 34 stage IA tumors developed recurrences. Despite this discouraging trend, these results are similar to those seen for incompletely staged malignancy at the time of laparotomy [64,65]. In the case of suspicious appearing masses, it seems appropriate that a surgeon who is capable of performing a complete staging procedure either manage or be readily available at the time of operation. Patients should be counseled adequately and prepared to undergo staging procedures in the event that a malignant mass is encountered.

Port site metastases

Beyond whether laparoscopy is feasible or adequate, some concern has been raised as to whether it is even appropriate and worth pursuing. Much of this concern is attributed to reports of port site metastases. In a review of cases, a reported incidence of port site metastases was reported in 1.1% to 16% of cases. Seven cases were attributed to borderline tumors and 37 to ovarian carcinomas [52]. Kruitwagen et al [66] reviewed 43 cases of ovarian cancer debulking and found that 7 (16%) developed trocar site disease. Similarly, Marquette et al [67] found a 10% rate of metastases among 173 cases performed with open laparoscopy technique. Van Dam et al [68] reported that port site recurrence occurred but had no affect on survival. Although no studies have been performed among gynecologic cancers for laparotomy, low rates of 1-1% to 5% abdominal wall recurrences after laparotomy have been reported in two large studies of gastrointestinal tumors.

In a MEDLINE search, Wang et al [69] found a 1.1% to 13.5% risk that was highest among operations for ovarian cancers with adenocarcinoma histology, peritoneal carcinomatosis, and ascites. Port site metastases were recorded as early as 1 week to 3 years. Port site metastases are not limited to ovarian cancer; they may occur in other gynecologic malignancies, including borderline tumors and endometrial and cervical cancers. The etiologic factors responsible for port site metastases are likely multifactorial. Possible factors include the use of carbon dioxide gas, local trauma to the skin surrounding the trocar, manipulation of the tumor, biologic aggressiveness of the tumor, trocar site hematomas, and leakage of ascites. Additional factors are related to surgical expertise and technique or an individual patient's local immune suppression. Recommendations to decrease the incidence of metastases include copious irrigation of the abdomen and pelvis and trocar sites, closure of underlying peritoneum, and use of endobags to remove specimens and wound protectors. The use of gasless laparoscopy or different inflation gases, such as helium, has been proposed. To avoid the chimney effect—a rapid deflation with subsequent seeding of the trocar sites—slow deflation is advocated. In cases of contamination with tumor specimens, excision of trocar sites may be necessary. Although the significance of port site metastases on overall prognosis and long-term survival is unknown, a few retrospective studies have failed to show any survival disadvantage [66–68].

Further study

Given the magnification that laparoscopy affords, staging of ovarian carcinomas does not necessarily mandate a laparotomy. GOG Protocol 9302 evaluates the feasibility and adverse effects of laparoscopic staging for incompletely staged ovarian, fallopian tube, and primary peritoneal carcinomas performed within ten weeks of initial surgery. To date, 70 patients have been entered. Novel techniques, such as photodynamic detection, to improve identification of microscopic implants are ongoing in animal models [70]. Sentinel node technology has yet to be used for ovarian cancer because of the difficulty in identifying stage I–II disease preoperatively and the lack of access to the tumor for lymphoscintigraphic injection.

Vulvar cancer

Approximately 10% to 26% of clinically confined malignancies to the vulva have disease spread to the inguinal lymph nodes [71]. Sentinel node mapping has been used in cervical and endometrial cancers in limited applications, but its use in vulvar cancers has generated particular interest. Vulvar cancer is the gynecologic malignancy most suited to sentinel node technology because of several factors. The lesion is easily accessible on the perineum. Most vulvar lesions are squamous cell carcinomas and typically spread in a methodical fashion to the inguinal lymph nodes before involving pelvic lymph nodes and systemic organs. The sentinel nodes can be removed easily through small groin incisions. For positive lymph nodes, radiotherapy is effective at reducing recurrence and morbidity, such as wound dehiscence, and lymphedema of the lower extremity is directly related to the number of lymph nodes removed.

Sentinel node technology

Although Ramon Cabanas first described sentinel node mapping techniques for penile cancers in 1977 [25], this technology generated interest when it was applied successfully to cutaneous melanomas [72,73]. In the first series to use sentinel node technology in vulvar cancers, Levenback et al [74] was able to identify seven sentinel nodes in nine patients using isosulfan blue. Two mutually independent techniques are used for mapping, The first relies on visual detection using a blue dye, such as isosulfan blue, which is used commonly in the United States, patent blue-V, and methylene blue. The first technique is relatively simple and inexpensive. With an intradermal injection, the dye is drained to the sentinel nodes by the superficial dermal lymphatics. Transit time is a quick 10 minutes or less, but the dye remains visible for approximately 45 minutes. The second technique uses a weak radioactive radionuclide, such as technetium 99m sulfur colloid, with nanoparticles that are detected using a handheld gamma probe. Although the application is more complicated, detection with the probe is more focused and requires a smaller dissection to sample the sentinel nodes than for the blue dye technique. Moore et al reported that sentinel nodes were detected in only 37.8% of cases using isosulfan blue dye compared with 97.6% with technetium 99m [75]. Using both techniques, however, improved detection to 100%. Other authors have reported similar 100% detection rates using either lymphoscintigraphy alone [76] or with blue dye [77]. The radioactive tracers facilitate the location of the sentinel nodes to begin the dissection.

Since the original series by Levenback et al, 18 studies have been reported with more than 300 patients. Sentinel nodes were detected in 97.5% of cases and 81.8% of dissected groins [78]. Metastases involve the sentinel nodes in 13% to 41% of reported series. In approximately 58% of cases, the sentinel node is the only positive lymph node. In three studies, however, false-negative sentinel nodes were found [74,79,80]. Approximately 6.5% of sentinel nodes initially reported to be negative are found to have metastases by ultrastaging.

Ultrastaging exceeds routine pathologic hematoxylin and eosin examination by performing serial sections that then undergo immunohistochemical staining for cytokeratin or polymerase chain reaction testing. It is estimated to increase identification of positive lymph nodes by 5% to 15%. In their series of 26 patients, Puig-Tintore et al [81] identified metastases in 30.8% of sentinel nodes; however, 37.5% were diagnosed only on the basis of ultrastaging. The management of patients with sentinel nodes with metastases only diagnosed by ultrastaging has not yet been addressed.

Failure to identify sentinel nodes has been seen in women with prior excisional biopsies or in cases of complete obliteration of lymph nodes by disease or extensive local inflammation [74]. A potential error can rest on the surgeon who is inexperienced. As in laparoscopy, surgical experience increases detection rates, as seen in sentinel node mapping in breast cancer [82]. Based on these studies, sentinel node mapping has been limited to women with International Federation of Gynecologic Oncology stage I–II squamous cell cancers or early-stage melanoma, with tumors measuring less than 4 cm in diameter and not involving the urethra, anus, or vagina.

Further study

Inguinal lymphadenectomy remains the standard of care for the management of vulvar cancers stage IB or more without obvious metastases. Sentinel node technology is investigational but presents a potentially minimally invasive surgical option to women with vulvar cancer. In 15 of 18 reported series, the negative predictive value is 100%. Currently, the Groningen International Sentinel Node in Vulvar Cancer study is a non-randomized trial investigating the natural course of patients with negative sentinel nodes. Other parallel studies are being performed in melanoma and breast cancer research that may assist with decision making in gynecologic malignancies.

Summary

In a study of laparoscopic complication rates, Chi et al [83] examined their 10-year experience and graded the procedures on the basis of the degree of difficulty. The most common procedures performed for malignancy were laparoscopic-assisted vaginal hysterectomy, bilateral salpingo-oophorectomy, and second-look laparoscopy. Although the complexity was greater for malignant cases, there was no statistically significant difference in complication rates (4% versus 1%). Conversion to laparotomy was actually inversely associated with more complex procedures. The most common complications were similar to laparotomy, including wound infection and incidental enterotomy or cystotomy.

Laparoscopy has been shown to be feasible, adequate, and reliable, although long-term data on disease impact and course are lacking. It is likely that data that favor laparoscopy may be biased by patient selection factors such as age, obesity, and prior surgical histories. Most published series also have been performed by expert laparoscopists. Studies have shown that laparoscopy has a high learning curve and that a minimum number of cases is necessary to become proficient in skills necessary to manage gynecologic malignancies (eg, retroperitoneal lymphadenectomy) [84,85]. Likewise, sentinel node mapping requires significant experience to harness its less morbid benefits.

Despite the enthusiasm for this minimally invasive technology, oncologists must be mindful that it remains an investigational tool and should be performed by appropriately experienced surgeons. It is unlikely that laparoscopy or sentinel node technology will make traditional laparotomy and lymphadenectomy obsolete. Instead, they should be viewed as a welcome complement rather than competitor to traditional surgical approaches. Laparoscopy or sentinel node technology is assuming an increasingly pertinent role in the diagnosis and staging of gynecologic malignancies. With the potential to perform a complete investigation of the abdomen, pelvis, and retroperitoneum and minimize postoperative adhesions and recovery times, laparoscopy has reintroduced surgical staging as another viable tool to aid oncologists in treating women with cancer.

References

[1] Namnoum AB, Murphy AA. Diagnostic and operative laparoscopy. In: Te Linde's operative gynecology. 8th edition. Philadelphia: Lippincott-Raven; 1997. p. 389–413.

[2] Hald T, Rasmussen F. Extraperitoneal pelvioscopy: a new aid in staging of lower urinary tract tumors. A preliminary report. J Urol 1980;124(2):245–8.

[3] Dargent D, Salvat J. Valeur des methods non invasives dans l'appreciation de l'etat des ganglions ilio-pelviens et lombo-aorticques. In: Dargent D, Salvat J, editors. L'envahissement ganglionnaire pelvien. Paris: Medsi McGraw Hill; 1989. p. 55.

[4] Querleu D, LeBlanc E, Castelain B. Laparoscopic pelvic lymphadenectomy in the staging of early carcinoma of the cervix. Am J Obstet Gynecol 1991;164(2):579–81.

[5] Childers JM, Hatch K, Surwit EA. The role of laparoscopic lymphadenectomy in the management of cervical carcinoma. Gynecol Oncol 1992;47(1):38–43.

[6] Chu KK, Chang SD, Chen FP, et al. Laparoscopic surgical staging in cervical cancer–preliminary experience among Chinese. Gynecol Oncol 1997;64(1):49–53.

[7] Fowler JM, Carter JR, Carlson JW, et al. Lymph node yield from laparoscopic lymphadenectomy in cervical cancer: a comparative study. Gynecol Oncol 1993;51(2):187–92.

[8] Nijman HW, Khalifa M, Covens A. What is the number of lymph nodes required for an "adequate" pelvic lymphadenectomy? Eur J Gynaecol Oncol 2004;25(1):87–9.

[9] Schlaerth JB, Spirtos NM, Carson LF, et al. Laparoscopic retroperitoneal lymphadenectomy followed by immediate laparotomy in women with cervical cancer: a gynecologic oncology group study. Gynecol Oncol 2002;85(1):81–8.

[10] Morrow CP, Curtin JP. Tumors of the cervix. In: Synopsis of gynecologic oncology. 5th edition. New York: Churchill-Livingston; 1998. p. 107–57.

[11] Downey GO, Potish RA, Adcock LL, et al. Pretreatment surgical staging in cervical carcinoma: therapeutic efficacy of pelvic lymph node resection. Am J Obstet Gynecol 1989;160(5 Pt 1):1055–61.

[12] Rotman M, Pajak TF, Choi K, et al. Prophylactic extended-field irradiation of para-aortic lymph nodes in stages IIB and bulky IB and IIA cervical carcinomas: ten-year treatment results of RTOG 79–20. JAMA 1995;274(5):387–93.

[13] Haie C, Pejovic MH, Gerbaulet A, et al. Is prophylactic para-aortic irradiation worthwhile in the treatment of advanced cervical carcinoma? Results of a controlled clinical trial of the EORTC radiotherapy group. Radiother Oncol 1988;11(2):101–12.

[14] Benedetti-Panici P, Maneschi F, Scambia G, et al. Lymphatic spread of cervical cancer: an anatomical and pathological study based on 225 radical hysterectomies with systematic pelvic and aortic lymphadenectomy. Gynecol Oncol 1996;62(1):19–24.

[15] Spirtos NM, Schlaerth JB, Spirtos TW, et al. Laparoscopic bilateral pelvic and paraaortic lymph node sampling: an evolving technique. Am J Obstet Gynecol 1995;173(1):105–11.

[16] Possover M, Plaul K, Krause N, et al. Left-sided laparoscopic para-aortic lymphadenectomy: anatomy of the ventral tributaries of the infrarenal vena cava. Am J Obstet Gynecol 1998;179(5):1295–7.

[17] Vasilev SA, McGonigle KF. Extraperitoneal laparoscopic para-aortic lymph node dissection. Gynecol Oncol 1996;61(3):315–20.

[18] Querleu D, Dargent D, Ansquer Y, et al. Extraperitoneal endosurgical aortic and common iliac dissection in the staging of bulky or advanced cervical carcinomas. Cancer 2000;88(8):1883–91.

[19] Downey GO, Potish RA, Adcock LL, et al. Pretreatment surgical staging in cervical carcinoma: therapeutic efficacy of pelvic lymph node resection. Am J Obstet Gynecol 1989; 160(5 Pt 1):1055–61.
[20] Dargent D, Ansquer Y, Mathevet P. Technical development and results of left extraperitoneal laparoscopic paraaortic lymphadenectomy for cervical cancer. Gynecol Oncol 2000;77(1):87–92.
[21] Vergote I, Amant F, Berteloot P, et al. Laparoscopic lower para-aortic staging lymphadenectomy in stage IB2, II, and III cervical cancer. Int J Gynecol Cancer 2002; 12(1):22–6.
[22] Panici PB, Scambia G, Baiocchi G, et al. Technique and feasibility of radical para-aortic and pelvic lymphadenectomy for gynecologic malignancies. J Gynecol Cancer 1991;1:133–40.
[23] Holcomb K, Abulafia O, Matthews RP, et al. The impact of pretreatment staging laparotomy on survival in locally advanced cervical carcinoma. Eur J Gynaecol Oncol 1999; 20(2):90–3.
[24] Noguchi H, Shiozawa I, Sakai Y, et al. Pelvic lymph node metastasis of uterine cervical cancer. Gynecol Oncol 1987;27(2):150–8.
[25] Cabanas RM. An approach for the treatment of penile carcinoma. Cancer 1977;39(2): 456–66.
[26] Levenback C, Coleman RL, Burke TW, et al. Intraoperative lymphatic mapping and sentinel node identification with blue dye in patients with vulvar cancer. Gynecol Oncol 2001;83(2): 276–81.
[27] Dargent D, Martin X, Mathevet P. Laparoscopic assessment of the sentinel lymph node in early stage cervical cancer. Gynecol Oncol 2000;79(3):411–5.
[28] Malur S, Krause N, Kohler C, et al. Sentinel lymph node detection in patients with cervical cancer. Gynecol Oncol 2001;80(2):254–7.
[29] Levenback C, Coleman RL, Burke TW, et al. Lymphatic mapping and sentinel node identification in patients with cervix cancer undergoing radical hysterectomy and pelvic lymphadenectomy. J Clin Oncol 2002;20(3):688–93.
[30] Lambaudie E, Collinet P, Narducci F, et al. Laparoscopic identification of sentinel lymph nodes in early stage cervical cancer: prospective study using a combination of patent blue dye injection and technetium radiocolloid injection. Gynecol Oncol 2003;89(1):84–7.
[31] Barranger E, Cortez A, Uzan S, Callard P, Darai E. Value of intraoperative imprint cytology of sentinel nodes in patients with cervical cancer. Gynecol Oncol 2004;94(1):175–80.
[32] Marchiole P, Beunerd A, Scoazec JY, et al. Sentinal lymph node biopsy is not accurate in predicting lymph status for patients with cervical carcinoma. Cancer 2004;100(10): 2154–9.
[33] Van Trappen PO, Gyselman VG, Lowe DG, et al. Molecular quantification and mapping of lymph-node micrometastases in cervical cancer. Lancet 2001;357(9249):15–20.
[34] Creasman WT, Morrow CP, Bundy BN, et al. Surgical pathologic spread patterns of endometrial cancer: a Gynecologic Oncology Group study. Cancer 1987;60(8Suppl): 2035–41.
[35] Childers JM, Surwit EA. Combined laparoscopic and vaginal surgery for the management of two cases of stage I endometrial cancer. Gynecol Oncol 1992;45(1):46–51.
[36] Childers JM, Brzechffa PR, Hatch KD, et al. Laparoscopically assisted surgical staging (LASS) of endometrial cancer. Gynecol Oncol 1993;51(1):33–8.
[37] Spirtos NM, Schlaerth JB, Gross GM, et al. Cost and quality-of-life analyses of surgery for early endometrial cancer: laparotomy versus laparoscopy. Am J Obstet Gynecol 1996; 174(6):1795–9; discussion 1799–800.
[38] Melendez TD, Childers JM, Nour M, et al. Laparoscopic staging of endometrial cancer: the learning experience. Journal of the Society of Laparoendoscopic Surgeons 1997;1(1):45–9.
[39] Malur S, Possover M, Michels W, et al. Laparoscopic-assisted vaginal versus abdominal surgery in patients with endometrial cancer: a prospective randomized trial. Gynecol Oncol 2001;80(2):239–44.

[40] Eltabbakh GH, Shamonki MI, Moody JM, et al. Laparoscopy as the primary modality for the treatment of women with endometrial carcinoma. Cancer 2001;91(2):378–87.
[41] Fram KM. Laparoscopically assisted vaginal hysterectomy versus abdominal hysterectomy in stage I endometrial cancer. Int J Gynecol Cancer 2002;12(1):57–61.
[42] Gemignani ML, Curtin JP, Zelmanovich J, et al. Laparoscopic-assisted vaginal hysterectomy for endometrial cancer: clinical outcomes and hospital charges. Gynecol Oncol 1999; 73(1):5–11.
[43] Childers JM, Spirtos NM, Brainard P, et al. Laparoscopic staging of the patient with incompletely staged early adenocarcinoma of the endometrium. Obstet Gynecol 1994;83(4): 597–600.
[44] Raspagliesi F, Ditto A, Kusamura S, et al. Hysteroscopic injection of tracers in sentinel node detection of endometrial cancer: a feasibility study. Am J Obstet Gynecol 2004;191(2):435–9.
[45] Burke TW, Levenback C, Tornos C, et al. Intraabdominal lymphatic mapping to direct selective pelvic and paraaortic lymphadenectomy in women with high-risk endometrial cancer: results of a pilot study. Gynecol Oncol 1996;62:169–73.
[46] Pelosi E, Arena V, Baudino B, et al. Preliminary study of sentinel node identification with 99mTc colloid and blue dye in patients with endometrial cancer. Tumori 2002;88:S9–10.
[47] Holub Z, Jabor A, Kliment L. Comparison of two procedures for sentinel lymph node detection in patients with endometrial cancer: a pilot study. Eur J Gynaecol Oncol 2002;23: 53–7.
[48] Bagley CM Jr, Young RC, Schein PS, et al. Ovarian carcinoma metastatic to the diaphragm–frequently undiagnosed at laparotomy: a preliminary report. Am J Obstet Gynecol 1973; 116(3):397–400.
[49] Querleu D. Laparoscopic paraaortic node sampling in gynecologic oncology: a preliminary experience. Gynecol Oncol 1993;49(1):24–9.
[50] Querleu D, LeBlanc E. Laparoscopic infrarenal paraaortic lymph node dissection for restaging of carcinoma of the ovary or fallopian tube. Cancer 1994;73(5):1467–71.
[51] Nezhat F, Nezhat C, Welander CE, et al. Four ovarian cancers diagnosed during laparoscopic management of 1011 women with adnexal masses. Am J Obstet Gynecol 1992; 167(3):790–6.
[52] Manolitsas TP, Fowler JM. Role of laparoscopy in the management of the adnexal mass and staging of gynecologic cancers. Clin Obstet Gynecol 2001;44(3):495–521.
[53] Canis M, Mage G, Pouly JL, et al. Laparoscopic diagnosis of adnexal cystic masses: a 12-year experience with long-term follow-up. Obstet Gynecol 1994;83(5 Pt 1):707–12.
[54] Canis M, Pouly JL, Wattiez A, et al. Laparoscopic management of adnexal masses suspicious at ultrasound. Obstet Gynecol 1997;89(5 Pt 1):679–83.
[55] Dottino PR, Levine DA, Ripley DL, et al. Laparoscopic management of adnexal masses in premenopausal and postmenopausal women. Obstet Gynecol 1999;93(2):223–8.
[56] Childers JM, Nasseri A, Surwit EA. Laparoscopic management of suspicious adnexal masses. Am J Obstet Gynecol 1996;175(6):1451–7; discussion 1457–9.
[57] Dembo AJ, Davy M, Stenwig AE, et al. Prognostic factors in patients with stage I epithelial ovarian cancer. Obstet Gynecol 1990;75(2):263–73.
[58] Sjovall K, Nilsson B, Einhorn N. Different types of rupture of the tumor capsule and the impact on survival in early ovarian carcinoma. Int J Gynecol Cancer 1994;4(5):333–6.
[59] Kadar N. Laparoscopic management of gynecological malignancies. Curr Opin Obstet Gynecol 1997;9(4):247–55.
[60] Maiman M, Seltzer V, Boyce J. Laparoscopic excision of ovarian neoplasms subsequently found to be malignant. Obstet Gynecol 1991;77(4):563–5.
[61] Crawford RA, Gore ME, Shepherd JH. Ovarian cancers related to minimal access surgery. Br J Obstet Gynaecol 1995;102(9):726–30.
[62] Lehner R, Wenzl R, Heinzl H, et al. Influence of delayed staging laparotomy after laparoscopic removal of ovarian masses later found malignant. Obstet Gynecol 1998;92(6): 967–71.

[63] LeBlanc E, Querleu D, Narducci F, et al. Laparoscopic restaging of early stage invasive adnexal tumors: a 10-year experience. Gynecol Oncol 2004;94(3):624–9.
[64] Young RC, Decker DG, Wharton JT, et al. Staging laparotomy in early ovarian cancer. JAMA 1983;250(22):3072–6.
[65] Averette HE, Hoskins W, Nguyen HN, et al. National survey of ovarian carcinoma: I. A patient care evaluation study of the American College of Surgeons. Cancer 1993;71(4 Suppl): 1629–38.
[66] Kruitwagen RF, Swinkels BM, Keyser KG, et al. Incidence and effect on survival of abdominal wall metastases at trocar or puncture sites following laparoscopy or paracentesis in women with ovarian cancer. Gynecol Oncol 1996;60(2):233–7.
[67] Marquette S, Amant F, Berteloot P, et al. Portsite metastases are frequent after open laparoscopy in patients with advanced ovarian carcinoma, but do not influence the survival: an analysis of 173 cases [abstract]. Int J Gynecol Cancer 2003;13:2.
[68] van Dam PA, DeCloedt J, Tjalma WA, et al. Trocar implantation metastasis after laparoscopy in patients with advanced ovarian cancer: can the risk be reduced? Am J Obstet Gynecol 1999;181(3):536–41.
[69] Wang PH, Yuan CC, Lin G, et al. Risk factors contributing to early occurrence of port site metastases of laparoscopic surgery for malignancy. Gynecol Oncol 1999;72(1): 38–44.
[70] Chan JK, Monk BJ, Cuccia D, et al. Laparoscopic photodynamic diagnosis of ovarian cancer using 5-aminolevulinic acid in a rat model. Gynecol Oncol 2002;87(1): 64–70.
[71] van der Velden J, Hacker NF. Prognostic factors in squamous cell cancer of the vulva and the implications for treatment. Curr Opin Obstet Gynecol 1996;8(1):3–7.
[72] Morton DL, Wen DR, Wong JH, et al. Technical details of intraoperative lymphatic mapping for early stage melanoma. Arch Surg 1992;127:392–9.
[73] Alex JC, Weaver DL, Fairbank JT, et al. Gamma-probe-guided lymph node localization in malignant melanoma. Surg Oncol 1993;2:303–8.
[74] Levenback C, Coleman RL, Burke TW, et al. Intraoperative lymphatic mapping and sentinel node identification with blue dye in patients with vulvar cancer. Gynecol Oncol 2001;83(2): 276–81.
[75] Moore RG, DePasquale SE, Steinhoff MM, et al. Sentinel node identification and the ability to detect metastatic tumor to inguinal lymph nodes in squamous cell cancer of the vulva. Gynecol Oncol 2003;89:475–9.
[76] De Cicco C, Sideri M, Bartolomei M, et al. Sentinel node biopsy in early vulvar cancer. Br J Cancer 2000;82:295–9.
[77] De Hullu JA, Hollema H, Piers DA, et al. Sentinel lymph node procedure is highly accurate in squamous cell carcinoma of the vulva. J Clin Oncol 2000;18:2811–6.
[78] Torne A, Puig-Tintore LM. The use of sentinel lymph nodes in gynaecological malignancies. Curr Opin Obstet Gynecol 2004;16(1):57–64.
[79] Ansink AC, Sie-Go DM, van der Velden J, et al. Identification of sentinel lymph nodes in vulvar carcinoma patients with the aid of a patent blue V injection: a multicenter study. Cancer 1999;86:652–6.
[80] Boran N, Kayikcioglu F, Kir M. Sentinel lymph node procedure in early vulvar cancer [letter]. Gynecol Oncol 2003;90:492–3.
[81] Puig-Tintore LM, Ordi J, Vidal-Sicart S, et al. Further data on the usefulness of sentinel lymph node identification and ultrastaging in vulvar squamous cell carcinoma. Gynecol Oncol 2003;88(1):29–34.
[82] Sanidas EE, de Bree E, Tsiftsis DD. How many cases are enough for accreditation in sentinel lymph node biopsy in breast cancer [review]? Am J Surg 2003;185:202–10.
[83] Chi DS, Abu-Rustum NR, Sonoda Y, et al. Ten-year experience with laparoscopy on a gynecologic oncology service: analysis of risk factors for complications and conversion to laparotomy. Am J Obstet Gynecol 2004;191(4):1138–45.

[84] Querleu D, Lanvin D, Elhage A, et al. An objective experimental assessment of the learning curve for laparoscopic surgery: the example of pelvic and para-aortic lymph node dissection. Eur J Obstet Gynecol Reprod Biol 1998;81(1):55–8.
[85] Occelli B, Narducci F, Lanvin D, et al. Learning curves for transperitoneal laparoscopic and extraperitoneal endoscopic paraaortic lymphadenectomy. J Am Assoc Gynecol Laparosc 2000;7(1):51–3.

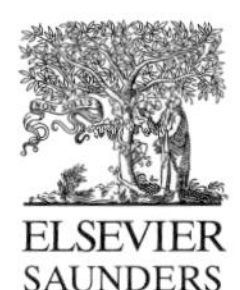
ELSEVIER
SAUNDERS

Surg Oncol Clin N Am
14 (2005) 289–300

SURGICAL
ONCOLOGY CLINICS
OF NORTH AMERICA

Pelvic Exenteration of Gynecologic Malignancy: Indications, and Technical and Reconstructive Considerations

Nicholas C. Lambrou, MD*, J. Matt Pearson, MD, Hervy E. Averette, MD

Department of Obstetrics and Gynecology, Division of Gynecologic Oncology, Jackson Memorial Hospital, Sylvester Comprehensive Cancer Center, University of Miami, 1475 NW 12th Avenue, Suite 33101, Miami, FL 33136, USA

Aside from radical hysterectomy, perhaps the single most defining surgical procedure for the practicing gynecologic oncologist is pelvic exenteration. The surgical skill and anatomic knowledge required to complete this radical procedure safely and successfully are a tribute to the teachings of our predecessors throughout the evolution of the subspecialty of gynecologic oncology. Through this teaching, we have improved the selection of candidates for exenteration and our ability to tailor the surgery for each candidate to provide the least morbid procedure without compromising the chance for cure. The availability of modern antibiotics, surgical intensive care units, and improvements in surgical reconstruction have decreased morbidity in patients undergoing pelvic exenteration and may improve overall survival in these patients [1–6].

Pelvic exenteration was developed by Dr. Alexander Brunschwig in the 1940s, primarily for palliative treatment of large pelvic cancers [7]. At that time, perioperative mortality was high and the patient selection was limited. Currently, potential candidates include women with cervical cancer, endometrial cancer, and ovarian cancer and other rarer pelvic neoplasms. In general, for patients who undergo pelvic exenteration for treatment of a gynecologic malignancy, the disease-free survival rate at 5 years approaches 50% [1,3,4,8]. Most of these patients are treated for central pelvic recurrence of cancer of the uterine cervix. Although data are limited, recent reports have demonstrated that adequate long-term survival can be achieved in

* Corresponding author.
E-mail address: nlambrou@med.miami.edu (N.C. Lambrou).

1055-3207/05/$ - see front matter
doi:10.1016/j.soc.2004.11.011

highly selected patients with recurrent endometrial cancer [1,3]. For patients with ovarian cancer, pelvic exenteration may be indicated to achieve optimal surgical debulking and improve the chances for long-term remission [9,10]. Finally, pelvic exenteration still may be considered in carefully selected patients for palliative purposes.

Postoperative management of patients after exenteration can be challenging and requires acute awareness of the potential complications that may arise as the patient recovers from the procedure. The psychological implications of disfiguring surgery, external appliances, and reconstructive surgery should be explored thoroughly with each patient before surgery; identifying adequate social and family support is of paramount importance. Carefully identifying the appropriate candidate for pelvic exenteration requires knowledge, not only of who will most likely benefit from the procedure but also who will best be able to endure the physical and emotional challenges throughout the recovery period and beyond. In this article, which is based on published data and our own experiences at the University of Miami and Jackson Memorial Hospital, we discuss patient selection and preoperative evaluation of candidates for pelvic exenteration, discuss the surgical techniques involved in performing the procedure, and describe management considerations in the postoperative setting.

Indications and preoperative evaluation

Cervical cancer

The indication for performing pelvic exenteration with curative intent in the setting of recurrent cancer remains specific to patients who have a histologically confirmed recurrence in the central pelvis after previous radiation therapy. Spread to the pelvic sidewall and metastatic disease are contraindications. As a general rule, unilateral obstructive uropathy, unilateral leg edema, and sciatic leg pain suggest pelvic sidewall disease that is unresectable. That said, it is often difficult on physical examination to differentiate between tumor extent and radiation fibrosis. Preoperative assessment with pelvic MRI may be helpful in evaluating the extent of recurrent tumor within the pelvis and predicting the likelihood of surgical resection. Whenever in doubt, however, the ultimate determination of tumor resection must be made in the operating theater.

Preoperatively, metastases outside of the pelvis should be ruled out using CT of the chest, pelvis, and abdomen. Recent interest in Flourodeoxyglucose (FDG) positron emission tomography has produced several compelling retrospective studies regarding its use in detecting metastatic disease in the setting of recurrent cervical cancer. In a review of 28 patients who underwent whole-body FDG positron emission tomography to evaluate for suspected recurrence, Havrilesky et al [11] demonstrated a sensitivity of 85.7% and specificity of 86.7% when correlated with histologic confirmation of disease. Unger et al [12] reviewed the charts of 44 patients who underwent FGD positron emission tomography to evaluate for recurrence. Sixty-seven percent of patients were symptomatic. They found that when correlated with either histologic confirmation or progression identified by serial CT scan, the sensitivity and specificity for detection of recurrence were 100% and 85.7%, respectively, in this group and 80% and 100%, respectively, in the asymptomatic patients. Any suspicious findings, such as hepatic lesions, enlarged lymph nodes, or pulmonary nodules, should be assessed with fine-needle aspiration or biopsy to exclude the presence of metastases before proceeding with exenteration.

Endometrial cancer

Barber and Brunschwig [13] were the first to report on the treatment of recurrent endometrial cancer with pelvic exenteration. In their series of 36 patients between 1947 and 1963, the absolute 5-year survival rate was 14%. Only 5 of the 36 patients, however, had localized disease. More recently, Morris et al [3] reported on 20 patients who underwent pelvic exenteration with curative intent for recurrent endometrial cancer. The study was a retrospective review of data from four institutions. All of the patients received pelvic irradiation before exenteration either as part of their primary treatment or after initial recurrence. For this group, the 5-year disease-free survival rate was 45%. Of 8 patients who had known recurrences, the median time to recurrence was 17 months.

Ovarian cancer

Modified posterior exenteration as described by Eisenkop et al [9] has been performed by some surgeons in an effort to achieve optimal primary cytoreduction of ovarian cancer that extensively involves the pelvic viscera [10]. At the University of Miami, Mirhashemi et al [14] published our experience on supralevator posterior exenteration in primary cytoreduction for extensive ovarian carcinoma in the pelvis and severe endometriosis with complete obliteration of the cul de sac. Our preference is to perform colorectal anastomosis to preserve bowel continuity and function in such cases. Angioli et al [15] found that in the nonirradiated pelvis, only 1 of 36 patients experienced anastomotic breakdown, and that patient was the only one in whom protective colostomy had been performed. Twenty-seven of these exenterations were performed for ovarian carcinoma, none of which had anastomotic failures.

Preoperative assessment

If results of the preoperative evaluation are negative, the patient should be counseled on the risks and benefits of undergoing this surgical procedure. The magnitude of physiologic stress and surgical risk associated with the surgery may be prohibitive for patients with major medical problems. The value of strong family or social support cannot be emphasized enough. The patient and her family must understand and accept all possible consequences of the surgery and be prepared for a prolonged hospitalization and home rehabilitation. At the University of Miami, we routinely arrange preoperative consultations for the patient and her family with our specialized team of social workers and ostomy nurses. They help educate the patient on the management of a colostomy and urinary diversion. Preoperative consultation with the psychology-oncology service is provided. It is important to consider the potential psychological and emotional impact of exenterative surgery and the physical changes that reconstructive procedures incur.

Surgical exploration

The first step in pelvic exenteration is the exploratory laparotomy. The pelvis and abdomen are thoroughly evaluated for evidence of disseminated disease. The presence of metastatic implants to the small or large bowel is a contraindication to the procedure. Direct involvement of small or large bowel that adheres in the pelvis may not represent systemic disease, however, and is not considered a contraindication for pelvic exenteration. At our institution, approximately 40% to 50% of exploratory laparotomies for exenterations were abandoned because of extrapelvic disease [2,4].

We routinely perform a pelvic lymphadenectomy as part of the initial surgical exploration. The presence of grossly positive pelvic lymph nodes is considered a contraindication to proceeding with exenteration. Long-term survival can be achieved in patients with microscopic positive pelvic lymph nodes, however [1]. When possible, we routinely perform a lymph node sampling from the lower para-aortic chain with a frozen section evaluation as part of the exploratory procedure. When para-aortic lymph nodes test positive for metastatic disease, it reflects systemic disease, and pelvic exenteration for curative purposes is abandoned.

The retroperitoneal spaces are then explored beginning with the pararectal and paravesical spaces to confirm the absence of sidewall involvement. For total pelvic exenterations, the space of Retzius and presacral and retrorectal spaces are dissected to ensure that complete resection of the pelvic tumor can be achieved. After dissection of the retroperitoneal spaces to confirm the absence of direct tumor extension to either of the bony boundaries, including the sidewall, sacrum, or pubis, the surgeon is ready to proceed with resection of pelvic organs.

Resection of pelvic organs

Although initially pelvic exenteration was synonymous with surgical removal of all pelvic organs, including bladder, uterus, cervix, vagina, rectosigmoid colon, and possibly the vulva in an en bloc specimen, a more complete description includes subdivision into an anterior and posterior component and an infralevator and supralevator component (Table 1) [16].

When disease is limited to the anterior lower genital tract, an anterior approach may be warranted, which spares the rectosigmoid colon and posterior vagina. Similarly, when disease is limited to the posterior lower genital tract, a posterior resection may be performed, which spares the bladder from resection. When performed with curative intent, it is of paramount importance to achieve negative surgical margins. Any tumor transection or incomplete tumor resection results in prompt recurrence and death. Although anterior and posterior exenterations are beneficial in sparing either the rectosigmoid colon or the bladder, complete excision of the tumor must be ensured.

It is also important to differentiate between infralevator and supralevator pelvic exenteration [16]. The supralevator pelvic exenteration includes removal of the bladder, upper vagina, cervix, uterus, and rectosigmoid colon while preserving the pelvic floor. When disease involves the lower part of the vagina, vulva, perineum, or anus, an infralevator pelvic exenteration must be performed with removal of pelvic floor muscles. Infralevator exenterations leave a large pelvic defect (Fig. 1), and reconstruction with myocutaneous flaps, omental flap, or dura mater has been described and is recommended [17–20].

The ureters are mobilized as far into the pelvis as possible and are transected at least 2 cm from the tumor. Care is taken to preserve the vascularized adventitia surrounding the ureters during mobilization. The rectosigmoid colon is mobilized and transected using standard stapling techniques. After the tumor has been mobilized circumferentially, attention is turned to the lateral dissection down to the levator muscles. This resection can be performed using GIA stapling device or large curved Heaney clamps and using other similar techniques. If an infralevator exenteration is required, the perineal phase is started at this point. If a supralevator exenteration is sufficient to excise the tumor adequately, then attention is turned to transection of the vagina and rectosigmoid colon individually using a roticulating thoracoabdominal (TA) stapling instrument.

The perineal phase of the procedure begins by marking the area on the vulva to be excised. If the tumor involves the vagina but does not involve the

Table 1
Classification of pelvic exenteration

Group	Type
Anterior	Supralevator
Posterior	Infralevator
Total	With vulvectomy

Adapted from Magrina JF, Stanhope CR, Weaver AL. Pelvic exenterations: supralevator, infralevator, and with vulvectomy. Gynecol Oncol 1997;64:131; with permission.

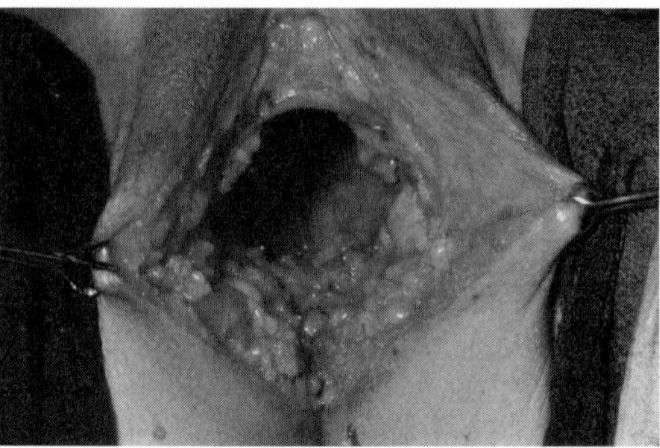

Fig. 1. Pelvic floor defect after total infralevator pelvic exenteration. (Courtesy of M. Penalver, MD, Miami, FL.)

introitus, a total vaginectomy and urethrectomy is performed and the vulva is spared. The skin is incised with a scalpel and carried down into the subcutaneous tissue with bovie electrocautery. Care must be taken to direct the incision medially toward the pubic bones until it reaches the pelvic floor. A tunnel is made in the pelvic floor to communicate with the paravaginal and pararectal spaces created from above. A combination of serial Heaney clamps along with sharp and blunt dissection may be used to ensure hemostatic detachment of paravaginal and perirectal attachments. The urethral meatus is dissected down from the pubic aponeurosis and the space is developed to connect with the paravaginal tunnels. Once the vagina and rectum are free from their surrounding attachments to the pelvic floor, the entire specimen is ready for removal through the perineal defect (Fig. 1).

Surgical reconstruction

As described by Sevin and Koechli [21], the reconstructive phase of pelvic exenteration includes four parts: (1) construction of a urinary diversion, (2) colostomy or low coloanal anastamosis, (3) pelvic floor reconstruction, and (4) vaginal reconstruction.

In general when choosing a urinary diversion, a choice is made between a conduit (noncontinent urinary diversion), which is faster and carries a smaller risk for complications, or a reservoir (continent urinary diversion), which is technically more challenging and is associated with more frequent complications but offers the benefit of urinary continence. Since 1988 at the University of Miami, we have used the continent ileocolonic reservoir—the Miami pouch—as the preferred method of continent urinary diversion [5] (Fig. 2). The Miami pouch offers an acceptable complication rate generally managed by conservative and noninvasive measures with a reliable continent urinary mechanism [22,23]. When the ileum is not available for

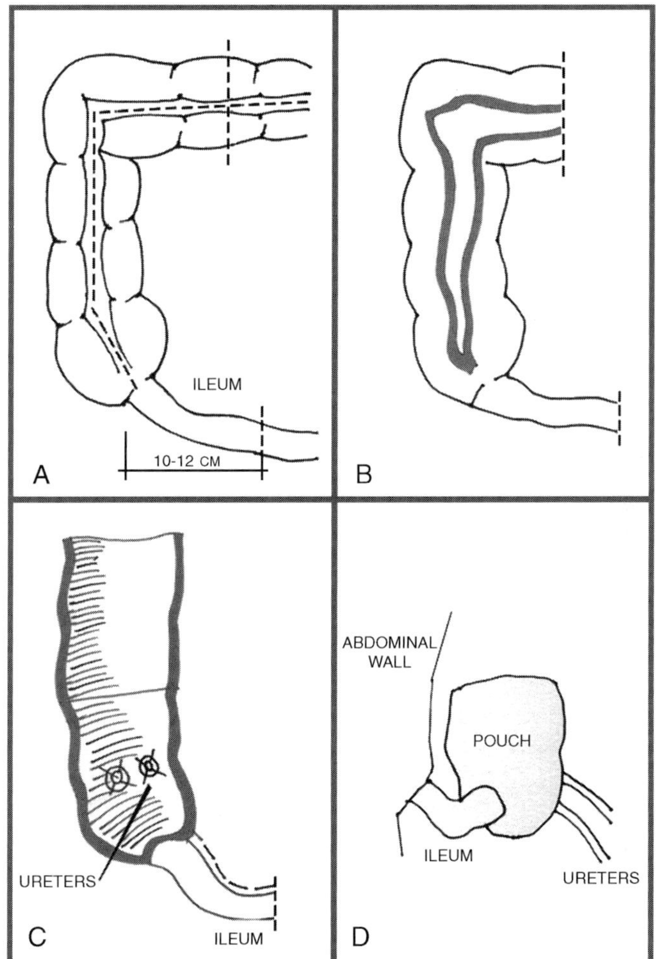

Fig. 2. Ileocolic continent urinary diversion with Miami Pouch technique. (*A*) Transection of distal ileum and transverse colon, followed by ileocolonic anastomosis. (*B*) Detubularization of the colon segment by incising with electrocautery along taenia libera. (*C*) Plication of ileum and insertion of ureters into posterior wall of reservoir. (*D*) Closure of pouch. Ileum is pulled through abdominal wall to create stoma.

reconstructive use because of severe radiation effects, the transverse colon is the preferred segment of bowel for the creation of a urinary conduit [24].

End colostomy is currently the standard procedure in patients who undergo total pelvic exenterations or posterior exenterations. Recent attempts have been made to perform a low rectal anastomosis in patients who have undergone a supralevator exenteration, however [14,15]. The rectal anastomosis is performed using standard circular stapling techniques, and an omental pedicle flap should be placed around the anastomosis when available.

Because of the high risk of fistula formation in patients with previous pelvic irradiation, a protective colostomy or ileostomy always should be performed and kept in place for approximately 3 months. Low rectal anastomosis is not an option for patients who undergo infralevator exenterations, because the distal rectum and anus are removed with the specimen.

Pelvic floor reconstruction or the creation of a neovagina should be contemplated in all patients who undergo exenteration. Neovaginas offer the potential for improving a patient's quality of life and decreasing surgical morbidity by filling the large pelvic defect with well-vascularized tissue. Several options are available for pelvic reconstruction. Miller et al [25] demonstrated a reduction in the incidence of intestinal fistula formation from 16% to less than 5% in patients who had an omental pedicle graft or a gracilis myocutaneous flap at the time of exenteration. Jurado et al [18] reported their results from a series of 16 patients who underwent vaginal reconstruction with a rectus abdominis myocutaneous flap, gracilis flap, or Singapore fasciocutaneous flap and demonstrated a significant reduction in postoperative pelvic abscess compared with patients who had no vaginal reconstruction. Other types of vaginal reconstruction include various uses of colon, skin grafts, and local flaps. More recent data are emerging on the use of rectus flaps [20,26]. Our preference at the University of Miami is to perform vaginal reconstruction with a rectus abdominis myocutaneous flap. The creation of a neovagina requires approximately 2 to 3 hours of additional operative time, a surgical team with the technical knowledge and experience to perform the reconstruction, and meticulous attention to postoperative care. Not all patients are good candidates for vaginal reconstruction, however.

Because of the large pelvic defect after an infralevator exenteration, the major risk has been the prolapse of pelvic organs, such as small bowel, and bowel fistulas. In these cases and especially when vaginal reconstruction is not an option, dura mater may be used to reconstruct the pelvic floor [27]. It is advisable to drape an omental pedicle flap over the dura and denuded area in the pelvis when an omental flap is possible and to place close-suctioned drains intraoperatively above and below the reconstructed pelvic floor.

Postoperative management

The postoperative management of exenteration patients begins in almost all cases in the surgical intensive care unit. This setting is optimal for monitoring the fluid shifts that occur postoperatively. Electrolytes and hematocrit should be checked, and replacement should be made when abnormalities are found. At our institution we maintain the hematocrit above 30%. Patients usually stay in the intensive care unit for 1 to 2 days, after which time they are transferred to the in-patient ward. The Miami pouch and stents are flushed at regular intervals (60 mL of normal saline every 8 hours) to ensure patency and adequate drainage. Broad-spectrum antibiotics are continued empirically until postoperative day 3 or 5, although this depends on the surgeon's preference. Anticoagulation for deep venous thrombosis prophylaxis is continued until patients are fully ambulatory. Nasogastric suctioning and dietary management are performed in the same manner as for patients with small bowel resection. Careful monitoring continues for approximately 14 days, at which time a CT scan or intravenous pyelogram is performed to check for leakage from the Miami pouch. The Foley catheter and ureteral stents are removed at bedside if there is no evidence of leakage on the imaging study. Ostomy education and psychological counseling occur throughout the postoperative stay, and appointments are made for continued follow-up before discharge from the hospital.

Complications

The types of complications encountered after pelvic exenteration depend largely on the specific procedures performed during the operation. Usual complications include fever, wound infection, ileus or small bowel obstruction, fistula formation, thromboembolic events, and pelvic or abdominal abscess. Anterior exenteration with reconstruction of the urinary tract by means of ileal conduit or ileocolonic reservoir increases the risk for urinary tract infection, ureteral stricture, stone formation, and urinary incontinence. Rectovaginal fistula and anastomotic leaks may occur after posterior exenteration with low colorectal anastomosis, especially in a previously irradiated pelvis. Significant reduction in rectovaginal fistula after low colorectal anastomosis in irradiated patients can be achieved with protective colostomy or ileostomy [23].

Salom et al [23] reviewed the University of Miami experience of continent ileocolonic reservoir (Miami pouch) over a period of 15 years. Seventy-one of the 90 patients presented had undergone total pelvic exenteration, and of these patients, 91% had a history of previous pelvic irradiation. The overall complication rate directly related to the Miami pouch was 53%. Complications were divided into early, which occurred within 60 days of surgery, and late, which occurred after 60 postoperative days. The most common early and late complication associated with the Miami pouch was urinary tract infection, 40% and 42%, respectively. Other early complications included pouch leak, ureteral stricture, difficult catheterization, and incontinence. Late complications included ureteral stricture, incontinence, pouch fistula, difficult catheterization, and urinary stone formation. Eighty percent of the complications encountered were managed successfully with nonsurgical conservative therapy.

Palliation

Pelvic exenteration for recurrent cancer should be performed with curative intent in most cases. Because of advances in the noninvasive or minimally invasive management of genitourinary and gastrointestinal consequences of recurrent disease, the use of pelvic exenteration as a palliative measure has been reduced. Specific groups of patients for whom palliative exenteration may be indicated still remain, however.

One such group includes patients with advanced pelvic disease with extensive fistula caused by tumor involvement of the bladder or rectum, in whom radiation is not initially safe or feasible. Urinary diversion or fecal diversion would be indicated initially. This might be followed by radiation or primary exenteration. There are also patients in whom pelvic irradiation has resulted in severe chronic hemorrhagic radiation cystitis, proctitis, or extensive fistulas. If attempts at conservative and minimally invasive management fail, these patients are candidates for anterior or posterior exenteration as palliation for their symptoms.

A final subset of patients includes those whose quality of life is so poor secondary to frank tumor extruding from the vagina, extensive necrosis of pelvic viscera, or unbearable malodorous discharge and unmanageable hygiene. For these patients, pelvic exenteration may be the only option for palliation for their symptoms. In a report by Magrina et al [16], palliative exenterations did not have an increase in perioperative complications; as expected, however, survival was lower than in patients who underwent exenteration for cure. Stanhope and Symmonds [28] retrospectively reviewed 59 patients at the Mayo Clinic who underwent pelvic exenteration for palliation between 1955 and 1981. They demonstrated a 46% 2-year survival rate and 23% 5-year survival rate with pelvic nodal involvement. Median survival for the total group was 19 months, with 47% surviving more than 2 years and 17% surviving more than 5 years.

Summary

Pelvic exenteration, whether for palliation or resection of primary or recurrent gynecologic cancer, is reserved for a highly specific group of patients. When performed appropriately, it may offer a marked improvement in survival and quality of life for these women. The variations in exenterative procedures discussed can offer tailored excision of disease while preserving selected organs and their function to minimize changes in lifestyle. Resection of the pelvic viscera and reconstruction of functional urinary and intestinal diversions can be technically challenging for surgeons and physically and emotionally demanding for patients. Appropriate patient selection and novel techniques have reduced complications and patient morbidity and improved quality of life for these patients.

References

[1] Barakat RB, Goldman NA, Patel DA, et al. Pelvic exenteration for recurrent endometrial cancer. Gynecol Oncol 1999;75:99–102.

[2] Averette HE, Lichtinger M, Sevin BU, et al. Pelvic exenteration: a 15-year experience in a general metropolitan hospital. Am J Obstet Gynecol 1984;150:179–84.
[3] Morris M, Alvarez R, Kinney W, et al. Treatment of recurrent adenocarcinoma of the endometrium with pelvic exenteration. Gynecol Oncol 1996;60:288.
[4] Penalver MA, Barreau G, Sevin BU, et al. Surgery for the treatment of locally recurrent disease. J Natl Cancer Inst Monogr 1996;21:117–22.
[5] Penalver MA, Benjany DE, Averette HE, et al. Continent urinary diversion in gynecologic oncology. Gynecol Oncol 1989;34:274–88.
[6] Morgan LS, Daly JW, Monif GR. Infectious morbidity associated with pelvic exenteration. Gynecol Oncol 1980;10:318–28.
[7] Brunschwig A. Complete excision of pelvic viscera for advanced carcinoma. Cancer 1948;1: 177–83.
[8] Rutledge FN, Smith JP, Wharton JT, et al. Pelvic exenteration: analysis of 296 patients. Am J Obstet Gynecol 1977;129(8):881–90.
[9] Eisenkop SM, Nalick RH, Teng NN. Modified posterior exenteration for ovarian cancer. Obstet Gynecol 1991;78(5–1):879–85.
[10] Scarabelli C, Gallo A, Franceschi S, et al. Primary cytoreductive surgery with rectosigmoid colon resection for patients with advanced epithelial ovarian carcinoma. Cancer 2000;88(2): 389–97.
[11] Havrilesky LJ, Wong TZ, Secord AA, et al. The role of PET scanning in the detection of recurrent cervical cancer. Gynecol Oncol 2003;90(1):186–90.
[12] Unger JB, Ivy JJ, Connor P, et al. Detection of recurrent cervical cancer by whole-body FDG PET scan in asymptomatic and symptomatic women. Gynecol Oncol 2004;94(1):212–6.
[13] Barber HRK, Brunschwig A. Treatment and results of recurrent cancer of corpus uteri in patients receiving anterior and total pelvic exenteration. Cancer 1968;22(5):949–55.
[14] Mirhashemi R, Averette H, Estape R, et al. Low colorectal anastamosis after radical pelvic surgery: a risk factor analysis. Am J Obstet Gynecol 2000;183(6):1375–80.
[15] Angioli R, Panici PB, Mirhashemi R, et al. Continent urinary diversion and low colorectal anastamosis after pelvic exenteration: quality of life and complication risk. Oncol Hematol 2003;48:281–5.
[16] Magrina JF, Stanhope CR, Weaver AL. Pelvic exenterations: supralevator, infralevator, and with vulvectomy. Gynecol Oncol 1997;64:130–5.
[17] Angioli R, Sevin B, Penalver M, et al. Pelvic floor reconstruction with dura mater allograft after pelvic exenteration: the University of Miami experience. Journal of Pelvic Surgery 1996;2:58–62.
[18] Jurado M, Bazan A, Elejageitia J, et al. Primary vaginal and pelvic floor reconstruction following pelvic exenteration: a study of morbidity. Gynecol Oncol 2000;77(2):293–7.
[19] Kusiak JF, Rosenblum NG. Neovaginal reconstruction after exenteration using an omental flap and split-thickness skin graft. Plast Reconstr Surg 1996;97:775–83.
[20] Smith HO, Genesen MC, Runowicz CD, et al. The rectus abdominis myocutaneous flap: modifications, complications, and sexual function. Cancer 1998;83(3):510–20.
[21] Sevin BU, Koechli OR. Pelvic exenteration. Surg Clin North Am 2001;81(4):771–9.
[22] Angioli R, Estape R, Cantuaria G, et al. Urinary complications of Miami pouch: trend of conservative management. Am J Obstet Gynecol 1998;179:343–8.
[23] Salom EM, Mendez LE, Schey D, et al. Continent ileocolonic reservoir (Miami pouch): the University of Miami experience over 15 years. Am J Obstet Gynecol 2004;190:994–1003.
[24] Hohenfellner R, Muller SC, Riedmiller H, et al. Continent urinary diversion: the Mainz pouch technique. In: Knapstein PG, Friedberg V, Sevin B, editors. Reconstructive surgery in gynecology. New York: Thieme Medical Publishers; 1990. p. 231–47.
[25] Miller B, Morris M, Gershenson DM, et al. Intestinal fistulae formation following pelvic exenteration: a review of the University of Texas M.D. Anderson Cancer Center Experience, 1957–1990. Gynecol Oncol 1995;56:207–10.

[26] Carlson JW, Soisson AP, Fowler JM, et al. Rectus abdominis myocutaneous flap for primary vaginal reconstruction. Gynecol Oncol 1993;51:323–9.
[27] Sevin B, Malinin T. Dura mater allograft in gynecologic reconstruction. In: Knapstein PG, Friedberg V, Sevin B, editors. Reconstructive surgery in gynecology. New York: Thieme Medical Publishers; 1990. p. 151–67.
[28] Stanhope CR, Symmonds RE. Palliative exenteration: what, when and why? Am J Obstet Gynecol 1985;152(1):12–6.

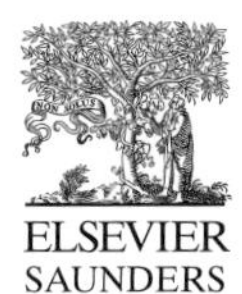
ELSEVIER
SAUNDERS

Surg Oncol Clin N Am
14 (2005) 301–319

SURGICAL
ONCOLOGY CLINICS
OF NORTH AMERICA

Surgical Management of Prostate Cancer: Optimizing Patient Selections and Clinical Outcome

Paul D. Maroni, MD[a], E. David Crawford, MD[b,*]

[a]*Division of Urology, Department of Surgery, University of Colorado Health Sciences Center, 4200 East Ninth Avenue, C-319, Denver, CO 80252, USA*

[b]*Departments of Surgery and Radiation Oncology, University of Colorado Health Sciences Center, 1665 North Ursula Street, Suite 1004, Aurora, CO 80010, USA*

Overview

The pleasure in multidisciplinary discussions about the treatment of prostate malignancy tends to disappear within minutes for the casual scientific observer. What may begin as a complicated clinical case often degenerates into the quoting of various poorly designed or executed studies that served more for territory protection than patient well-being. If the observer is displeased, one may only imagine the terror a patient must feel when presented with the vast uncertainty that remains. With an estimated 230,000 newly diagnosed cases of prostate cancer and nearly 30,000 deaths in 2004, the ambiguity cannot be blamed on the rarity or insignificance of the condition [1]. Lamentably, the sophistication of prostate cancer treatment evidence lags far behind breast and cervical cancer algorithms, the reasons for which are complicated [1]: the long period of time for patients to achieve meaningful endpoints, particularly for localized disease [2], the discontinuity in providers of the various treatments, which introduces bias and disincentive for stringent clinical evaluation [3], the variability in outcome with the plethora of different physicians, techniques, and modalities, and the generally unavoidable morbidities associated with therapy [4]. Largely because of our inability to get organized and team up, patients are left to hear incomplete advice, read biased and possibly false literature, and rely on familiar anecdote.

* Corresponding author. University of Colorado Health Sciences Center, 1665 North Ursula Street, Suite 1004, Aurora, CO 80010.

E-mail address: david.crawford@uchsc.edu (E.D. Crawford).

doi:10.1016/j.soc.2004.11.009 ***surgonc.theclinics.com***

Most physicians dread when a patient with clinically localized prostate cancer asks them directly, "What would you do?" or "What is the best therapy?" The following thought process and discussion revolves around calculable and incalculable variables. With calculable variables such as prostate-specific antigen (PSA), clinical stage, and Gleason grade, we can use numerous validated nomograms and long-term retrospective studies to give patients a rough but decent idea of preoperative cancer extent, long-term control, and expected rates of side effects with the various options [2–6]. Intangibles, such as the relative values patients place in those outcomes, present an entirely different problem. The calculable variables factor into good treatment/medicine, whereas careful attention to the intangibles defines patient satisfaction, parenthetically the more important outcome. This article addresses both conditions but focuses on selecting appropriate patients for exenterative surgical management with radical prostatectomy (RP) based on available data of clinical outcomes.

Patient selection

Natural history

The primary goal of choosing appropriate patients for surgical management of clinically localized prostate cancer should be to achieve complete eradication of disease in patients who would experience morbidity and mortality from cancer progression. Although cure is the initial aim, radical surgery also provides excellent local control of disease and avoids urologic morbidity from symptoms of urinary tract obstruction, pain, azotemia, and hematuria or clot retention. Implicit in the previous comment is the attempted avoidance of treatment in individuals who otherwise would not experience morbidity from prostate cancer because of the high rates of treatment-related side effects. Contrary to experience with faster growing malignancies, many men diagnosed with prostate cancer die from unrelated causes before symptomatic progression of disease. Overdiagnosis that leads to treatment of clinically "insignificant" prostate cancer may be "significant" if one considers that approximately 70% of patients with low-grade disease in watchful waiting protocols do not progress or require treatment before death from other causes [7]. With the proliferation of PSA screening since 1986, this number undoubtedly has increased, but so have the number of organ-confined tumors in patients with all grades of disease, which suggests intervention at a time when cure is possible. A study by Albertson et al [8] estimated that localized disease reduces life expectancy by 0 to 8 years, and it depends heavily on the histologic grade of the tumor. Gleason [9] initially observed that men with poorly differentiated tumor (Gleason scores 7–10) experienced ten times the mortality of patients with lower grade disease (Gleason scores 2–6).

Analysis of large groups of patients who selected watchful waiting protocols provides the bulk of data regarding the natural history of prostate cancer. Chodak et al [10] compiled a large database of international nonrandomized studies, including 828 patients with clinically localized disease who entered observation protocols with medical or surgical castration on progression. Grade of tumor clearly was shown to impact long-term outcome, with prostate cancer causing mortality in 13%, 13%, and 66% of patients with grade 1 (Gleason 2–4), 2 (Gleason 5–6), and 3 (Gleason 7–10) disease, respectively. Distant metastases also occurred in 19%, 42%, and 74% of patients with grades 1 through 3 at 10 years. The authors concluded that patients with low-grade disease might not benefit substantially from "aggressive treatment," and the benefit of local therapy in patients with high-grade disease was unknown. Johansson et al's [7,11] analysis of their long-term cohort found similar results 15 years after diagnosis, but longer follow-up of this group has suggested that men who live longer than 15 years triple their risk of dying of prostate cancer even with lower grades. Unfortunately, only approximately 25% of men survived to the 15-year time point, with many of them (84%) dying of other diseases. This group has been criticized heavily because the average age at diagnosis was 72, which is already considered by many surgeons to be beyond the age of surgical treatment. Modern series of RP suggest higher disease-specific survival rates, with a large multi-institutional series demonstrating 10-year disease-specific survival rates that compare favorably to watchful waiting protocols (grade 1, 94%; grade 2, 80%; grade 3, 77%) [12].

Many numerical and statistical exercises have tried to identify the patients most likely to benefit from intervention. In a highly controversial study about watchful waiting, Fleming et al [13] cited that local therapy (prostatectomy or radiation) disadvantaged cancer patients in almost all instances when applying quality-adjusted life years. (Briefly, calculations of quality-adjusted life years try to estimate survival by treatment based on current data and incorporate a variable for treatment-related side effects. Also, the calculations identify average benefit, which means that some patients may suffer from treatment while others gain greater than the specified time.) Although this study highlights the "most important" question in prostate cancer, it has been criticized heavily because of outdated assumptions on rates of progression, which would change the conclusions of the analysis to favor surgery in some instances [14,15]. With contemporary information, Bhatnagar et al [16] used quality-adjusted life years with a similar model and found surgical benefits of 1 to 3 years with Gleason score 7 to 10 cancer but suggested treatment detriment in patients with lesser grades (Fig. 1). Younger patients tended to derive greater survival, but even 75-year-old patients might recoup a few years. The use of group level assessments for quality-adjusted life years neglects individual utilities for given outcomes (eg, a man already impotent at diagnosis would view treatment-related sexual dysfunction differently from a potent patient)

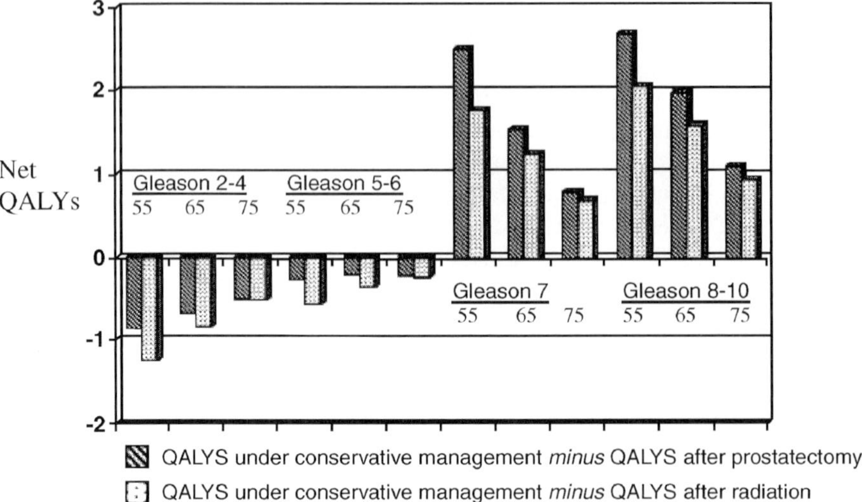

Fig. 1. Net quality-adjusted life years at ages 55, 65, and 75 after prostatectomy or radiation treatment relative to quality-adjusted life years under conservative management. (*From* Bhatnagar V, Stewart ST, Bonney WW, et al. Treatment options for localized prostate cancer: quality-adjusted life years and the effects of lead-time. Urology 2004;63:106; copyright 2004 with permission from Elsevier.)

[17]. This major point has limited clinical application of these types of analysis.

In the late 1980s, the Swedish Cancer Society and the Scandinavian Prostatic Cancer Group Study Number 4 started an ambitious project to determine the impact of RP on survival compared with watchful waiting [18]. Approximately 350 patients were randomized to both groups, with a high number being compliant with the treatment recommendations for a median follow-up of 6.2 years. RP did reduce disease-specific deaths (16 versus 31), with a trend toward effecting overall mortality (53 versus 62). Rates of local progression and metastasis also strongly favored the surgical arm. Proponents of watchful waiting highlight the impact on overall survival (no difference), the low yield of impact on disease (number needed to treat = 17 for one life saved at 8 years), and the relatively short increase in disease-specific survival (less than 1 year). Although not as robust a difference as expected, experts hope the difference will expand with further follow-up, because the separation between the arms increased by 4% from the 5- to 8-year follow-up groups. The fact that many of the patients enrolled in this study had disease diagnosed in the pre-PSA era should be kept in mind. Risk stratification and the designation of the true beneficiaries of treatment should aid in patient and physician decision making with further analysis.

The complicated natural history of prostate cancer creates the conundrum of optimal individualized treatment and has been reviewed elsewhere [19]. The cancer-related outcome depends directly on two trajectories for which only actuarial estimates are possible: cancer progression and progression of other disease to death within the individual. The goals of traditional teaching and practice have been to offer radical surgery to patients with clinically localized disease and a life expectancy of more than 10 years. This approach generally has been corroborated by Albertson et al's observations [20] that local therapy tends not to provide survival or progression benefit to patients with significant comorbid illness. Urologists were found to be acceptably accurate in face-to-face determinations of medical fitness in a retrospective study of patients who received surgical treatment, but the scientific basis of this limit has not been investigated fully [21]. More accurate methods of comorbidity estimation exist, such as the Charlson index, and practical application to patients during consultation seems prudent. Until information from randomized trials such as the Prostate Intervention versus Observation Trial and longer follow-up on the Scandinavian study is available, more precise risk stratification will be difficult. In broad strokes, the data would support surgical treatment in patients with more than 15 years of life expectancy with Gleason ≤ 6 disease and 10-year life expectancies in patients with high-grade disease. Using actuarial tables, the average gentleman aged 66 would survive 15 years [22]. A consideration for repeat or extended biopsy should be made for patients with low-grade cancer because prostatectomy upgrades disease 22% to 25% of the time with whole mount sectioning [23,24].

Clinical categorization and staging

An elevated PSA level or abnormal digital rectal examination indicates a need for prostate biopsy. With the addition of the Gleason score, when histologic cancer is established these three parameters function in risk stratification for many clinical staging systems. Numerous other parameters have been proven to be helpful in determining patients at high risk for disease progression, recurrence after local therapy, or death (Box 1). The quantity of cancer in the biopsy specimen as indicated by percentage of cores with cancer (number of positive cores/number of cores) or percent of biopsy with cancer (length of positive section/total length) have been proven significant in predicting pathologic stage after prostatectomy and disease recurrence [25–27]. The rate of PSA rise over time also has been shown to be clinically significant; particularly in men with a PSA increase of 2 ng/dL or more the year before prostatectomy [28]. Few patients with T1a prostate cancer (incidental finding of $\leq$ 5% of transurethral resection of prostate [TURP] specimen) experience progression and might be best served by serial PSA measurement with active intervention in younger patients with a rising PSA [29]. Patients with T1b prostate cancer ($>$ 5% of TURP specimen) have similar—if not less favorable—rates of organ confined disease than palpable cancers and should be approached as stage T2a. For localized

Box 1. Preoperative prognostic factors

Independent variables

- Clinical stage
- Gleason grade
- PSA
- Percentage of biopsy involved with cancer
- Preoperative PSA velocity

Future variables

- Molecular markers
  EZH2:ECAD (pathologic specimen)
  HA-HYAL-1, HYAL-1 (pathologic specimen)
  Interleukin-6 soluble receptor, transforming growth factor-beta1 (serum)

disease, large variability in rates of progression, development of metastatic disease, and survival make individual predictions difficult. Although PSA, tumor volume on biopsy, and clinical stage all predict cancer recurrence, tumor grade seems to be the strongest predictor for achieving any of the outcomes showing the lasting utility of Gleason's observations made 30 years ago. Several molecular markers have been described as having prognostic significance, and we continue to hold great hope that these basic science advances will become clinical reality [30–33].

Tables and nomograms are available for predicting pathologic stage and recurrence-free survival based on the mentioned criteria. Partin tables, Kattan's nomograms, and calculations of pathologic stage using artificial neural networks are readily available on the Internet (www.urology.jhu.edu/prostate/partintables.php; www.nomograms.org; www.prostatecalculator.org). Kattan's nomogram also can calculate pretreatment 5-year progression-free probabilities based on treatment and can be downloaded for use on a personal digital assistant. Another nomogram can give the probability that a patient has an indolent tumor [34]. The use of these tables is straightforward and recommended, but fewer groupings make categorization more practical for clinical trial management. D'Amico et al [35] defined risk groups for recurrence that have less precision than tables but may use a nomenclature more easily interpreted by some patients. Individuals may be categorized as low-risk (1992 American Joint Committee on Cancer stage T1c or T2a, Gleason $\leq$ 6, and PSA $\leq$ 10), intermediate risk (T2b, Gleason 7, or PSA 10 to $\leq$ 20), or high risk (T2c, Gleason 8–10, or PSA $>$ 20) with significant prognostic appeal. Although not a randomized trial, this study showed significant benefit of prostatectomy over seed implantation in patients from the intermediate- and high-risk groups.

Indications for lymph node dissection

In the pre-PSA era (before 1985) cancer deposits in lymph nodes were encountered up to 56% of the time at pelvic exploration, and most surgeons would abort the prostatectomy with frozen section confirmation [36,37]. With the increasing use of PSA and improved imaging technology, cancerous lymph node rates are less than 8% [38]. The addition of a bilateral obturator node dissection adds operative time and cost and contributes to the morbidity of the procedure, with some patients requiring lymphocele drainage and a slightly higher risk of deep venous thrombosis [39]. Permanent androgen blockade in patients with positive nodes prolongs survival, but this result does not seem durable if the prostate is left in situ [40,41]. Some authors suggest improved cancer staging by doubling positive lymph node detection rates with an extended node dissection, including the external and common iliac nodes, but this practice is not widely accepted and might result in more complications [42,43].

Numerous reviews present parameters for prostatectomy with lymphadenectomy. Most reviews set a PSA limit at 10, Gleason component of 4 or more in the biopsy specimen, or the palpable extent of disease (T2b or more) as indications for performing a pelvic node dissection [44]. Bishoff et al [38] examined a contemporary series of RP and developed easy-to-use probability tables based on clinical stage, PSA, and Gleason score. Approximately 50% of patients in their series would have avoided lymph node dissection if patients with less than a 5% chance of positive nodes underwent RP only. Partin tables, the Kattan nomogram, and artificial neural networks also estimate the likelihood of positive lymph nodes. Meng and Carroll [45] used decision analysis interpolating risk/benefit utilities and judged that lymph node biopsy should proceed only if the probability of positive nodes was 18% or more, but small changes in parameters (eg, morbidity of lymph node dissection) might change this number considerably. The use of postoperative androgen ablation also was not calculated in the decision tree. A sensible approach would be to evaluate a patient's risk of positive lymph nodes using an accepted nomogram, present the risk of 5% additional morbidity and benefits of the procedure, including the possibility for lifetime androgen blockade, and guide the patient to a decision.

Anatomic (nerve-sparing) radical prostatectomy

RP in its original description did not include resection of tissue that was later found to contain the nerves responsible for erections, but lack of anatomic understanding routinely led to surgical injury of these structures. Postoperative erectile dysfunction was the rule, with impotence rates up to 85% [46]. Largely through the efforts of Walsh, the vascular and nervous anatomy were defined in a fashion that refined the dissection and spared the cavernosal nerves, thus reducing a man's risk of postoperative impotence to as low as 10% in certain populations (less than 50 years old) [47]. These rates increase to 25% for patients up to age 60, 42% for patients aged 60 to 70, and 75% for men over age 70. More advanced clinical stage also suggests worse outcome with attempts to retain potency. The indications for nerve-sparing prostatectomy are somewhat controversial. Few researchers argue that men with low-risk features (eg, PSA less than 10, minimal unilateral palpable disease, and Gleason score less than 7) are candidates, but many accomplished surgeons base nerve-sparing procedures on intraoperative findings in patients with adverse tumor characteristics and achieve excellent clinical outcomes [29]. Induration around or near the neurovascular bundle or fixation of the bundle to the prostate during dissection indicates wide excision. Others have been more selective, only considering young potent patients with low-risk features [48]. Preoperatively, careful assessment of a patient's potency status, digital rectal exam, and Gleason grade can give a patient a decent idea if nerve sparing is at risk.

Perineal prostatectomy

An RP was first reported using this approach nearly 100 years ago by Young [49]. The perineal approach was largely abandoned for the more painful—but more versatile—retropubic approach because of the ability to sample the local lymph nodes simultaneously. This procedure returned to favor somewhat with the decreased need for lymph node dissection, but most urologists still use the more familiar anterior approach. A few patient groups might benefit, however, based on certain qualities of the operation that facilitate prostate removal in hostile circumstances (eg, prior pelvic surgery). Patients who categorically refuse blood transfusions also may benefit because this operation typically incurs less risk of hemorrhage than a retropubic prostatectomy. These patients must be able to lie in an exaggerated lithotomy position in the office to ensure proper positioning on the day of surgery, and gland sizes more than 100 g make the procedure difficult [50].

Laparoscopic prostatectomy

Any patient who is considered for RP is also a candidate for laparoscopic prostatectomy. Lymph node dissections and nerve-sparing procedures can be performed. The actual technique of prostate removal is similar to the open procedure, and early cancer control rates are comparable [51–54]. A few academic centers and private hospitals have used robotic devices to shorten the learning curve associated with the advanced laparoscopic techniques required for the free-hand procedure [55]. Ultimately, results with the robot likely will be more reproducible in a trained urologist's hands. Arguably, the magnified view provides superior visualization, and studies that determine cancer control and side-effect rates are promising [52,56,57]. Although promising, the downsides are the relative lack of surgeons trained in this technique, the huge capital outlay hospitals must make to purchase and maintain a robotic device, and the learning curve that invariably harms many patients until the equipment and ability become mainstream.

Salvage prostatectomy

RP after radiation failure for prostate cancer has been performed successfully in certain circumstances [58]. Confirmation by transrectal ultrasound biopsy or rectal examination progression with a rising PSA may give the caregiver more certainty that the disease remains in the prostate. An absolute criterion for consideration is that a patient must have had localized disease that would have been curable with surgical therapy at the outset (T1-2). The technique is more demanding secondary to scar tissue and disruption of tissue planes, and the perineal approach has been found to be beneficial for the dissection between the prostate and rectum. The tenfold rates of side effects relative to nonradiated controls and low (15%–33%) local control rates generally mitigate recommendation for salvage prostatectomy [59].

Clinical outcome

Cancer control

Assessing the effect of RP on important clinical outcomes relative to other therapies, including watchful waiting, can be difficult. Most trials have difficulty estimating the impact on overall survival (the “ultimate endpoint”) largely because of the incredibly long lead time in screen-detected, clinically localized cancer. Unlike other malignancies, some studies may require 15 to 20 years of follow-up to find meaningful differences in local progression (eg, hematuria, obstruction, renal failure), development of metastatic disease, and survival. Investigators and funding agencies hesitate to use resources in protracted endeavors because technologic advances in two decades may obviate the studied treatment. Surrogate endpoints (eg, laboratory tests) that precede meaningful endpoints by measurable amounts of time can be useful, however. A handy endpoint used by most retrospective reviews is PSA progression defined after surgery as more than 0.4 ng/mL or more than 0.2 ng/mL. Although PSA doubling time may be a more useful surrogate of possessing deadly disease, most large series of RP imply any PSA progression as evidence of surgical failure.

Many men with clinically localized disease at surgery do not have organ-confined cancer on final pathologic examination. Between 32% and 49% of them have extracapsular extension, and 11% to 24% have extension with positive surgical margins based on large reviews from experienced centers (Table 1) [4,6,60–63]. Previously mentioned nomograms have proven validity in preoperative prediction of adverse pathologic characteristics

Table 1
Short-and long-term radical prostatectomy results from experienced institutions in the PSA era

Institution	*N*	Follow-up	Positive organ confined margins (%)	PSA limit	Biochemical progression-free survival			Metastasis-free survival			Death from disease		
					5-y (%)	10-y (%)	15-y (%)	5-y (%)	10-y (%)	15-y (%)	5-y (%)	10-y (%)	15-y (%)
Baylor [63]	1000	4 (median)	60	13 > 0.4	78	75		90	84		1	2.5	
Cleveland Clinic [60]	1034	5 (median)	58	16 > 0.2	81								
Duke (Perineal prostatectomy) [61]	1319	4 (median)	53	24 > 0.5	70						1–3		
Johns Hopkins [4]	2404	6 (mean)	51	11 > 0.2	84	74	66	96	90	82	1	4	10
Mayo Clinic [62]	2782	6–7 (median)	68	>0.4	76	60							
Washington Univ/ Northwestern [6]	3478	5–6 (mean)	68	19 > 0.2	80	68						3	

and progression-free survival based on postoperative characteristics. Ten-year progression-free probabilities with organ-confined disease are 80% to 93%, with successive decreases to roughly 50% for extracapsular extension, 26% to 30% for positive seminal vesicles, and 10% to 12% for positive lymph nodes. Even so, mortality from prostate cancer remains low in prostatectomy series, with 3% to 4% dying from disease at 10 years, but results from the Scandinavian trial are closer to 7% at 8 years, probably because of more advanced disease at diagnosis in this population (eg, 47% with PSA > 10) [18]. The pathologic Gleason grade and preoperative PSA value also have prognostic significance, with higher Gleason grade and higher PSA demonstrating worse outcomes.

Although specialized academic centers produce most available comparative data, some authors have suggested that the community may not enjoy similar outcomes. A nomogram developed from data at experienced centers tends to overestimate progression-free survival when compared with a community cohort [64]. Numerous reviews from community health systems and databases demonstrate similar rates of cancer control, however [65–67]. Although it seems that the community may be able to emulate universities in terms of cancer control, this may not be true for all urologists. The surgeon and surgical volume have been shown to be independent variables in predicting margin status [68]. High-volume hospitals and surgeons (> 20 RP/y) can lower postoperative and urinary complications by up to 9% [69].

Complications and side effects

Surgical removal of the prostate should not be presented to patients as trivial or benign. Although substantial advances in technique have moved us from the massive hemorrhage of elective ("trauma") prostatectomy to the delicate dissection required of the anatomic technique, treatment-related side effects generate the controversy in how to approach prostate cancer. Hypothesizing near-zero rates of side effects would lead nearly every man to choose treatment unless saddled with the burden of payment. Perioperative complications are relatively rare events with modern surgical management (Box 2). These important complications tend not to overly concern a patient during preoperative consultation. Men fear replacing prostate cancer with a social cancer (eg, disabling urinary incontinence) and the emasculation of impotence. Metrics that evaluate these symptoms exist, but varying definitions of incontinence and erectile dysfunction make critical evaluation difficult. Patients probably respond to concrete parameters better, but complicated scoring indexes may be ideal for detecting subtle differences between treatments during clinical trials. The Expanded Prostate Index Composite and European Organization for Research and Treatment of Cancer QLQ-C30 are two of many accepted surveys that assess quality-of-life issues that surround prostate cancer [70]. Independent analyses are preferred

Box 2. Complications of radical prostatectomy

Perioperative
Hermorrhage (variable, depends on surgeon)
Rectal injury (approximately 1%)
Ureteral injury (< 1%)
Pulmonary emboli (approximately 1%)
Myocardial infarction (< 1%)
Ileus (3%)
Infection (8%)

Postoperative
Impotence (10%–90%)
Incontinence (2%–10%)
Hernia (up to 21%)
Bladder neck contracture (2%–17%)

to eliminate the potential bias from surgeon-directed questioning. Unfortunately, practical considerations prevent the well-meaning urologist interested in good patient outcomes from obtaining uninfluenced information. Although extended surveys may be helpful, rapid assessments of continence and potency can be performed with candid questioning about use of incontinence pads, bother by incontinence episodes, ability to achieve an erection satisfactory for penetration with complete intercourse, and bother by erectile dysfunction.

Large institutional reviews of urinary incontinence report varying rates of continence after RP. Walsh et al [29,71] reported that 92% of men demonstrate complete urinary control, with 6% of men wearing one pad per day and no patients being totally incontinent. Men older than age 70 fare somewhat less well, with 86% being completely dry. Other high-volume surgeons reported similar results [72,73]. The Prostate Cancer Outcomes Study, a cross-sectional analysis from diverse health care settings and probably more representative of community experience, suggested rates of total incontinence after prostatectomy of near 10%, with almost 30% wearing pads to stay dry, with an overall bother rate of 11% [74]. Time to continence varies, but further improvement after 1 year is unlikely [75]. Surgeon preference probably plays a large role (Table 2). Bowel bother and fecal incontinence are probably underemphasized to patients preoperatively, with significant numbers experiencing bowel issues after surgery, some of which may be lasting [76].

Postoperative impotence results follow similar trends of excellent reported rates from academic centers, with poorer results from independent examiners of heterogeneous populations. Potency rates are 60% to 90% for younger men (< 60 years) with age-related decreases in return of erectile

Table 2
Complications and bother from experienced surgeons and the Prostate Cancer Outcomes Study

Outcomes	12–24 mo
Continence (%)	
Experienced surgeons	
No pads [71,73]	92–93
Bother (no/small) [71]	98
General results [76]	
No pads	60
Bother (no/small)	70
Sexual function (%)	
Experienced surgeons	
Potent [71,73]	68–86
Bother (no/small) [71]	76–84
General results [76]	
Potent	44
Bother (no/small)	32–36

function after RP [29,72]. Excision of one neurovascular bundle may decrease return of erections by up to 20%. The Prostate Cancer Outcomes Study reported impotence after 18 months in 56% of bilateral nerve-sparing techniques, 59% of unilateral nerve-sparing techniques, and 65% of non–nerve-sparing procedures, with more than 40% experiencing at least moderate sexual bother [77]. Improving on potency is clearly an area of great interest. The anatomic technique described by Walsh is reproducible, but an adequate explanation for the high impotence rates in patients with "nerve-sparing surgery" is lacking. Young men who likely benefit the most from RP also experience lower rates of complications and side effects, which encourages urologists to appraise other options carefully in older patients with localized disease [72].

Quality of life

The ultimate dictum of use of treatment is patient satisfaction. A satisfactory experience and return to preoperative functioning depend on numerous factors that nomograms cannot calculate precisely. An interesting analysis of the CaPSURE database surveyed men and searched for factors that predicted return to baseline functioning [78]. Patients younger than 65 years old and in excellent health with no comorbidities most often returned to a preoperative level by 1 year. Unfortunately, only approximately 66% returned to baseline urinary function, 20% to sexual function, 80% to physical function, and 86% to mental function by 12 months after surgery. Although almost unmentionable, higher socioeconomic status seems directly related to quality-of-life outcomes in patients with prostate cancer [79]. Cancer anxiety plays a large role in a patient pursuing treatment, and most of us lack the time and savvy to soothe tension over disease. Strict criteria or improved laboratory instruments for determining indolent cancer would be helpful to talk some patients out of treatment, but current nomograms still miss unacceptable numbers of significant cancers [34].

Late benefits

Recently, large database assessment has suggested that patients who undergo RP may fare better in terms of progression and death after disease recurrence than patients who have other therapies. An analog of this concept exists in other tumor treatment, in particular the surgical treatment of minimally metastatic renal cancer. One study and a meta-analysis of that study combined with a European study concluded that nephrectomy and immunochemotherapy provide a short but real survival advantage over immunochemotherapy alone [80,81]. Several studies of ovarian cancer suggest that operative debulking may be beneficial [82–84]. Although the small benefits noted in renal cancer create controversy, potential increases in survival in slower growing malignancies, such as prostate cancer, may be more appreciable. In a reanalysis of Southwest Oncology Group 8894 originally designed to examine maximal androgen blockade in patients with metastatic disease, groups were stratified by original treatment (if any) for localized disease [85]. Of the 1286 patients evaluated, survival was higher in the 148 patients who had undergone previous prostatectomy. A few theories exist: (1) removal of the primary tumor and the attendant debulking of the largest volume of disease in patients with undiagnosed micrometastatic disease, although not curative, resets the time period of progression to death to benefit the patient; (2) a large metastasis-producing depot is removed with RP; (3) local progression is less likely after prostatectomy and more easily detected by examination, which begets earlier intervention; (4) residual disease after radiation is almost always high grade; and (5) detection of PSA recurrence is less ambiguous, which allows earlier treatment. Although an interesting side note about prostatectomy, a lack of high-level evidence exists, which precludes this information from being presented confidently to patients.

Multispecialty treatment

A sensible approach to a patient with newly diagnosed prostate cancer requires careful review of clinical staging information with the option of multispecialty tumor board review. Although delay in treatment may make a patient anxious, this time may be used wisely by the patient to learn about the disease from reputable well-designed publications and Websites. No studies or trials have demonstrated a change in survival from waiting several weeks or months to formulate a treatment plan satisfactory to the patient. Groups, hospitals, and institutions should develop evidence-based treatment algorithms compiled by oncologists, urologists, and radiation oncologists. When possible, patients should be offered enrollment in clinical studies, particularly men with high-risk prostate cancer for whom many available adjuvant chemotherapy trials are currently underway.

References

[1] American Cancer Society. Cancer facts and figures 2004. Available at: www.cancer.org. Accessed August 1, 2004.
[2] Partin AW, Mangold LA, Lamm DM, et al. Contemporary update of prostate cancer staging nomograms (Partin tables) for the new millennium. Urology 2001;58(6):843–8.
[3] Kattan MW, Eastham JA, Stapleton AM, et al. A preoperative nomogram for disease recurrence following radical prostatectomy for prostate cancer. J Natl Cancer Inst 1998; 90(10):766–71.
[4] Han M, Partin AW, Pound CR, et al. Long-term biochemical disease-free and cancer-specific survival following anatomic radical retropubic prostatectomy: the 15-year Johns Hopkins experience. Urol Clin North Am 2001;28(3):555–65.
[5] Hull GW, Rabbani F, Abbas F, et al. Cancer control with radical prostatectomy alone in 1,000 consecutive patients. J Urol 2002;167(2 Pt 1):528–34.
[6] Roehl KA, Han M, Ramos CG, et al. Cancer progression and survival rates following anatomical radical retropubic prostatectomy in 3,478 consecutive patients: long-term results. J Urol 2004;172(3):910–4.
[7] Johansson J-E, Holmberg L, Johansson S, et al. Fifteen-year survival in prostate cancer: a prospective, population-based study in Sweden. JAMA 1997;277(6):467–98.
[8] Albertson PC, Fryback DG, Storer BE, et al. Long-term survival among men with conservatively treated localized prostate cancer. JAMA 1995;274:626–31.
[9] Gleason DF. Histologic grading and clinical staging of carcinoma of the prostate. In: Tannenbaum M, editor. Urologic pathology. Philadelphia: Lea & Febiger; 1977. p. 171–98.
[10] Chodak GW, Thisted RA, Gerber GS, et al. Results of conservative management of clinically localized prostate cancer. N Engl J Med 1994;330(4):242–8.
[11] Johansson J-E, Andren O, Andersson S-O, et al. Natural history of early, localized prostate cancer. JAMA 2004;291(22):2713–9.
[12] Gerber GS, Thisted RA, Scardino PT, et al. Results of radical prostatectomy in men with clinically localized prostate cancer: multi-institutional pooled analysis. JAMA 1996;276(8): 615–9.
[13] Fleming C, Wasson JH, Albertson PC, et al. A decision analysis of alternative treatment strategies for clinically localized prostate cancer. JAMA 1993;269(20):2650–8.
[14] Kattan MW, Cowen ME, Miles BJ. A decision analysis for treatment of clinically localized prostate cancer. J Gen Intern Med 1997;12:299–305.
[15] Beck JR, Kattan MW, Miles BJ. A critique of the decision analysis for clinically localized prostate cancer. J Urol 1994;152:1894–9.
[16] Bhatnagar V, Stewart ST, Bonney WW, et al. Treatment options for localized prostate cancer: quality-adjusted life years and the effects of lead-time. Urology 2004;63:103–9.
[17] Cowen ME, Miles BJ, Cahill DF, et al. The danger of applying group-level utilities in decision analyses of the treatment of localized prostate cancer in individual patients. Med Decis Making 1998;18(4):376–80.
[18] Holmberg L, Bill-Axelson A, Helgesen F, et al. A randomized trial comparing radical prostatectomy with watchful waiting in early prostate cancer. N Engl J Med 2002;347(11): 781–9.
[19] Kessler B, Albertson P. The natural history of prostate cancer. Urol Clin North Am 2003;30: 219–26.
[20] Albertson PC, Fryback DG, Storer BE, et al. The impact of co-morbidity on life expectancy among men with localized prostate cancer. J Urol 1996;156:127–32.

[21] Koch MO, Miller DA, Butler R, et al. Are we selecting the right patients for treatment of localized prostate cancer? Results of an actuarial analysis. Urology 1998;51(2):197–202.
[22] Calculated life expectancy with Palm Prostogram v3.0. Available at: www.nomograms.org. Accessed August 15, 2004.
[23] San Francisco IF, DeWolf WC, Rosen S, et al. Extended prostate needle biopsy improves concordance of Gleason grading between prostate needle biopsy and radical prostatectomy. J Urol 2003;169(1):136–40.
[24] King CR, McNeal JE, Gill H, et al. Extended prostate biopsy scheme improves reliability of Gleason grading: implications for radiotherapy patients. Int J Radiat Oncol Biol Phys 2004; 59(2):386–91.
[25] D'Amico AV, Whittington R, Malkowicz SB, et al. Clinical utility of the percentage of positive prostate biopsies in defining biochemical outcome after radical prostatectomy for patients with clinically localized prostate cancer. J Clin Oncol 2000;18(6):1164–72.
[26] Grossklaus DJ, Coffey CS, Shappell SB, et al. Percent of cancer in the biopsy set predicts pathological findings after prostatectomy. J Urol 2002;167(5):2032–5.
[27] Lotan Y, Shariat SF, Khoddami SM, et al. The percent of biopsy cores positive for cancer is a predictor of advanced pathologic stage and poor clinical outcomes in patients treated with radical prostatectomy. J Urol 2004;171(6 Pt 1):2209–14.
[28] D'Amico AV, Chen MH, Roehl KA, et al. Preoperative PSA velocity and the risk of death from prostate cancer alter radical prostatectomy. N Engl J Med 2004;351(2):125–35.
[29] Walsh PC. Radical prostatectomy: a procedure in evolution. Semin Oncol 1994;21(5):662–71.
[30] Moul JW, Merseburger AS, Srivastava S. Molecular markers in prostate cancer: the role in preoperative staging. Clin Prostate Cancer 2002;1(1):42–50.
[31] Posey JT, Soloway MS, Ekici S, et al. Evaluation of the prognostic potential of hyaluronic acid and hyaluronidase (HYAL1) for prostate cancer. Cancer Res 2003;63(10):2638–44.
[32] Rhodes DR, Sanda MG, Otte AP, et al. Multiplex biomarker approach for determining risk of prostate-specific antigen-defined recurrence of prostate cancer. J Natl Cancer Inst 2003; 95(9):661–8.
[33] Kattan MW, Shariat SF, Andrews B, et al. The addition of interleukin-6 soluble receptor and transforming growth factor beta1 improves a preoperative nomogram for predicting biochemical progression in patients with clinically localized prostate cancer. J Clin Oncol 2003;21(19):3573–9.
[34] Kattan MW, Eastham JA, Wheeler TM, et al. Counseling men with prostate cancer: a nomogram for predicting the presence of small, moderately differentiated, confined tumors. J Urol 2003;170(5):1792–7.
[35] D'Amico AV, Whittington R, Malkowicz SB, et al. Biochemical outcome after radical prostatectomy, external beam radiation therapy, or interstitial radiation therapy for clinically localized prostate cancer. JAMA 1998;280(11):969–74.
[36] Grossman IC, Carpiniello V, Greenberg SH, et al. Staging pelvic lymphadenectomy for carcinoma of the prostate: review of 91 cases. J Urol 1980;124(5):632–4.
[37] Donohue RE, Fauver HE, Whitesel JA, et al. Prostatic carcinoma: influence of tumor grade on results of pelvic lymphadenectomy. Urology 1981;17(5):435–40.
[38] Bishoff JT, St Clair SR, Reyes A, et al. Pelvic lymphadenectomy can be omitted in selected patients with carcinoma of the prostate: development of a system of patient selection. Urology 1995;45(2):270–4.
[39] Augustin H, Hammerer P, Graefen M, et al. Intraoperative and perioperative morbidity of contemporary radical retropubic prostatectomy in a consecutive series of 1243 patients: results of a single center between 1999 and 2002. Eur Urol 2003;43(2):113–8.
[40] Messing EM, Manola J, Sarosdy M, et al. Immediate hormonal therapy compared with observation after radical prostatectomy and pelvic lymphadenectomy in men with node-positive prostate cancer. N Engl J Med 1999;341(24):1781–8.
[41] Schroder FH, Kurth KH, Fossa SD, et al. Early versus delayed endocrine treatment of pN1–3 M0 prostate cancer without local treatment of the primary tumor: results of European

Organisation for the Research and Treatment of Cancer 30846: a phase III study. J Urol 2004;172(3):923–7.
[42] Heidenreich A, Von Knobloch R, Varga Z, et al. Extended pelvic lymphadenectomy in men undergoing radical prostatectomy: an update on more than 300 cases. J Clin Oncol 2004; 212:4612.
[43] Clark T, Parekh DJ, Cookson MS, et al. Randomized prospective evaluation of extended versus limited lymph node dissection in patients with clinically localized prostate cancer. J Urol 2003;169(1):145–7.
[44] Ekman P. Predicting pelvic lymph node involvement in patients with localized prostate cancer. Eur Urol 1997;32(Suppl 3):60–4.
[45] Meng MV, Carroll PR. When is pelvic lymph node dissection necessary before radical prostatectomy? A decision analysis. J Urol 2000;164:1235–40.
[46] Fowler JE Jr, Clayton M, Sharifi R, et al. Early experience with Walsh technique of radical retropubic prostatectomy. Urology 1987;29(3):242–6.
[47] Quinlan DM, Epstein JI, Carter BS, et al. Sexual function following radical prostatectomy: influence of preservation of neurovascular bundles. J Urol 1991;145(5):998–1002.
[48] Sokoloff MH, Brendler CB. Indications and contraindications for nerve-sparing radical prostatectomy. Urol Clin North Am 2001;28(3):535–43.
[49] Young HH. The early diagnosis and radical cure of carcinoma of the prostate: being a study of 40 cases and presentation of a radical operation which was carried out in four cases. Bull Johns Hopkins Hosp 1905;16:315–21.
[50] Gibbons RP. Radical perineal prostatectomy. In: Walsh PC, Retik AB, Vaughan ED, et al, editors. Campbell's urology. 8th edition. Philadelphia: WB Saunders; 2002. p. 3131–46.
[51] Salomon L, Levrel O, Anastasiadis AG, et al. Outcome and complications of radical prostatectomy in patients with PSA < 10 ng/ml: comparison between the retropubic, perineal and laparoscopic approach. Prostate Cancer Prostatic Dis 2002;5(4):285–90.
[52] Menon M, Tewari A, Baize B, et al. Prospective comparison of radical retropubic prostatectomy and robot-assisted anatomic prostatectomy: the Vattikuti Urology Institute experience. Urology 2002;60(5):864–8.
[53] Guillonneau B, el-Fettouh H, Baumert H, et al. Laparoscopic radical prostatectomy: oncological evaluation after 1,000 cases at Montsouris Institute. J Urol 2003;169(4): 1261–6.
[54] Rassweiler J, Schulze M, Teber D, et al. Laparoscopic radical prostatectomy: functional and oncological outcomes. Curr Opin Urol 2004;14(2):75–82.
[55] Menon M, Shrivastava A, Tewari A, et al. Laparoscopic and robot assisted radical prostatectomy: establishment of a structured program and preliminary analysis of outcomes. J Urol 2002;168(3):945–9.
[56] Anastasiadis AG, Salomon L, Katz R, et al. Radical retropubic versus laparoscopic prostatectomy: a prospective comparison of functional outcome. Urology 2003;62(2): 292–7.
[57] Su LM, Link RE, Bhayani SB, et al. Nerve-sparing laparoscopic radical prostatectomy: replicating the open surgical technique. Urology 2004;64(1):123–7.
[58] Eastham JA, DiBlasio CJ, Scardino PT. Salvage radical prostatectomy for recurrence of prostate cancer after radiation therapy. Curr Urol Rep 2003;4(3):211–5.
[59] Catalona WJ, Ramos CG, Carvalhal GF. Contemporary results of anatomic radical prostatectomy. CA Cancer J Clin 1999;49(5):282–96.
[60] Kupelian PA, Potters L, Khuntia D, et al. Radical prostatectomy, external beam radiotherapy < 72 Gy, external beam radiotherapy ≥ 72 Gy, permanent seed implantation, or combined seeds/external beam radiotherapy for stage T1–2 prostate cancer. Int J Radiat Oncol Biol Phys 2004;58(1):25–33.
[61] Iselin CE, Box JW, Vollmer RT, et al. Surgical control of clinically localized prostate carcinoma is equivalent in African-American and white males. Cancer 1998;83: 2353–60.

[62] Amling CL, Blute ML, Bergstralh EJ, et al. Long-term hazard of progression after radical prostatectomy for clinically localized prostate cancer: continued risk of biochemical failure after 5 years. J Urol 2000;164:101–5.
[63] Hull GW, Rabbani F, Abbas F, et al. Cancer control with radical prostatectomy alone in 1,000 consecutive patients. J Urol 2002;167:528–34.
[64] Greene KL, Meng MV, Elkin EP, et al. Validation of the Kattan preoperative nomogram for prostate cancer recurrence using a community based cohort: results from cancer of the prostate strategic urological research endeavor (capsure). J Urol 2004;171(6 Pt 1):2255–9.
[65] Moul JW, Connelly RR, Lubeck DP, et al. Predicting risk of prostate specific antigen recurrence after radical prostatectomy with the Center for Prostate Disease Research and Cancer of the Prostate Strategic Urologic Research Endeavor databases. J Urol 2001;166(4): 1322–7.
[66] Tol-Fakkar M, Hermansson CG, Hugosson J, et al. Radical prostatectomy: long-term oncological outcome from a community hospital. Scand J Urol Nephrol 2003;37(5):376–81.
[67] Zhang Y, Glass A, Bennett N, et al. Long-term outcomes after radical prostatectomy performed in a community-based health maintenance organization. Cancer 2004;100(2): 300–7.
[68] Eastham JA, Kattan MW, Riedel E, et al. Variations among individual surgeons in the rate of positive surgical margins in radical prostatectomy specimens. J Urol 2003;170(6 Pt 1): 2292–5.
[69] Begg CB, Riedel ER, Bach PB, et al. Variations in morbidity after radical prostatectomy. N Engl J Med 2002;346(15):1138–44.
[70] Penson DF, Litwin MS, Aaronson NK. Health related quality of life in men with prostate cancer. J Urol 2003;169(5):1653–61.
[71] Walsh PC, Marschke P, Ricker D, et al. Patient-reported urinary continence and sexual function after anatomic radical prostatectomy. Urology 2000;55(1):58–61.
[72] Eastham JA, Kattan MW, Rogers E, et al. Risk factors for urinary incontinence after radical prostatectomy. J Urol 1996;156(5):1707–13.
[73] Catalona WJ, Carvalhal GF, Mager DE, et al. Potency, continence and complication rates in 1,870 consecutive radical retropubic prostatectomies. J Urol 1999;162(2):433–8.
[74] Potosky AL, Legler J, Albertsen PC, et al. Health outcomes after prostatectomy or radiotherapy for prostate cancer: results from the Prostate Cancer Outcomes Study. J Natl Cancer Inst 2000;92(19):1582–92.
[75] Wahle GR. Urinary incontinence after radical prostatectomy. Semin Urol Oncol 2000;18: 66–70.
[76] Bishoff JT, Motley G, Optenberg SA, et al. Incidence of fecal and urinary incontinence following radical perineal and retropubic prostatectomy in a national population. J Urol 1998;160:454–8.
[77] Stanford JL, Feng Z, Hamilton AS, et al. Urinary and sexual function after radical prostatectomy for clinically localized prostate cancer: the Prostate Cancer Outcomes study. JAMA 2000;283(3):354–60.
[78] Hu JC, Elkin EP, Pasta DJ, et al. Predicting quality of life after radical prostatectomy: results from CaPSURE. J Urol 2004;171(2 Pt 1):703–7.
[79] Penson DF, Stoddard ML, Pasta DJ, et al. The association between socioeconomic status, health insurance coverage, and quality of life in men with prostate cancer. J Clin Epidemiol 2001;54:350–8.
[80] Flanigan RC, Salmon SE, Blumenstein BA, et al. Nephrectomy followed by interferon alpha-2b compared with interferon alpha-2b alone for metastatic renal-cell cancer. N Engl J Med 2001;345(23):1655–9.
[81] Flanigan RC, Mickisch G, Sylvester R, et al. Cytoreductive nephrectomy in patients with metastatic renal cancer: a combined analysis. J Urol 2004;171(3):1071–6.
[82] Bristow RE, Montz FJ, Lagasse LD, et al. Survival impact of surgical cytoreduction in stage IV epithelial ovarian cancer. Gynecol Oncol 1999;72:278–87.

[83] Liu PC, Benjamin I, Morgan MA, et al. Effect of surgical debulking on survival in stage IV ovarian cancer. Gynecol Oncol 1997;64:4–8.
[84] Curtin JP, Malik R, Venkatraman ES, et al. Stage IV ovarian cancer: impact of surgical debulking. Gynecol Oncol 1997;64:9–12.
[85] Thompson IM, Tangen C, Basler J, et al. Impact of previous local treatment for prostate cancer on subsequent metastatic disease. J Urol 2002;168(3):1008–12.

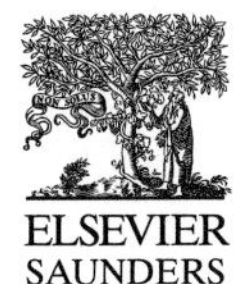

Surg Oncol Clin N Am
14 (2005) 321–352

SURGICAL
ONCOLOGY CLINICS
OF NORTH AMERICA

Bladder Cancer—Resection/Ablation

Federico A. Corica, MD, Thomas E. Keane, MB, FRCSI*

Department of Urology, Medical University of South Carolina, 96 Jonathan Lucas Street, CSB 644, PO Box 250620, Charleston, SC 29425, USA

Superficial bladder cancer is a misnomer commonly associated with a heterogeneous group of tumors that have not yet involved the detrusor muscle of the bladder (muscularis propria; stage T2) and includes stages Ta (no penetration of the lamina propria), Tis (carcinoma in situ [CIS]), and T1 (invasion of lamina propria into submucosa) of any grade. The treatment and prognosis of these tumors are different. Most superficial tumors present as Ta (70%), followed by T1 (20%) and CIS (10%).

Superficial bladder tumor recurrence and progression are influenced by tumor grade and stage. Currently, two grading systems are commonly in use and are often used interchangeably. The standard World Health Organization (WHO) grading system includes lesions graded as 1, 2, and 3, depending on the degree of differentiation. The International Society of Urologic Pathologists (ISUP) adopted a new grading system in 1998, which also attempted to include the biologic aggressiveness of superficial tumors. This grading system includes three classes: papillary neoplasms of low malignant potential, low-grade lesions, and high-grade lesions. Although low-grade Ta lesions frequently recur (50%–70%), they progress (5%) less often than high-grade T1 lesions (80% recurrence, 50% progression) within 3 years of resection [1]. Currently, there is no uniform system for grading superficial bladder cancer. Despite the recommended WHO/ISUP classification system, most pathologists still use the traditional numeric grading system (Table 1).

Tumor grade is a more important predictor of progression than stage because grade 3 tumors are 5 times more likely to progress than grade 1, compared with only twice the risk of progression for T1 stage tumors compared with lower stage Ta lesions [2]. CIS of the bladder is a high-grade, flat, noninvasive form of transitional cell cancer (TCC) which is associated

* Corresponding author. 96 Jonathan Lucas Street, CSB 644, Charleston, SC 29425.
E-mail address: keanet@musc.edu (T.E. Keane).

doi:10.1016/j.soc.2004.11.001 ***surgonc.theclinics.com***

Table 1
1998 World Health Organization/International Society of Urologic Pathologists classifications of superficial transitional cell cancer

Cancer type	Traditional system	WHO/ISUP classification
Papilloma	Grade 0	Papilloma
Well-differentiated TCC	Grade 1	Papillary urothelial neoplasia of low malignant potential
Moderately differentiated TCC	Grade 2	Low-grade urothelial carcinoma
Poorly differentiated TCC	Grade 3	High-grade urothelial carcinoma

with the highest recurrence (70%–80%) and progression (>50%) rates of any superficial bladder tumor [3]. The malignant potential of this lesion was frequently underestimated in the past, and it is still frequently misnamed as high-grade dysplasia. As can be seen in Table 2, it is ranked in the highest risk group in terms of recurrence, progression, and death [4].

Diagnosis

More than 80% of patients present with gross hematuria or irritative lower urinary tract symptoms. The standard workup of gross hematuria has classically included cystoscopy, upper urinary tract imaging, and urine cytology. Urine cytology is highly specific but poorly sensitive for the most common (low grade and stage) superficial bladder cancers. Its sensitivity ranges from 25% to 30% for low-grade to 75% to 80% for high-grade tumors.

Several biologic tumor markers have recently been characterized (Table 3). Their main advantage seems to be an improved sensitivity over standard urine cytology. Their degree of sensitivity, however, does not allow for replacement of cystoscopy at this time. Recent data from the current authors' institution suggest that fluorescence in situ hybridization (FISH) may detect molecular changes in urinary urothelial cells specific for cancer long before the disease is either visibly manifest or detectable by cytology. The sensitivity and specificity for FISH versus cytology were 100% and 11% and 60% and 100%, respectively, using histology as the gold standard. Furthermore, analysis of 95 patients with atypical cytologic findings revealed that 20% of patients ultimately developed TCC of the bladder. From the current authors'

Table 2
Superficial transitional cell cancer risk groups

Risk groups	Tumor types	5-y recurrence (%)	5-y progression (%)	5-y mortality (%)
1	TaG1, single T1G1	35	0	0
2	TaG2, single T1G2, and multifocal T1G1	45	1.8	0.73
3	Multifocal T1G2, CIS, and Ta/T1G3	54	15	9.5

Table 3
Urinary markers used in diagnosis of superficial bladder cancer

Urinary tumor marker [6]	Sensitivity (%)	Specificity (%)
Cytology	34	99
NMP-22	73	80
BTA TRAK	69	90
FISH [7–9]	73	91
Telomerase	77	99
HA-HAase [10]	88	81
Survivin [11]	64	93

experience and that of others it would seem that FISH is a significantly superior diagnostic tool than cytology for bladder cancer [5–11].

Treatment

Transurethral resection (TUR), the hallmark of treatment and staging of superficial bladder cancer, entails tumor resection under direct visualization with a loop electrocautery resectoscope or cold cup biopsy forceps. Diagnostic accuracy of superficial TCC by TUR is challenged by the inter-observer variability in pathologic assessment and the inadequacy of a single resection. Significant reclassification of high-risk superficial tumors with upstaging to invasive disease after central pathology review has been reported among patients participating in various European Organization for Research and Treatment of Cancer (EORTC) trials (Table 4) [12]. These results highlight the importance of central pathology review.

Repeat TUR enables the reappraisal of tumor stage and grade. Several reports have shown the value of second TUR as a staging tool, especially for high-risk tumors and in cases of incomplete tumor resection and absence of detrusor muscle (muscularis propria) in the initial biopsy specimen. Herr [13] reported a 76% residual tumor rate and significant tumor downstaging and upstaging (especially in the absence of detrusor muscle on the original specimen) in repeat TUR specimens. Upstaging resulted in a cystectomy being recommended for 20% of such patients (Table 5). A second biopsy reading is recommended in cases of high-risk superficial disease when aggressive treatment is entertained.

Table 4
Inter observer variability in pathologic assessment of high-grade/stage superficial bladder tumors

	Pathology review		
Initial diagnosis	Reclassified	Upstaged to invasive	Downstaged
T1G3	50%	10.6%	39.6%

Table 5
Pathologic outcomes of repeat transurethral resection

Stage at first TUR	Residual tumor (%)	CIS/Ta (%)	T1 (%)	T2 (%)	Upstaging (%)	Downstaging (%)
CIS	70	40	20	10	30	—
Ta	72	39	28	5	33	—
T1 w/o muscle	74	31	29	14	14	31
T1 w/muscle	83	17	17	49	49	17

Dalbagni et al [14] further studied the accuracy of a second TUR among 15 patients who underwent immediate cystectomy for high-risk T1 disease. Despite a significant residual tumor rate, no case of understaging was reported, suggesting that no further TURs are needed for patients whose bladders may be spared as a consequence of pathologic understaging of their disease (Table 6) [14].

The role of random bladder biopsies (RBBs) of normal-appearing bladder mucosa is controversial. Proponents argue that RBB findings influence tumor recurrence, progression rates, and therapeutic decisions. Opponents claim they add little to the prognostic factors for any individual tumor. RBBs of normal-appearing bladder mucosa show tumor in only 8% to 14% of cases [15,16]. May et al [16] reported 7% and 10.5% upstaging and therapy change rates, respectively, among 1033 patients undergoing RBBs during resection of primary tumors, mainly caused by incidental CIS. Mufti and Singh [17] reported an increased 5-year tumor recurrence rate if an RBB was positive (48% versus 16%); Kiemeney et al [18] noted increased 3-year tumor progression if an RBB showed CIS (31% versus 7%), and Fujimoto et al [19] concluded that positive urine cytology predicted CIS in RBBs.

Contrary to these findings, van der Meijden et al [15] concluded from data collected from EORTC trials 30863 and 30911 that RBBs do not contribute to therapy or staging of superficial bladder cancer.

Other forms of treatment of superficial bladder tumors include laser and photodynamic therapy. Laser (Nd:YAG) TUR is advocated by some groups because of minimal bleeding, the absence of obturator reflex, and reports of fewer recurrence rates than TUR in the treated area (5% versus 32%) [20]. Increased cost, lack of tissue for pathologic diagnosis, and the risk of perforation and injury of adjacent bowel have limited its acceptance, however.

Table 6
Impact of second transurethral resection for Ta–T1 transitional cell cancer[a]

	Cystectomy specimen		
	Residual tumor	Upstaging to invasive	Understaging
Second TUR (Ta–T1 w/CIS)	80%	6.7%	0%

[a] n = 15.

Photodynamic therapy involves the administration of an intravenous photosensitizing agent (a porphyrin derivative) followed by intravesical activation 48 hours later achieved by whole-bladder red-laser therapy for 15 to 20 minutes. Although the treatment is easy to deliver, significant early morbidity ensues, including hematuria (85%), irritative urinary symptoms (99%), bladder contracture (16%), and dermal sensitivity (19%). Also, treated patients must avoid direct sunlight for 6 to 8 weeks. In the only prospective randomized study, 33% of treated patients experienced recurrence at 13 months versus 83% of patients in the observation group 3 months after TUR [21].

Intravesical therapy

Despite predominately low grade and stage at diagnosis, superficial cancer is associated with high recurrence rates after TUR alone. This finding may be because of panurothelial instability leading to increased urothelial risk of malignant transformation or microscopic implantation of tumor cells following TUR. Recurrent papillary TCC is high grade in 15% to 30% of patients [22].

As mentioned previously, CIS is a high-grade, flat, and noninvasive form of TCC whose aggressive nature is frequently underestimated. Until quite recently, this lesion was frequently misnamed as high-grade dysplasia. Witjes [3] showed the malignant nature of this disease by reporting that in his series, within 5 years of TUR, 9 of 10 patients who received no adjuvant therapy experienced recurrence and 5 of 10 experienced progression of their disease.

Intravesical therapy is offered as an adjunct to TUR in an attempt to decrease recurrence, prevent progression, and eradicate residual disease after resection, particularly in intermediate- and high-risk tumors. Lower recurrence rates reduce or eliminate the need for further TUR and lower rates of progression, may reduce the need for radical cystectomy.

Common indications for intravesical therapy include the following: multiple primary tumors, frequent tumor recurrences, T1G3 tumors, tumor size greater than 3 cm, post-TUR positive urine cytology, and CIS in the pathologic specimen [22]. Several agents optimized for intravesical administration have been studied, including bacille Calmette-Guérin (BCG), thiotepa, mitomycin C (MMC), doxorubicin, epirubicin, and valrubicin.

Intravesical chemotherapy

Most of the agents in use are intercalating or alkylating agents that act by interrupting nucleic acid replication or other processes, resulting in cell death. Although toxicity can be a problem with all the agents, tissue trauma from the procedure and infection can disrupt the integrity of the urothelium with resultant systemic absorption of low-molecular-weight agents and significant toxicity if used in the immediate postoperative period. Such agents (eg, thiotepa) are therefore not recommended for immediate post-TUR use. Mitomycin and doxorubicin, however, have proved safe for immediate post-TUR instillation. Contraindications to immediate instillation include the following: allergy to the agent, previous systemic absorption, and suspected bladder perforation following TUR.

MMC seems to be the most effective intravesical chemotherapeutic agent [23]. According to Huncharek et al's [24] recent meta-analysis, MMC prophylaxis is associated with a 38% decrease in recurrence. A single, immediate post-TUR instillation has been found to be as efficacious as a year-long, every-3-month regimen (5-y recurrence rates of 47% versus 36%, respectively; $P = 0.14$) [25]. Moreover, Kaasinen et al [26] showed a twofold higher risk of tumor recurrence if the immediate MMC instillation was given later than the day of the TUR. The efficacy of MMC may be further enhanced by hyperthermia (Table 7) [27]. For CIS, however, MMC is not first-line treatment because it is associated with only a 50% response rate compared with rates of 70% to 75% following BCG [3]. Increasing dose concentration (lower instillation volume), limiting urine production, and alkalinizing the urine are all strategies which have been utilized to increase treatment efficacy [28–30]. Multiple weekly therapies do not add efficacy and maintenance intravesical chemotherapy has not been shown to be effective [22].

MMC is associated with mild to moderate lower urinary symptoms (because of chemical cystitis), contact dermatitis commonly presenting as palmar or perineal desquamation, and, rarely, bladder contracture [22]. Controversy remains as to the exact role for intravesical chemotherapy because most meta-analyses and long-term reviews show little, if any, benefit in terms of recurrence and progression versus TUR alone.

Intravesical immunotherapy

BCG, a live, attenuated mycobacterium initially developed as a tuberculosis vaccine, is considered the most effective form of intravesical therapy. It is currently used as adjuvant treatment for CIS, residual papillary TCC (ablative therapy), and prophylaxis for recurrent superficial cancer. BCG is tumoricidal, and it is considered to have two mechanisms of action: (1) a direct binding to normal and malignant urothelial cells, leading to cytokine secretion and decreased tumor proliferation, and (2) activation of cellular immunity. Cytokines attract mononuclear cells, including mono-

Table 7
Summary of relevant mitomycin C treatment option outcomes

2-y outcome	TUR alone (%) [29]	TUR + immediate MMC (%) [29]	TUR + 12-mo MMC (%) [25]	TUR + MMC + hyperthermia (%) [30]
Recurrence	34.3	15.8 (low-risk TCC) [29]; 38 (all TCC) [25]	30	7 (low-risk TCC); 24.6
Progression	1.5	1.7	1.5	0

cytes, dendritic cells, and T-helper (Th) lymphocytes, leading to granuloma formation. Antigen-presenting cells interact with CD4+ lymphocytes and natural killer (NK) cells by means of γ-interferon (IFN-γ), interleukin 2 (IL-2), and IL-12 (Th-1 cytokines), resulting in BCG-activated killer (BAK; activated NK cell) cells and tumoricidal γ-IFNs. BAK cells exert their tumorcidal effect by means of perforins [31].

BCG therapy yields better results than chemotherapeutic agents for high-grade TCC (Table 8). A number of meta-analysis of randomized trials [32–34] showed that BCG was superior to MMC in preventing tumor recurrences, particularly the BCG maintenance arm, irrespective of tumor risk status.

Randomized prospective studies in the 1980s, comparing BCG to various chemotherapeutic intravesical protocols, have shown an average 40% and 14% reduction in tumor recurrence and progression respectively, when compared with TUR alone (Tables 9 and 10) [35,36]. Encouraging results from early BCG randomized trials were later tempered by data from long-term studies suggesting that, although BCG delays tumor recurrence, it does not prevent tumor progression (see Table 10; Table 11) [36,37]. Extravesical recurrences occur in up to 1 in 5 patients, either in the upper urinary tract (21%) or the prostatic urethra (19%) [37].

Cookson et al [37] reported a median time to cystectomy of 8 and 24 months in the TUR alone and TUR plus BCG groups, respectively. At 15 years, 35% of patients had died of TCC, and cancer-specific survival was 63%.

Maintenance BCG therapy was the logical next step to improve on the early successes of BCG induction. The objective of maintenance therapy is to extend the benefits of induction BCG by delaying the first recurrence in hopes of prolonging time to disease progression. Lamm et al [38] reported the results of the Southwest Oncology Group trial (SWOG-8507) comparing BCG induction versus maintenance therapy. With the exception of cancer-specific survival, lower rates of recurrence and progression were reported in the BCG maintenance arm (Table 12). Maintenance BCG (up to 3 y) is advocated for CIS and Ta/T1 TCC associated with CIS.

A significant problem of BCG maintenance has been treatment toxicity. A significant 84% of patients failed to complete the full BCG maintenance protocol because of toxicity in SWOG-8507 [38]. This figure contrasts with a rate of only 20% in BCG maintenance discontinuation in a recent EORTC trial [39], which used the same BCG dose and schedule as in SWOG-8507. Furthermore, 70% of dropouts in the EORTC trial occurred during BCG induction or shortly afterwards [39]. Stricter indications for discontinuation of BCG therapy in the SWOG trial seem to have accounted for the difference in BCG maintenance completion rates.

Because of BCG-related toxicity, reduced-dose schedules have been tested. Martinez-Pineiro et al [40] noted similar recurrence, progression, and cancer-specific survival in the reduced-dose arm compared with the standard

Table 8
Meta-analyses of randomized trials of intravesical bacille Calmette-Guérin and mitomycin C [32]

First author	n	Trials included	Follow-up (y)	For recurrence	For progression	Toxicity
Bohle [32]	1421	11	2	BCG maintenance (38%) >BCG induction > MMC (46%) Full-dose BCG = reduced-dose BCG	—	BCG maintenance = BCG induction
Shelley [33]	1527	6	2–7	BCG>MMC (31% advantage) Full-dose BCG = reduced-dose BCG	BCG = MMC	BCG = MMC
Bohle [34]	1277	9	2	—	BCG maintenance (7.6%) > BCG induction > MMC (9.4%)	—

Abbreviations: =, similar to; >, better than; <, worse than.

Table 9
Recurrence after transurethral resection alone versus transurethral resection + bacille Calmette-Guérin [35]

5-y outcome	TUR alone (%)	TUR + BCG (%)
Recurrence-free	10	48
Progression-free	53	78

dose. Because of a nonstatistically significant trend toward better specific survival rates in the standard-dose group, however, these authors advised against a reduced-dose schedule for high-risk patients. A dose of 27 mg of BCG was less effective than the standard dose in patients with three or more tumors (Table 13).

All BCG strains used in different trials seem to be equally effective [41], and lower doses, in patients with toxicity to full doses, have shown similar efficacy [42]. Incomplete BCG induction, however, seems to be associated with an increased risk of tumor recurrence [43]. According to the European Association of Urology Working Groups on Oncological Urology, BCG administration is discouraged for patients with low-risk TCC because its efficacy does not outweigh the potential toxicity [44]. Prophylactic isoniazid also is not recommended because it does not reduce the incidence of side effects [45] and animal studies have shown decreased BCG efficacy [46]. Contraindications to BCG administration include previous BCG sepsis, active urinary tract infection, gross hematuria, and immunosuppression.

Contrary to popular belief, Sylvester et al [47] reported that the degree of local or systemic BCG toxicity is not related to a lower risk of recurrence.

Complications of bacille Calmette-Guérin therapy

During BCG therapy, 70% to 90% of patients complain of some degree of dysuria, hematuria, and irritative lower urinary symptoms. Malaise, fatigue, and lethargy are reported by up to 20% of patients. More severe complications are rare (Table 14). Uncommon complications include the following: conversion to purified protein derivative (PPD)+ state, symptomatic granulomatous prostatitis, hepatitis, and contracted bladder.

Table 10
Progression after transurethral resection alone versus transurethral resection + bacille Calmette-Guérin [36]

Progression-free at	TUR alone (%)	TUR + BCG (%)
5 y	54	78
5–10 y	45	65
15 y	25	60

Table 11
Long-term recurrence and progression rates [37]

Treatment	Recurrence (%) 2 y	Recurrence (%) 15 y	Progression (%) 2 y	Progression (%) 6 y	Progression (%) 15 y
TUR alone	37	100	35	35*	53
TUR + BCG	0	100	7	28*	53

* $P > 0.05$.

Second-line intravesical chemotherapy

Before salvage intravesical therapy is considered, the physician has to define when superficial TCC is refractory to BCG. Herr and Dalbagni [48] suggested waiting for at least 6 months after BCG therapy to label a tumor refractory. They argued that labeling a tumor refractory before 6 months will artificially inflate the successes of second-line intravesical therapy. Greenberg and Ignatoff [49] defined BCG-refractory TCC as that which persists or recurs following two courses of BCG or BCG plus chemotherapy. Second-line intravesical chemotherapy strategies include repeat BCG, BCG plus IFN, and valrubicin. Either second-induction or maintenance BCG therapy following failure after single-induction therapy has been reported to effect significant response rates. A third BCG course following failed a second BCG course is associated with much lower response rates [50].

IFN is a biologic response modifier found to act synergistically with BCG by potentiating Th-lymphocyte response by means of inhibition of IL-10 production. Initial small-scale, nonrandomized studies provided evidence of acceptable recurrence-free survival rates for the combination of BCG plus IFN-α as salvage for BCG failure [51–53]. The current authors' experience has mirrored the previously described findings and suggests that patients who have failed two or more courses of BCG may frequently respond to the combination therapy. Those patients who did progress to cystectomy were not disadvantaged by the therapy in terms of disease stage [54]. Interim 2-year data analysis from an ongoing randomized trial of BCG plus IFN-α attests to its safety, but data are still immature to assess outcomes (Table 15) [55]. This therapy may prove particularly useful in patients who have

Table 12
Outcomes of bacille Calmette-Guérin maintenance therapy from the Southwest Oncology Group trial 8507 [38]

5-y outcome	No BCG maintenance	BCG maintenance
Recurrence-free	41%	60%*
Progression-free	70%	76%*
Cancer-specific survival	78%	83%
Time to recurrence	36 mo	77 mo

* $P < 0.05$.

Table 13
Outcome of reduced-dose bacille Calmette-Guérin therapy [40]

5-y outcome	Reduced BCG, 27 mg (%)	Standard BCG, 81 mg (%)
Recurrence-free	69	70*
Progression-free	86	88*
Cancer-specific survival	7.5	7.9*

* $P > 0.05$.

experienced toxic side effects of BCG because a dose reduction to one third or even one tenth of the standard BCG dose has achieved equivalent results.

Valrubicin is approved by the US Food and Drug Administration for the treatment of BCG-refractory CIS in patients who could not undergo immediate cystectomy. Steinberg et al [56] treated 90 patients with BCG-refractory CIS with six weekly instillations of valrubicin (800 mg). A complete response was noted in 19 patients (21%), which lasted a median of 18 months. Progression to stage T2 disease occurred in two (3%) patients. Half of the nonresponders underwent cystectomy, of whom six (15%) had pathologic stage T3 or greater disease. Four (5%) of the nonresponders died of bladder cancer. The authors favored radical cystectomy only for those with T1 and worse recurrences, particularly because of the relatively low valrubicin response rate and the availability of more effective modified bladder-sparing protocols. This therapy is therefore rarely used in the management of this high-risk population.

Table 14
bacille Calmette-Guérin complications and treatment

BCG toxicity	Hospitalization	Treatment	Discontinue BCG?	Resume BCG?
Dysuria, hematuria	No	Phenazopyridine, anticholinergics	No	—
Temperature				
>101.5°F for <24 h	No	NSAIDs	No	—
>101.5°F for >24 h	Maybe	INH (300 mg orally) for 3 mo	Yes	When asymptomatic
>103°F and/or BCG sepsis	Yes	Blood cultures Immediate prednisolone 40 mg IV + cycloserine or quinolones (bactericidal within 24 h) INH + RIF ± ETH for 6 mo (bactericidal within 7 d)	Yes	Never again

Abbreviations: ETH, ethambutol; INH, isoniazid; NSAIDs, nonsteroidal anti-inflammatory drugs; RIF, Rifampin.

Table 15
Outcomes and toxicity of bacille Calmette-Guérin + interferon-α in the BCG-failure group[a] [55]

Recurrence	Progression to T2	Metastasis	Cystectomy	Cancer-specific mortality	Toxicity	Treatment termination
52%	4.3%	2.3%	3.9%	0.83%	3.9%	12.6%

[a] n = 231.

Prognostic factors

Multiple prognostic factors for recurrence have been reported in the literature. Millan-Rodriguez et al [4] derived prognostic factors from one of the largest series of superficial TCC (> 1500 patients; Table 16). High-grade TCC was associated with the highest risk for progression and mortality but not recurrence. Furthermore, tumor stage was not an independent prognostic factor in multivariate analysis. Only 25% of the patients received BCG. The prognosis after intravesical immunotherapy is affected by several factors. Importantly, tumor grade was predictive of progression but not recurrence [4]; incomplete BCG induction was predictive of both (Tables 17 and 18) [43,57]. With the advances in molecular biology, a new generation of potential progression markers is under investigation and includes p53, p21, Ki-67,CK-20, E-cadherin expression, and EGFR and VEGF expression.

Cystectomy for superficial transitional cell cancer

Cystectomy for superficial bladder cancer is a treatment typically reserved for high-risk (T1, high grade, with or without CIS; failure of local therapies, including resection/ablation and adjuvant strategies) patients who do not wish to run the risk of progression of their disease beyond the confines of the bladder. Experts who advocate this procedure for high-risk or recurrent CIS/papillary tumor after BCG will do so typically [49] for technically unresectable tumors [58] and in the case of concomitant CIS, which causes higher risk of invasive cancer [59]. The rationale for this approach is based on the fact that tumor progression after BCG failure is 50% (82% among those that recur within 3 mo, and 25% among those

Table 16
Multivariate analysis prognostic factors following transurethral resection [4]

Prognostic factors	5-y recurrence	5-y progression	5-y mortality
High-grade (G3) tumor	No	Yes (RR, 19.9)	Yes (RR, 14)
Tumor multifocality	Yes (RR, 2)	Yes (RR, 1.9)	No
Concomitant CIS	Yes (RR, 1.65)	Yes (RR, 2.1)	Yes (RR, 3)
Tumor size >3 cm	Yes (RR, 1.65)	Yes (RR, 1.7)	No
Previous BCG therapy	Yes (RR, 0.39)	Yes (RR, 0.3)	No

Abbreviation: RR, relative risk.

Table 17
Multivariate analysis of predictors of poor outcome following transurethral resection + bacille Calmette-Guérin [43,57]

Recurrence	Progression	Mortality
Male gender	Previous TUR	Urethral invasion
Previous TUR	Tumor onset within last 12 mo	Solid/sessile tumor
High grade (G3)	High-grade tumor (G3)	
Multifocality	Presence of T1 and/or CIS tumor	
p53 Overexpression	Tumor size	
Incomplete BCG induction	p53 Overexpression	
No BCG maintenance	Incomplete BCG induction	
	Positive cytology at first surveillance	
	CIS and/or T1 tumor at first surveillance	

whose cancers recur later); the 10-year survival rate after cystectomy for superficial TCC ranges from 67% and 92%. Finally, in patients with intact bladders, the rate of T1 disease recurrence is 50%, with a 30% rate of cancer-related deaths over 15 years [37]. Another area of controversy is the timing of cystectomy. Herr and Sogani [60] reported a 92% 15-year cancer-specific survival rate after BCG failure provided cystectomy was undertaken within the first 2 years, compared with a rate of only 56% among those whose bladder was removed after 2 years. In contrast, Thalmann et al [61] reported better 5-year cancer-specific survival rates among the delayed cystectomy group (80% versus 69%). A significant problem is that currently there are no reliable markers for prediction of tumor progression or mortality.

Follow-up after bacille Calmette-Guérin

The follow-up for patients diagnosed with superficial bladder cancer has been controversial, with many studies looking for alternatives to cystoscopy, particularly in the area of urinary markers. Despite much progress, to date no urinary test has yet been proved to have the sensitivity or specificity to replace regular cystoscopy. Typically, initial follow-up has included cystoscopy at 3 months and at three monthly intervals for 2 years, then six monthly intervals for another 2 years, and then yearly for another year. Urinary markers are checked at each cystoscopy. If the patient has completed an induction course of BCG, then a cystoscopy and RBBs are

Table 18
Multivariate analysis of predictors of poor outcome following transurethral resection + bacille Calmette-Guérin if first surveillance cystoscopy is negative [43]

Recurrence	Progression
Male gender	Stage T1
Incomplete BCG induction	Incomplete BCG induction
No BCG maintenance	

undertaken 6 weeks after completion of BCG and the previously described follow-up plan is then implemented.

For patients with low-risk disease, recommended follow-up can include cystoscopy at 9 months, if initial cystoscopy is negative, and can be continued for at least 5 years. In this situation, three monthly cytologies are recommended, although, at the current authors' institution, FISH has replaced cytology because of its better sensitivity and specificity. In these circumstances, the assumption has been made that because the initial disease was low risk, any recurrence will be similar, and even if not picked up by urinary markers, a cystoscopy interval of 9 months will still allow curative management by local endoscopic resection.

For patients with high-risk disease, cystoscopy and cytology are recommended every 3 months during the first year, and every 3 to 6 months during the second year. Cystoscopy is undertaken every 6 months thereafter for 5 years, and then yearly. Cytologies and or other urinary markers should be examined at each cystoscopy [62]. Skemp and Fernandes [63] have suggested that in patients with Ta or T1 disease without CIS initial follow-up after BCG therapy, with office cystoscopy is acceptable if cytology is negative; however, the authors still favor biopsies. It is important to realize that superficial TCC of the bladder may recur or progress many years after diagnosis (Table 19) [64,65].

Tumor prophylaxis and bacille Calmette-Guérin

Following complete resection of T1 and high-grade Ta lesions, BCG treatment decreases recurrence rates when compared with TUR alone by approximately 40%. Progression rates have varied depending on the series, from 4% to 40%, which shows the need to define more accurate prognostic markers than just pathologic features, tumor number and size, and presence of CIS [36,66]. Although recurrence is significantly reduced with the addition of BCG, the question of preventing progression is more controversial. In the short term, there has been evidence to support a reduction in progression [67]; however, as follow-up is continued to more than 10 years, the delay in progression rates and concomitant reduction in cystectomy rates may be diminished, and further long-term studies are required [37].

Table 19
Timeline of recurrence and progression of Ta and T1 transitional cell cancer

Years after initial treatment	Recurrence (%) [64]	Progression (%) [65]
0–5 y	43	1
5–10 y	22	4
10–15 y	2	3
15–20 y	—	1

Invasive bladder cancer

Approximately 20% to 25% of bladder cancers are muscle-invasive at presentation. Despite diagnostic advances, the incidence of de novo muscle-invasive TCC has remained unchanged over the last 15 years (27%–29%) [68]. When cystectomy series are considered, however, de novo muscle-invasive TCC has decreased in frequency as an indication for surgery (from 85% to 57%) [69]. Currently, 70% of invasive bladder cancers present de novo, and 30% progress from superficial TCC [70]. Women are more likely to present with invasive bladder cancer than men (Table 20) [69].

Radical cystectomy remains the standard of care for invasive TCC. It allows assessment of risk of recurrence and mortality and, with pelvic lymphadenectomy, is the only therapy to date providing the best local disease control and long-term disease-free survival. This approach has been extensively reported in the United States and in the world literature, and it has proved highly successful in disease control and long-term survival. Recent improvements in nerve-sparing techniques and orthotopic neobladder diversion, including better understanding of the associated metabolic complications, have improved patient functionality and quality of life (QOL), which has been reported similar to age-matched control subjects [71]. Furthermore, recent advances in surgical technique, anesthesia care, and postoperative management have reduced the morbidity and mortality of the procedure. Current perioperative mortality rates are less than 2% [72].

Diagnosis

TUR and bimanual examination under anesthesia constitute the initial diagnostic approach.

The metastatic workup commonly includes CT scan or MRI of the abdomen and pelvis with contrast, chest radiograph, liver function tests, and, unusually, a bone scan. Suspicious chest radiographs are followed by CT scan of the chest. Staging CT scan of the pelvis should be scheduled before TUR biopsy to avoid the confounding artifact produced by the endoscopic resection. Pathologic understaging of invasive bladder TCC in TUR specimens approaches 45% [73], a figure that almost doubles in cases of incomplete tumor resection. Radiologic staging is also suboptimal because of low imaging yields.

Despite outperforming TUR and bimanual examination, CT scan has limited accuracy for detection of extravesical tumor extension and pelvic

Table 20
Gender differences in presentation of muscle-invasive bladder cancer [69]

Cancer type	Male (%)	Female (%)
De novo invasive TCC	51	85

lymph node (LN) and distant metastasis. Specifically, CT scan is unable to detect microscopic or small-volume extravesical and pelvic LN tumor invasion, resulting in significant understaging. Paik et al [74] noted that CT scan provides limited additional staging information (9.8%), alters management in a small group of patients (3.7%), and, rarely, avoids unnecessary surgery (1.2%; Table 21) [74]. Some experts advocate limiting the use of preoperative CT scanning to cases in which advanced local or metastatic cancer are suspected. MRI does not offer significant staging advantage over CT scan, except in cases of iodinated contrast allergy or renal insufficiency [75,76].

Treatment

Surgical approaches include radical or partial cystectomy, bladder conservation therapies, and adjunctive chemo- or radiotherapy.

Partial cystectomy

Partial cystectomy is a procedure reserved for highly selected patients and only rarely indicated. Approximately 6% to 9% of patients with invasive TCC undergo partial cystectomy [77]. The classic indications include tumors at the bladder dome or inside a diverticulum without associated CIS. Associated CIS, pelvic LN metastasis, tumor multifocality, and positive frozen surgical margins are associated with an increased risk of tumor recurrence. A recent report of 58 patients who underwent partial cystectomy revealed a 69% recurrence-free survival rate at 33 months. Tumor recurred in 56% of the cases, 50% locally and the rest distantly. No operative mortality was recorded, the mean hospital stay was 6 days, and 12% of patients experienced minor morbidity [77].

Radical cystectomy

Radical cystectomy is the standard therapy for invasive cancer bladder for various reasons. If untreated, invasive bladder cancer kills four of five patients within 2 years of diagnosis [78]. Radio- and chemotherapy are not as effective as surgical tumor removal [79], and bladder-sparing approaches, such as partial cystectomy or repeated TUR, result in delayed cystectomy for tumor progression in almost 50% of cases [80]. Last, morbidity and mortality of radical cystectomy have substantially declined over the past two decades [81].

Table 21
Staging value of CT scan in invasive bladder cancer

Staging CT scan [1]	Overall (%)	Extravesical extension (%)	LN metastasis (%)	Distant metastasis (%)
Accuracy	54.9	4.9	4.9	2.4
Understaging	39	20–35 [74,76]	20–25 [74,76]	0

Besides the bladder, the prostate is removed in men, and the uterus, broad ligaments, and anterior half of the vagina are removed in women (ie, anterior pelvic exenteration). Recent technical improvements include nerve, prostate, and seminal vesicle-sparing cystectomy to preserve urine continence, potency, and fertility. The performance of these techniques seems not to compromise cancer control when compared with nonsparing surgery. A total recovery rate of 43% of sexual function has been reported [82]. Nerve-sparing surgery may have more impact on urine continence than on potency. Older men may benefit the most from improved continence and younger men, having stronger urinary sphincters, benefit from better potency rates. The preservation of the neurovascular bundle opposite to the tumor side has been advocated [81].

In women, the removal of the anterior half of the vagina has been noted to be associated with higher blood loss during surgery (1.4 L versus 0.5 L), requiring more blood transfusion and longer ICU stay compared with their male counterparts [83]. The preservation of the anterior vaginal wall has been advocated by Schoenberg et al [84] to improve urinary continence following orthotopic urinary diversion. TCC extension into the vagina is rare (1%–3% of cases) and easily identified during surgery in almost all cases [85].

The final commitment to orthotopic neobladder cannot be made until intraoperative frozen-section analysis shows the distal urethral margin to be free of tumor. The presence of bladder cancer at the bladder neck in women is predictive of urethral TCC and constitutes a relative contraindication for orthotopic diversion (Table 22) [86].

Intraoperative analysis of ureteral margins before the urinary diversion is completed is standard practice. Residual TCC, especially CIS, can involve the ureter. Schoenberg et al [87] reported that six patients with positive ureteral margin for TCC were free of recurrence 41 months after surgery. Silver et al [88] noted a 10% rate of upper tract recurrence among 30 patients with CIS at the ureteral margin on final pathology, 17% of which were not identified on intra-operative frozen section. Upper urinary tract recurrence was not associated with positive ureteral margin status, and expectant management was recommended. The false-negative rate of frozen pathology, minimal morbidity, and apparent lack of prognostic significance of a positive ureteral margin call into question the value of intraoperative analysis of ureteral margins.

Table 22
Intraoperative prediction of transitional cell cancer of the urethra [86]

Bladder neck TCC	Likelihood of urethral tumor (%)
Yes	50*
No	0*

* $P < 0.05$.

The indications for radical cystectomy, not its efficacy, are presently the subject of intense debate. The impetus is placed in broadening the indications for bladder-sparing therapy and tailoring treatment to the individual patient.

Pelvic lymphadenectomy

Another area of controversy is the role of pelvic lymphadenectomy as a staging and therapeutic adjunct to radical cystectomy. Cystectomy for cancer cures 60% to 80% of patients with cancer confined to the bladder wall, 40% to 50% of those invading the perivesical fat, and 20% to 30% of those with node-positive disease [89]. The risk of LN involvement performing standard pelvic lymphadenectomy is directly related to tumor stage. Stages pT2 and pT3 are associated with pelvic LN metastasis in 10% to 30% and 30% to 65% of cases, respectively [90].

The total number of LNs removed, total number of positive LNs, and density of positive LNs seem to be directly correlated with recurrence and survival [91]. Several reports [92–94] have shown that patients whose LN dissection included more than 11 LNs enjoyed a significantly lower recurrence rate and longer survival. Poulsen et al [95] noted that extending the boundaries of standard LN dissection effected an improved survival among patients undergoing cystectomy, regardless of LN status. More than eight positive LNs are believed to be associated with worse survival [94]. Last, LN density, defined as the number of positive LNs divided by the total number of LNs removed, is also associated with prognosis. Those patients with more than 20% positive LN density are at increased risk for tumor recurrence [94].

Increased node removal is beneficial to survival; however, is this benefit from the increased number of nodes resected or because of the retrieval of metastatic nodes outside the bounds of the standard dissection, which would otherwise have been left behind? Sanderson et al [96] have recently examined this issue and concluded that in view of the unpredictable lymphatic drainage of the bladder, skip lesions in the pelvic nodes, and the frequent presence of nodal metastases above the iliac bifurcation, the benefit is the result of a more comprehensive bilateral resection of metastatic disease, which would not otherwise have been removed. These authors further pointed out that many patients undergoing radical cystectomy do not receive an adequate node dissection despite the fact that in patients with advanced local disease, local control, prevention of distant metastases, and survival can all be influenced by extended surgical resection. Those patients with presumed low-stage disease are also negatively impacted because many of these patients do not receive any node dissection, which, given the 5% incidence of occult nodal disease in this group, denies them an opportunity for cure [97].

Lymphadenectomy should include the obturator, external, and common iliac lymph nodes, with the proximal boundary being the distal aorta, laterally, the genitofemoral nerve and distally the circumflex iliac vein and lymph node of Cloquet. More limited dissections proximally and laterally have been used [98]. Because patients with nodal involvement may experience extended survival even without adjuvant therapy [99], however, more extensive dissections, including dissection of the aorta and inferior vena cava distal to the inferior mesenteric artery that includes resection of the left para-aortic, interaortic, and right para caval and presacral nodes along with the common and external iliac and obturator nodes, have been advocated [99].

Role of extended lymphadenectomy

Extended lymphadenectomy has been advocated for several reasons. Accurate pathologic staging is only possible after lymphadenectomy because one in four to five patients have clinically unsuspected LN metastasis. Approximately 20% to 30% of patients with LN involvement experience survival rates of 5 years or more by surgery alone. Last, a more anatomic and safer cystectomy is possible after careful lymphadenectomy [81]. No standard for pelvic lymphadenectomy has been defined or accepted. The extended approach to this procedure recovers 38% more LNs than the standard approach (Table 23) [97,100]. The incidence of LN involvement above the aortic bifurcation increases with pathologic stage [101]. Of patients with stage pT3-4 disease, 16% to 18%, as opposed to only 3% with pT2 bladder cancer, are found to have LN metastasis outside the boundaries for standard lymphadenectomy [97,101]. Despite skip pelvic LN metastasis, the periaortic or common iliac nodes are infrequently involved [97]. Extended lymphadenectomy requires up to 60 minutes longer to perform compared with the standard procedure, and it should be performed bilaterally, regardless of tumor location. Opposite LNs are involved in 10% to 40% of cases [97,102]. The number of LNs removed is inversely associated with risk of progression and directly associated with survival (Table 24) [92]. A finding of more than 11 (if LN-negative status) and 13 (if LN-positive status) removed LNs is associated with improved survival [92]. Finally, Brossner et al [103] noted that extended lymphadenectomy is not associated with higher complication rates than is standard lymphadenectomy (Table 25).

Chemotherapy

Surgical failure to control bladder cancer results from occult metastatic disease present at the time of surgery. Current imaging modalities are

Table 23
Median number of lymph nodes removed by standard versus extended lymphadenectomy [101]

Standard (range)	Extended (range)
13 (1–46)	34 (3–96)

Table 24
Treatment outcome by number of nodes removed [94]

No. nodes examined	5-y recurrence (%)	5-y survival (%)
<11	12.7	38.5*
≥11	5.5	76*

* $P < 0.05$.

suboptimally sensitive, and no reliable serum biomarker for this disease exists. Initial studies showed that combination chemotherapy is more effective than single-agent treatment [104]. The chemotherapeutic combination of methotrexate, vinblastine, adriamycin, and cisplatin (MVAC) emerged as the standard of treatment for patients with metastatic disease, outperforming other regimens [105]. Although MVAC significantly delays progression and improves survival, few patients achieve cure, and the side effects of this regimen are significant. A recent randomized trial proved the gemcitabine/cisplatin (GC) combination to be as effective as MVAC but associated with less toxicity [106]. Although underpowered to prove equivalence of GC to MVAC, this 405-patient trial showed equivalent complete and partial responses rates associated with a lower death rate, fewer infections, and less mucositis.

Efforts at integrating chemotherapy to cystectomy for bladder cancer have been sought. The rationale for this approach is that patient performance status is optimal and the burden of metastatic disease is minimal.

Neoadjuvant chemotherapy

The goal of this approach is to render bladder cancer resectable and to reduce the burden of micrometastatic disease before surgery. The risks of overtreating organ-confined disease and delaying surgery must be accounted for, however. Although preceded by three randomized trials showing no survival advantage of this approach over cystectomy alone, Grossman et al [107] reported a significant survival benefit in the neoadjuvant MVAC arm of the study. A total of 317 patients were randomized to MAVC (3 cycles) followed by cystectomy or to cystectomy alone. Median survival time was

Table 25
Morbidity of extended lymphadenectomy compared with the standard approach [104]

Morbidity	Standard	Extended
Overall complication rate	37%	43%*
Surgery for complications	9%	11%*
Blood transfusion (No. units)	3.2	0.7*
Lymphocele	None	None

* $P > 0.05$.

77 months and 46 months in the combination and cystectomy-alone groups, respectively ($P = 0.06$), accounting for a 25% reduction in the risk of death. The survival benefit of neoadjuvant MVAC seemed to be related to tumor downstaging: 38% of patients in this group had stage pT0 disease compared with only 15% of patients in the cystectomy-alone arm ($P < 0.001$). A recent meta-analysis of randomized neoadjuvant chemotherapy trials reported by the Medical Research Council Clinical Trials Unit [108] revealed a 13% reduction in the risk of death and an absolute survival benefit of 5% at 5 years, from 45% to 50%, compared with cystectomy alone. Neoadjuvant chemotherapy has been advocated for patients for clinical pT3-4 disease with or without suspected regional LN metastasis. This treatment scheme may also benefit patients with micrometastatic disease involving LNs above the bifurcation of the common iliac arteries.

Perioperative chemotherapy, neo- plus adjuvant chemotherapy, has been devised to limit precystectomy complications and the risk of overtreating organ-confined disease. Millikan et al [109] randomized 140 patients to either 2 cycles of neochemotherapy followed by 3 adjuvant cycles of MVAC or 5 cycles postoperatively. Similar time to recurrence, overall and cancer-specific survival, protocol noncompletion rates (12.8% and 10%, $P > 0.05$), and chemotherapy deaths (9%) were reported. Clinical understaging was significant (23%), especially in the presence of lymphovascular invasion (61%). The latter was predictive of higher pathologic stage, but it was not associated with poorer survival, which was a mean of 6.8 years following therapy.

Adjuvant chemotherapy

The goal of this therapy scheme is to tailor chemotherapy to those patients likely to benefit the most based on the more reliable pathologic staging and to reduce the complications of cystectomy following chemotherapy. Treatment of micrometastatic disease is delayed, assessment of objective response becomes impossible because there is no measurable disease, and debilitated patients following surgery may never receive chemotherapy, however. Millikan et al [109] reported similar protocol noncompletion rates. The authors reported that 9 of 70 patients (12.8%) did not complete the chemotherapy regimen following surgery and 7 of 70 (10%) did not undergo surgery following neoadjuvant chemotherapy ($P > 0.05$) [109].

Few randomized trials have assessed the efficacy of adjuvant chemotherapy. Skinner et al [110] randomized 91 patients to cystectomy plus cisplatin cyclophosphamide adriamycin (CISCA) versus cystectomy alone. Three-year recurrence and cancer-specific death rates were significantly improved over cystectomy alone (30% and 50%, respectively; $P < 0.05$). Subsequent statistical analysis of the data only showed significant benefit in delaying recurrence without affecting survival [111]. Stockle et al [112] reported significant 5-year progression delay and survival improvement rates in a series of 83 patients receiving MVAC or methotrexate, vinblastine, etoposide, and cisplatin, or MVEC, following cystectomy. These results are difficult to interpret because of selection bias. Randomization to either combination therapy or cystectomy alone was closed at 3 years because of significant advantage for the combination therapy arm and the later inclusion of nonrandomized patients render the data difficult to interpret. Freiha et al [113] randomized 55 patients with locally advanced bladder cancer to cisplatin, methotrexate, and vinblastine (CMV; 4 cycles) followed by cystectomy or surgery alone. Tumor recurrence was significantly delayed (37 and 12 mo, respectively; $P < 0.05$), but no survival advantage could be assessed. Possibly, survival was not affected because patients in the observation arm were given CMV at the time of relapse. In summary, data from randomized trials are insufficient to recommend chemotherapy immediately following surgery. An ongoing randomized trial (EORTC 30994) is set to recruit more than 1000 patients to either adjuvant or salvage chemotherapy following cystectomy. An ongoing SWOG trial is evaluating the effects of adjuvant MVAC (3 cycles) on patients with altered p53 expression.

Salvage chemotherapy

MVAC remains the gold standard for metastatic disease. Newer combination chemotherapies have been tested. A recent phase 3 trial comparing MVAC to GC [106] showed similar overall survival, but patients in the GC arm experienced less toxicity. As a result, the GC regimen is considered an acceptable standard regimen for metastatic and locally advanced bladder cancer. Taxanes in combination with GC also have been studied [114]. In addition, omitting cisplatin to reduce renal complications among patients with impaired renal function has been explored (Table 26) [115,116].

Radiotherapy

To the current authors' knowledge, there are no randomized trials comparing surgery to radiotherapy alone in the literature. A meta-analysis of randomized trials comparing neoadjuvant radiotherapy to radiotherapy

Table 26
Newer chemotherapeutic regimens for metastatic bladder cancer

Regimen	Complete response (%)	Partial response (%)	Survival (mo)	Time to progression (mo)	Toxicity
MVAC [107]	11.9	33.8	15	7.4	3% deaths, 12% sepsis
GC [107]	12.2	37.2	14	7.4	1% deaths, 1% sepsis
GC + paclitaxel [115]	27	50	24	N/R	2% deaths
G + paclitaxel [116]	7	47	14	9	2% deaths
G + docetaxel [117]	7.5	26	13	5	No deaths or sepsis

Abbreviations: C, cisplatin; G, gemcitabine.

with salvage cystectomy was recently reported [117]. Analysis of the data suggested better survival among those undergoing immediate surgery than salvage surgery.

Bladder-preservation protocols

Although controversial, the concept of bladder-sparing therapy is extremely attractive to patients, and evidence from retrospective or small series demonstrates its efficacy. Most of these trials, however, have included highly selected patients. There are few, if any, ongoing randomized controlled trials comparing radical cystectomy to bladder-preserving protocols. Although the overall 5-year survival for radical cystectomy and trimodality therapy is approximately 50%, those patients with pure T2 disease frequently achieve 5-year survival rates approaching 70% [72,118,119].

Several significant questions must be considered when bladder-preserving protocols are being contemplated. First, the stalwart of bladder preservation has been the assertion that QOL is considerably improved in this group of patients as compared with the radical cystectomy series. Improvements in surgical technique and postoperative care, however, have resulted in current perioperative mortality rates of less than 2% [72,119] and potency rates of up to 64% after nerve-sparing radical cystectomy [120]. Furthermore, recent reports show similar subjective QOL in patients after orthotopic urinary diversion compared with matched control subjects [71] and a similar rate of patient-reported urine incontinence compared with those who underwent trimodality therapy (local endoscopic resection, chemotherapy, and radiation; 18% versus 19%) [121]. Second, bladder cancer staging is inaccurate and may result in significant understaging of T1 (75%) and T2 (55%) cancers on TUR specimens [119,122,123]. Such patients would be denied the opportunity of a beneficial surgical approach with LN dissection were they to undergo a bladder-preserving protocol. Third, evidence from nonrandomized studies suggests that subtotal TUR [123] and noncompletion or reduced-dose completion of chemo/radiation protocols are associated with poorer survival [124,125]. Recent series report noncompletion rates of 15% to 20% [126–128], up to 30% dose reduction, and mortality rates of 4% to 5% during induction therapy because of toxicity [128]. In addition, cancer may progress during chemoradiation in up to 10% of patients [128]. Finally, the reported local invasive recurrence rate after complete response to trimodality therapy of 15% [126] exposes patients to the risk of metastasis that would have been eliminated by primary cystectomy. Fourth, salvage cystectomy rates, even with the most up-to-date treatment protocols, remain at approximately 20% to 30% [126,128], primarily because of failure to control disease but also because of treatment complications (up to 10%) [129]. The mortality rate of salvage cystectomy is close to 8% [129] and has remained stable. The procedure is typically more difficult with fewer reconstructive options available, particularly as they relate to continent orthotopic neobladders. Fifth, the cost and time commitment required for multimodality bladder-preserving strategies, including diagnosis, treatment, and surveillance, greatly surpasses that of radical cystectomy. Zietman et al [130] admits that such strategies require the coordinated efforts of at least three specialties and more than 6 months to complete, incurring costs twice that of radical cystectomy. Patients are committed to intensive, lifelong surveillance for cancer recurrence, which may arise 10 to 15 years later.

Although survival with current multimodality, bladder-sparing approaches does seem comparable to radical cystectomy, considerations such as complexity, cost, and morbidity of bladder-sparing approaches must be taken into account and compared with the putative increase of QOL achieved with bladder retention. Current advances in surgical approaches must also be taken into consideration.

Finally, although bladder-preserving strategies are an extremely attractive option for patients wishing to retain their bladders in the face of muscle-invasive bladder cancer, these patients should be aware that the chemotherapeutic protocols being undertaken have achieved, at best, modest success when applied to more advanced forms of this disease and that the ideal combination of chemotherapy and radiation has yet to be devised. With the development of newer, more effective chemo- and radiotherapeutic protocols, it may be that such a strategy will prove ultimately successful, but, at the present time, the standard of care should remain a radical surgical approach.

In the absence of definitive data, such as that provided by a randomized trial, the debate will continue, using retrospective small analyses to scrutinize outcome. Protagonists will claim that bladder-conservation strategies deal adequately with a potentially fatal disease with enhanced QOL through bladder preservation. Antagonists will claim that the bladder-sparing strategy places patients' lives at unnecessary risk because QOL has considerably improved with the development of nerve-sparing orthotopic neobladder techniques. Presently, both strategies are appropriate, but only provided that the patient is fully educated as to the risks and benefits of each strategy. Unlike prostate cancer, where time to death is frequently measured in decades, a considerable number of patients will die within 5 years. Some might not if they had undergone standard treatment with radical cystectomy because no study to date has suggested an improved outlook with bladder-sparing protocols.

Follow-up after cystectomy

Long-term surveillance is warranted for possible tumor recurrence and complications related to the interposition of bowel in the urinary tract. Distant metastasis occurs more frequently than local recurrence (Table 27)

Table 27
Rates of local recurrence and distant metastasis in recent cystectomy series [132]

Pathologic stage	Local recurrence rate (%)	Distant metastasis rate (%)
T2	3–6	25
T3	7–10	11–50
T4	20	50–70
LN positive	25–45	70–80

[131]. Local and distant recurrences occur mostly within the first 2 and 3 years, respectively. Concomitant local and distant recurrences are identified in 30% to 50% of patients.

Prognostic factors for local recurrence include tumor stage, LN-positive disease, extent of the LN dissection, and whether perioperative chemotherapy was received. Prognostic factors for distant recurrence include tumor stage and LN-positive disease. Commonly involved locations include bone, lung, and liver.

Both local and distant recurrences are treated with systemic chemotherapy [131].

Tumor surveillance

Abdominopelvic CT scan, chest radiograph, IVP, urethral stump and upper tract cytology, and electrolytes and liver function tests should be obtained at months 3, 6, 12, 18, and 24, and years 3, 4, and 5 following cystectomy. Importantly, tumor surveillance should be performed every other year past year 5 [131].

In summary, this article has discussed most of the current controversies in superficial and invasive TCC of the bladder while trying to incorporate the issues of whether resection or ablation is the most appropriate strategy. The issues in bladder cancer are becoming more defined, and therefore it is likely that some progress in the future will be seen. In the superficial area, there is an urgent need for better and less invasive diagnostic methods. Improved pathologic assessment and prognostic indicators are required, and the development of better adjuvant strategies may improve what are disappointing recurrence and progression rates. For invasive and advanced disease, surgery, as a component of multimodality therapy, clearly has a role. The objective, however, must be to improve these therapies such that dependence on extirpative therapies can be reduced and physicians can focus more on the molecular level to correct the basic defects that have led to the disease state. In this regard, novel therapeutic strategies combining immune system stimulants or genetic manipulation with the newer generation of cytotoxic agents after cytoreductive therapy deserves further study. The answer to these problems lies neither in the clinic nor in the laboratory but in the continuing cooperation of both.

References

[1] Epstein JI, Amin MB, Reuter VR, Mostofi FK. The World Health Organization/International Society of Urological Pathology consensus classification of urothelial (transitional cell) neoplasms of the urinary bladder. Bladder Consensus Conference Committee. Am J Surg Pathol 1998;22:1435–48.

[2] Chopin DK, Gattegno B. Superficial bladder tumors. Eur Urol 2002;42:533–41.

[3] Witjes JA. Bladder carcinoma in situ in 2003: state of the art. Eur Urol 2004;45:142–6.

[4] Millan-Rodriguez F, Chechile-Toniolo G, Salvador-Bayarri J, Palou J, Algaba F, Vicente-Rodriguez J. Primary superficial bladder cancer risk groups according to progression, mortality and recurrence. J Urol 2000;164:680–4.

[5] Ramakumar S, Bhuiyan J, Besse JA, et al. Comparison of screening methods in the detection of bladder cancer. J Urol 1999;161:388–94.

[6] Lotan Y, Roehrborn CG. Sensitivity and specificity of commonly available bladder tumor markers versus cytology: results of a comprehensive literature review and meta-analyses. Urology 2003;61:109–18.

[7] Friedrich MG, Toma MI, Hellstern A, et al. Comparison of multitarget fluorescence in situ hybridization in urine with other noninvasive tests for detecting bladder cancer. BJU Int 2003;92:911–4.

[8] Placer J, Espinet B, Salido M, Sole F, Gelabert-Mas A. Clinical utility of a multiprobe FISH assay in voided urine specimens for the detection of bladder cancer and its recurrences, compared with urinary cytology. Eur Urol 2002;42:547–52.

[9] Sarosdy MF, Schellhammer P, Bokinsky G, et al. Clinical evaluation of a multi-target fluorescent in situ hybridization assay for detection of bladder cancer. J Urol 2002;168:1950–4.

[10] Schroeder GL, Lorenzo-Gomez MF, Hautmann SH, et al. A side by side comparison of cytology and biomarkers for bladder cancer detection. J Urol 2004;172:1123–6.

[11] Shariat SF, Casella R, Khoddami SM, et al. Urine detection of survivin is a sensitive marker for the noninvasive diagnosis of bladder cancer. J Urol 2004;171:626–30.

[12] van der Meijden A, Sylvester R, Collette L, Bono A, Ten Kate F. The role and impact of pathology review on stage and grade assessment of stages Ta and T1 bladder tumors: a combined analysis of 5 European Organization for Research and Treatment of Cancer trials. J Urol 2000;164:1533–7.

[13] Herr HW. The value of a second transurethral resection in evaluating patients with bladder tumors. J Urol 1999;162:74–6.

[14] Dalbagni G, Herr HW, Reuter VE. Impact of a second transurethral resection on the staging of T1 bladder cancer. Urology 2002;60:822–4.

[15] van der Meijden A, Oosterlinck W, Brausi M, Kurth KH, Sylvester R, de Balincourt C. Significance of bladder biopsies in Ta, T1 bladder tumors: a report from the EORTC Genito-Urinary Tract Cancer Cooperative Group. EORTC-GU Group Superficial Bladder Committee. Eur Urol 1999;35:267–71.

[16] May F, Treiber U, Hartung R, Schwaibold H. Significance of random bladder biopsies in superficial bladder cancer. Eur Urol 2003;44:47–50.

[17] Mufti GR, Singh M. Value of random mucosal biopsies in the management of superficial bladder cancer. Eur Urol 1992;22:288–93.

[18] Kiemeney LA, Witjes JA, Heijbroek RP, Debruyne FM, Verbeek AL. Dysplasia in normal-looking urothelium increases the risk of tumour progression in primary superficial bladder cancer. Eur J Cancer 1994;30:1621–5.

[19] Fujimoto N, Harada S, Terado M, Sato H, Matsumoto T. Multiple biopsies of normal-looking urothelium in patients with superficial bladder cancer: are they necessary? Int J Urol 2003;10:631–5.

[20] Beisland HO, Seland P. A prospective randomized study on neodymium-YAG laser irradiation versus TUR in the treatment of urinary bladder cancer. Scand J Urol Nephrol 1986;20:209–12.

[21] Dugan M, Crawford E, Nseyo UO. A randomized trial of observation versus photodynamic therapy after TUR for superficial papillary bladder cancer. Proc Am Soc Clin Oncol 1991;10:173.

[22] Bird VG, Soloway MS. Intravesical therapy option for bladder malignancy. Contemp Urol 2003;May(Suppl):3–13.

[23] Smith JA Jr, Labasky RF, Cockett AT, Fracchia JA, Montie JE, Rowland RG. Bladder cancer clinical guidelines panel summary report on the management of non-muscle invasive bladder cancer (stages Ta, T1 and TIS). The American Urological Association. J Urol 1999; 162:1697–701.

[24] Huncharek M, McGarry R, Kupelnick B. Impact of intravesical chemotherapy on recurrence rate of recurrent superficial transitional cell carcinoma of the bladder: results of a meta-analysis. Anticancer Res 2001;21:765–9.

[25] Tolley DA, Parmar MK, Grigor KM, et al. The effect of intravesical mitomycin C on recurrence of newly diagnosed superficial bladder cancer: a further report with 7 years of follow up. J Urol 1996;155:1233–8.

[26] Kaasinen E, Rintala E, Hellstrom P, et al. Factors explaining recurrence in patients undergoing chemoimmunotherapy regimens for frequently recurring superficial bladder carcinoma. Eur Urol 2002;42:167–74.

[27] Colombo R, Da Pozzo LF, Salonia A, et al. Multicentric study comparing intravesical chemotherapy alone and with local microwave hyperthermia for prophylaxis of recurrence of superficial transitional cell carcinoma. Journal of Chemical Oncology 2003;21:4270–6.

[28] Au JL, Badalament RA, Wientjes MG, et al. International Mitomycin C Consortium. Methods to improve efficacy of intravesical mitomycin C: results of a randomized phase III trial. J Natl Cancer Inst 2001;93:597–604.

[29] Solsona E, Iborra I, Ricos JV, Monros JL, Casanova J, Dumont R. Effectiveness of a single immediate mitomycin C instillation in patients with low risk superficial bladder cancer: short and long-term followup. J Urol 1999;161:1120–3.

[30] van der Heijden AG, Kiemeney LA, Gofrit ON, et al. Preliminary European results of local microwave hyperthermia and chemotherapy treatment in intermediate or high risk superficial transitional cell carcinoma of the bladder. Urology 2004;46:65–71.

[31] Bohle A, Brandau S. Immune mechanisms in bacillus Calmette-Guerin immunotherapy for superficial bladder cancer. J Urol 2003;170:964–9.

[32] Bohle A, Jocham D, Bock PR. Intravesical bacillus Calmette-Guerin versus mitomycin C for superficial bladder cancer: a formal meta-analysis of comparative studies on recurrence and toxicity. J Urol 2003;169:90–5.

[33] Shelley MD, Wilt TJ, Court J, Coles B, Kynaston H, Mason MD. Intravesical bacillus Calmette-Guerin is superior to mitomycin C in reducing tumour recurrence in high-risk superficial bladder cancer: a meta-analysis of randomized trials. BJU Int 2004;93:485–90.

[34] Bohle A, Bock PR. Intravesical bacille Calmette-Guerin versus mitomycin C in superficial bladder cancer: formal meta-analysis of comparative studies on tumor progression. Urology 2004;63:682–7.

[35] Patard JJ, Moudouni S, Saint F, et al. Tumor progression and survival in patients with T1G3 bladder tumors: multicentric retrospective study comparing 94 patients treated during 17 years. Urology 2001;58:551–6.

[36] Herr HW. Tumor progression and survival in patients with T1G3 bladder tumors: 15-year outcome. Br J Urol 1997;80:762–5.

[37] Cookson MS, Herr HW, Zhang ZF, Soloway S, Sogani PC, Fair WR. The treated natural history of high risk superficial bladder cancer: 15-year outcome. J Urol 1997;158:62–7.

[38] Lamm DL, Blumenstein BA, Crissman JD, et al. Maintenance bacillus Calmette-Guerin immunotherapy for recurrent TA, T1 and carcinoma in situ transitional cell carcinoma of the bladder: a randomized Southwest Oncology Group Study. J Urol 2000;163:1124–9.
[39] van der Meijden AP, Sylvester RJ, Oosterlinck W, Hoeltl W, Bono AV. Maintenance bacillus Calmette-Guerin for Ta T1 bladder tumors is not associated with increased toxicity: results from a European Organization for Research and Treatment of Cancer Genito-Urinary Group phase III trial. Eur Urol 2003;44:429–34.
[40] Martinez-Pineiro JA, Flores N, Isorna S, et al. Long-term follow-up of a randomized prospective trial comparing a standard 81 mg dose of intravesical bacille Calmette-Guerin with a reduced dose of 27 mg in superficial bladder cancer. BJU Int 2002;89: 671–80.
[41] Sylvester RJ, van der Meijden AP, Lamm DL. Intravesical bacillus Calmette-Guerin reduces the risk of progression in patients with superficial bladder cancer: a meta-analysis of the published results of randomized clinical trials. J Urol 2002;68:1964–70.
[42] Martinez-Pineiro JA, Martinez-Pineiro L, Solsona E, et al. Comparison of standard BCG dose (81mg) versus three-fold reduced dose (27mg) in high-risk superficial bladder cancer (T1G3, Tis). A Cueto prospective randomized study #95012 [abstract 752]. Eur Urol 2003; 2(Suppl):190.
[43] Andius P, Holmang S. Bacillus Calmette-Guerin therapy in stage Ta/T1 bladder cancer: prognostic factors for time to recurrence and progression. BJU Int 2004;93:980–4.
[44] Oosterlink W, Solsona E, van der Meijden AP, et al. European Association of Urology. EAU guidelines on diagnosis and treatment of upper urinary tract transitional cell carcinoma. Eur Urol 2004;46:147–54.
[45] van der Meijden AP, Brausi M, Zambon V, Kirkels W, de Balincourt C, Sylvester R. Intravesical instillation of epirubicin, bacillus Calmette-Guerin and bacillus Calmette-Guerin plus isoniazid for intermediate and high risk Ta, T1 papillary carcinoma of the bladder: a European Organization for Research and Treatment of Cancer genito-urinary group randomized phase III trial. J Urol 2001;166:476–81.
[46] De Boer EC, Steerenberg PA, van der Meijden AP, et al. Impaired immune response by isoniazid treatment during intravesical BCG administration in the guinea pig. Prog Clin Biol Res 1992;378:81–93.
[47] Sylvester RJ, van der Meijden AP, Oosterlinck W, Hoeltl W, Bono AV. The side effects of bacillus Calmette-Guerin in the treatment of Ta T1 bladder cancer do not predict its efficacy: results from a European Organization for Research and Treatment of Cancer Genito-Urinary Group phase III trial. Eur Urol 2003;44:423–8.
[48] Herr HW, Dalbagni G. Defining bacillus Calmette-Guerin refractory superficial bladder tumors. J Urol 2003;169:1706–8.
[49] Greenberg RE, Ignatoff JM. Intravesical therapy for refractory transitional cell cancer in situ. Contemp Urol 2003;May(Suppl):14–9.
[50] Joudi FN, O'Donnell MA. Second-line intravesical therapy versus cystectomy for bacille Calmette-Guerin (BCG) failures. Curr Opin Urol 2004;14:271–5.
[51] O'Donnell MA, Krohn J, DeWolf WC. Salvage intravesical therapy with interferon-alpha 2b plus low dose bacillus Calmette-Guerin is effective in patients with superficial bladder cancer in whom bacillus Calmette-Guerin alone previously failed. J Urol 2001; 166:1300–4.
[52] Stricker P, Pryor K, Nicholson T, et al. Bacillus Calmette-Guerin plus intravesical interferon alpha-2b in patients with superficial bladder cancer. Urol 1996;48:957–61.
[53] Bercovich E, Deriu M, Manferrari F, Irianni G. BCG vs. BCG plus recombinant alpha-interferon 2b in superficial tumors of the bladder. Arch Ital Urol Androl 1995;67: 257–60.
[54] Keane TE, Eldaieef SM, Clarke HS, Daily PP. Combination intravesical immunotherapy (BCG plus interferon alpha -2B) in high-grade recurrent superficial transitional cell carcinoma [abstract 48]. SEAUA 2003;Mar.

[55] O'Donnell MA, Lilli K, Leopold C. Interim results from a national multicenter phase II trial of combination bacillus Calmette-Guerin plus interferon alfa-2b for superficial bladder cancer. J Urol 2004;172:888–93.
[56] Steinberg G, Bahnson R, Brosman S, Middleton R, Wajsman Z, Wehle M. Efficacy and safety of valrubicin for the treatment of bacillus Calmette-Guerin refractory carcinoma in situ of the bladder. The Valrubicin Study Group. J Urol 2000;163:761–7.
[57] Saint F, Salomon L, Quintela R, et al. Do prognostic parameters of remission versus relapse after bacillus Calmette-Guerin (BCG) immunotherapy exist? Analysis of a quarter century of literature. Eur Urol 2003;43:351–60.
[58] Soloway M, Sofer M, Vaidya A. Contemporary management of stage T1 transitional cell carcinoma of the bladder. J Urol 2002;167:1573–83.
[59] Masood S, Sriprasad S, Palmer JH, Mufti GR. T1G3 bladder cancer—indications for early cystectomy. Int Urol Nephrol 2004;36:41–4.
[60] Herr HW, Sogani PC. Does early cystectomy improve the survival of patients with high-risk superficial bladder tumors? J Urol 2001;166:1296–9.
[61] Thalmann GN, Markwalder R, Shahin O, Burkhard FC, Hochreiter WW, Studer UE. Primary T1G3 bladder cancer: organ preserving approach or immediate cystectomy? J Urol 2004;172:70–5.
[62] Oosterlink W, Lobel B, Jakse G, Malmstrom PU, Stockle M, Sternberg C. European Association of Urology (EAU) Working Group on Oncological Urology. Guidelines on bladder cancer. Eur Urol 2002;41:105–12.
[63] Skemp NM, Fernandes E. Routine bladder biopsy after BCG treatment: is it necessary? Urology 2002;59:224–6.
[64] Morris SB, Gordon EM, Shearer RJ, Woodhouse CR. Superficial bladder cancer: for how long should a tumour-free patient have check cystoscopies? Br J Urol 1995;75:193–6.
[65] Fujii Y, Fukui I, Kihara K, Tsujii T, Kageyama Y, Oshima H. Late recurrence and progression after a long tumor-free period in primary Ta and T1 bladder cancer. Eur Urol 1999;36:309–13.
[66] Gohji K, Nomi M, Okamoto M. Conservative therapy for stage T1b grade 3 transitional cell carcinoma of the bladder. Urology 1999;53:308–13.
[67] Lamm DL, Blumenstein BA, Crawford ED. A randomized trial of intravesical doxorubicin and immunotherapy with BCG for transitional cell carcinoma of the bladder. N Engl J Med 1991;325:1205–9.
[68] Schellhammer PF. Superficial bladder cancer-insight and expertise. Contemp Urol 2004; May(Suppl):3–24.
[69] Vaidya A, Soloway MS, Hawke C. De novo muscle invasive bladder cancer: is there a change in trend? J Urol 2001;165:45–50.
[70] Grossman HB. Contemp Urol 2004;(Suppl):10.
[71] Henningsohn L, Steven K, Kallestrup EB, Steineck G. Distressful symptoms and well-being after radical cystectomy and orthotopic bladder substitution compared with a matched control population. J Urol 2002;168:168–74.
[72] Rosario DJ, Becker M, Anderson JB. The changing pattern of mortality and morbidity from radical cystectomy. BJU Int 2000;85:427–30.
[73] Lee SE, Jeong IG, Ku JH, Kwak C, Lee E, Jeong JS. Impact of transurethral resection of bladder tumor: analysis of cystectomy specimens to evaluate for residual tumor. Urology 2004;63:873–7.
[74] Paik ML, Scolieri MJ, Brown SL, Spirnak JP, Resnick MI. Limitations of computerized tomography in staging invasive bladder cancer before radical cystectomy. J Urol 2000;63: 1693–6.
[75] Kim B, Semelka RC, Ascher SM, Chalpin DB, Carroll PR, Hricak H. Bladder tumor staging: comparison of contrast-enhanced CT, T1- and T2-weighted MR imaging, dynamic gadolinium-enhanced imaging, and late gadolinium-enhanced imaging. Radiology 1994; 193:239–45.

[76] Jalon-Monzon A, Fernandez Gomez JM, Garcia Rodriguez J, et al. Utility of computerized tomography in determining the extent of infiltrating bladder tumors: our experience. Arch Esp Urol 2003;56:133–8.
[77] Holzbeierlein JM, Lopez-Corona E, Bochner BH, et al. Partial cystectomy: a contemporary review of the Memorial Sloan-Kettering Cancer Center experience and recommendations for patient selection. J Urol 2004;172:878–81.
[78] Prout GR, Marshall VF. The prognosis with untreated bladder tumors. Cancer 1956;9: 551–8.
[79] Holmang S, Hedelin H, Borghede G, Johansson SL. Long-term follow-up of a bladder carcinoma cohort: questionable value of radical radiotherapy. J Urol 1997;157:1642–6.
[80] Kim HL, Steinberg GD. The current status of bladder preservation in the treatment of muscle invasive bladder cancer. J Urol 2000;164:627–32.
[81] Madersbacher S, Studer UE. Contemporary cystectomy and urinary diversion. World J Urol 2002;20:151–7.
[82] Schoenberg MP, Walsh PC, Breazeale DR, Marshall FF, Mostwin JL, Brendler CB. Local recurrence and survival following nerve sparing radical cystoprostatectomy for bladder cancer: 10-year followup. J Urol 1996;155:490–4.
[83] Lee K, et al. During cystectomy men and women are not equal. Urology Times 2004; February 15.
[84] Schoenberg M, Hortopan S, Schlossberg L, Marshall FF. Anatomical anterior exenteration with urethral and vaginal preservation: illustrated surgical method. J Urol 1999;161:569–72.
[85] Chang SS, Cole E, Smith JA Jr, Cookson MS. Pathological findings of gynecologic organs obtained at female radical cystectomy. J Urol 2002;168:147–9.
[86] Stein JP, Esrig D, Freeman JA, et al. Prospective pathologic analysis of female cystectomy specimens: risk factors for orthotopic diversion in women. Urology 1998;51:951–5.
[87] Schoenberg MP, Carter HB, Epstein JI. Ureteral frozen section analysis during cystectomy: a reassessment. J Urol 1996;155:1218–20.
[88] Silver DA, Stroumbakis N, Russo P, Fair WR, Herr HW. Ureteral carcinoma in situ at radical cystectomy: does the margin matter? J Urol 1997;158:768–71.
[89] Stein JP, Lieskovsky G, Cote R, et al. Radical cystectomy in the treatment of invasive bladder cancer: long-term results in 1,054 patients. J Clin Orthod 2001;19:666–75.
[90] Konety BR, Joslyn SA, O'Donnell MA. Extent of pelvic lymphadenectomy and its impact on outcome in patients diagnosed with bladder cancer: analysis of data from the Surveillance, Epidemiology and End Results Program data base. J Urol 2003;169: 946–50.
[91] Queck ML, Stein JP, Skinner DG. Current strategies for managing locally advanced bladder cancer. Contemp Urol 2004;16:44–55.
[92] Herr HW. Extent of surgery and pathology evaluation has an impact on bladder cancer outcomes after radical cystectomy. Urology 2003;61:105–8.
[93] Leissner J, Hohenfellner R, Thuroff JW. Lymphadenectomy in patients with transitional cell cancer of the urinary bladder. BJU Int 2000;85:817–23.
[94] Stein JP, Cai J, Groshen S, Skinner DG. Risk factors for patients with pelvic lymph node metastases following radical cystectomy with en bloc pelvic lymphadenectomy: concept of lymph node density. J Urol 2003;170:35–41.
[95] Poulsen AL, Horn T, Steven K. Radical cystectomy: extending the limits of pelvic lymph node dissection improves survival for patients with bladder cancer confined to the bladder wall. J Urol 1998;160:2015–9.
[96] Sanderson KM, Stein JP, Skinner DG. The evolving role of pelvic lymphadenectomy in the treatment of bladder cancer. Urol Oncol 2004;22:205–13.
[97] Leissner J, Ghoneim H, Abol-Enein J, et al. Extended radical lymphadenectomy in patients with urothelial bladder cancer: results of a prospective multicenter study. J Urol 2004;171: 139–44.

[98] Wishnow KI, Johnson DE, Ro J, Swanson DA, Babaian RJ, von Eschenbach AC. Incidence, extent and location of unsuspected pelvic lymph node metastasis in patients undergoing radical cystectomy for bladder cancer. J Urol 1987;137:408–10.

[99] Herr HW, Donat SM. Outcomes of patients with grossly node positive bladder cancer after pelvic node dissection and cystectomy. J Urol 2001;165:62–4.

[100] Herr HW. Improving outcome after bladder cancer surgery. Contemp Urol 2003;15: 23–9.

[101] Vazina A, Dugi D, Shariat SF, Evans J, Link R, Lerner SP. Stage specific lymph node metastasis mapping in radical cystectomy specimens. J Urol 2004;171:1830–4.

[102] Mills RD, Turner WH, Fleischmann A, Markwalder R, Thalmann GN, Studer UE. Pelvic lymph node metastases from bladder cancer: outcome in 83 patients after radical cystectomy and pelvic lymphadenectomy. J Urol 2001;166:19–23.

[103] Brossner C, Pycha A, Toth A, Mian C, Kuber W. Does extended lymphadenectomy increase the morbidity of radical cystectomy? BJU Int 2004;93:64–6.

[104] Loeher SR, Einhorn LH, Elson PJ, et al. A randomized comparison of cisplatin alone or in combination with methotrexate, vinblastine, and doxorubicin in patients with metastatic urothelial carcinoma: a cooperative group study. J Clin Oncol 1992;10:1066–73.

[105] Logothetis CJ, Dexeus FH, Finn L, et al. A prospective randomized trial comparing MVAC and CISCA chemotherapy for patients with metastatic urothelial tumors. J Clin Orthod 1990;8:1050–5.

[106] von der Maase H, Hansen SW, Roberts JT, et al. Gemcitabine and cisplatin versus methotrexate, vinblastine, doxorubicin, and cisplatin in advanced or metastatic bladder cancer: results of a large, randomized, multinational, multicenter, phase III study. J Clin Orthod 2000;18:3068–77.

[107] Grossman HB, Natale RB, Tangen CM, et al. Neoadjuvant chemotherapy plus cystectomy compared with cystectomy alone for locally advanced bladder cancer. N Engl J Med 2003; 349:859–66.

[108] Stadler WM, Lerner SP. Neoadjuvant chemotherapy in invasive bladder cancer: a systematic review and meta-analysis. Lancet 2003;361:1927–34.

[109] Millikan R, Dinney C, Swanson D, et al. Integrated therapy for locally advanced bladder cancer: final report of a randomized trial of cystectomy plus adjuvant M-VAC versus cystectomy with both preoperative and postoperative M-VAC. J Clin Orthod 2001;19: 4005–13.

[110] Skinner DG, Daniels JR, Russell CA, et al. The role of adjuvant chemotherapy following cystectomy for invasive bladder cancer: a prospective comparative trial. J Urol 1991;145: 459–64.

[111] Raghavan D. Editorial comment re: Skinner DG, Daniels JR, Russell CA, et al. The role of adjuvant chemotherapy following csytectomy for invasive bladder cancer: a prospective comparative trial. J Urol 1991;145:465–6.

[112] Stockle M, Meyenburg W, Wellek S, et al. Adjuvant polychemotherapy of nonorgan-confined bladder cancer after radical cystectomy revisited: long-term results of a controlled prospective study and further clinical experience. J Urol 1995;153:47–52.

[113] Freiha F, Reese J, Torti FM. A randomized trial of radical cystectomy versus radical cystectomy plus cisplatin, vinblastine and methotrexate chemotherapy for muscle invasive bladder cancer. J Urol 1996;155:495–9.

[114] Bellmunt J, Guillem V, Paz-Ares L, et al. Phase I-II study of paclitaxel, cisplatin, and gemcitabine in advanced transitional-cell carcinoma of the urothelium. Spanish Oncology Genitourinary Group. J Clin Oncol 2000;18:3247–55.

[115] Meluch AA, Greco FA, Burris HA III, et al. Paclitaxel and gemcitabine chemotherapy for advanced transitional-cell carcinoma of the urothelial tract: a phase II trial of the Minnie Pearl Cancer Research Network. J Clin Oncol 2001;19:3018–24.

[116] Gitlitz BJ, Baker C, Chapman Y, et al. A phase II study of gemcitabine and docetaxel therapy in patients with advanced urothelial carcinoma. Cancer 2003;98:1863–9.

[117] Shelley MD, Wilt TJ, Barber J, Mason MD. A meta-analysis of randomized trials suggests a survival benefit for combined radiotherapy and radical cystectomy compared with radical radiotherapy for invasive bladder cancer: are these data relevant to modern practice? Clin Oncol 2004;16:166–71.

[118] Madersbacher S, Hochreiter W, Burkhard F, et al. Radical cystectomy for bladder cancer today—a homogeneous series without neoadjuvant therapy. J Clin Orthod 2003;21:690–6.

[119] Pagano F, Bassi P, Galetti TP, et al. Results of contemporary radical cystectomy for invasive bladder: a clinicopathological study with an emphasis on the inadequacy of the TNM classification. J Urol 1991;145:45–50.

[120] Brendler CB, Steinberg GD, Marshall FF, Mostwin JL, Walsh PC. Local recurrence and survival following nerve-sparing cystoprostatectomy. J Urol 1990;144:1137–40.

[121] Zietman AL, Sacco D, Skowronski U, et al. Organ conservation in invasive bladder cancer by transurethral resection, chemotherapy and radiation: results of a urodynamic and quality of life study on long-term survivors. J Urol 2003;170:1772–6.

[122] Cheng L, Neumann RM, Weaver AL, et al. Grading and staging of bladder carcinoma in transurethral resection specimens-correlation with 105 matched cystectomy specimens. Am J Surg Pathol 2000;113:275–9.

[123] Dunst J, Sauer R, Schrott M, Kuhn R, Wittekind C, Altendorf-Hofmann A. Organ-sparing treatment in advanced bladder cancer: a 10-year experience. Int J Radiat Oncol Biol Phys 1994;30:261–6.

[124] Kaufman DS, Shipley WU, Griffin PP, Heney NM, Althausen AF, Efird JT. Selective bladder preservation by combination treatment of invasive bladder cancer. N Engl J Med 1993;329:1377–82.

[125] Sauer R, Birkenhake S, Kuhn R, Wittekind C, Schrott KM, Martus P. Efficacy of radiochemotherapy with platin derivatives compared to radiotherapy alone in organ-sparing treatment of bladder cancer. Int J Radiat Oncol Biol Phys 1998;40:121–7.

[126] Rodel C, Grabenbauer GG, Kuhn R, et al. Combined modality treatment and selective organ preservation in invasive bladder cancer: long-term results. J Clin Orthod 2002;20: 3061–71.

[127] Hussain SA, Stocken DD, Peake DR, et al. Long-term results of a phase II study of synchronous chemoradiotherapy in advanced muscle invasive bladder cancer. Br J Cancer 2004;90:1–6.

[128] Hagan MP, Winter KA, Kaufman DS, et al. RTOG 97-06: initial report of a phase I-II trial of selective bladder conservation using TURBT, twice-daily accelerated irradiation sensitized with cisplatin, and adjuvant MCV combination chemotherapy. Int J Radiat Oncol Biol Phys 2003;57:665–72.

[129] Chahal R, Sundaram SK, Iddenden R, Forman DF, Weston PM, Harrison SC. A study of the morbidity, mortality and long-term survival following radical cystectomy and radical radiotherapy in the treatment of invasive bladder cancer in Yorkshire. Eur Urol 2003;43: 246–57.

[130] Zietman AL, Shipley WU, Kaufman DS, et al. A phase I/II trial of transurethral surgery combined with concurrent cisplatin, 5-fluorouracil, and twice daily radiation followed by selective bladder preservation in operable patients with muscle invading bladder cancer. J Urol 1998;160:1673–7.

[131] Bochner BH, Montie JE, Lee CT. Follow-up strategies and management of recurrence in urologic oncology bladder cancer: invasive bladder cancer. Urol Clin North Am 2003;30: 777–89.

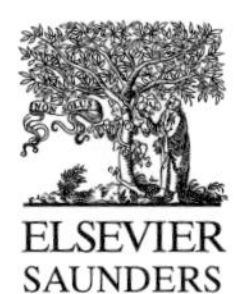
ELSEVIER
SAUNDERS

Surg Oncol Clin N Am
14 (2005) 353–365

SURGICAL
ONCOLOGY CLINICS
OF NORTH AMERICA

Laparoscopic Lymph Node Dissection in Urologic Cancer

Eliecer Kurzer, MD, MPH*, Raymond J. Leveillee, MD

Division of Endourology and Laparoscopy, Department of Urology, University of Miami School of Medicine, PO Box 016960 (M814), Miami, FL 33101, USA

The union of laparoscopic surgery and urology has been brief—barely a decade old—but several advances have been made during this short time. Laparoscopic pelvic lymph node dissection (L-PLND) was the first procedure that popularized these surgical techniques and introduced the necessary skills to the urologic community. L-PLND became the "gallbladder" equivalent for urologists to acquire laparoscopic skills and advance to more complex extirpative and reconstructive procedures. Currently, laparoscopy is performed routinely by urologists for radical and partial nephrectomies, radical prostatectomy, pyeloplasty, radiofrequency ablation, and even radical cystectomy. An important yet somewhat limited role for laparoscopic lymph node dissection exits in urology, primarily with respect to prostate and testicular cancer, with a lesser role in other urologic malignancies (ie, bladder and penile cancer). Whether performed for curative or diagnostic purposes, lymphadenectomy can be divided into pelvic and retroperitoneal areas depending on the principle organ involved. This article describes the indication, techniques, and complications for laparoscopic pelvic and retroperitoneal lymph node dissections (RPLND).

Laparoscopic pelvic lymphadenectomy

Prostate cancer

Indications

Selection of who should undergo pelvic lymph node dissection in prostate cancer is controversial (Box 1). The most common indication for performing

* Corresponding author.
E-mail address: ekurzer@yahoo.com (E. Kurzer).

doi:10.1016/j.soc.2004.11.013 **surgonc.theclinics.com**

Box 1. Contraindications to laparoscopic pelvic lymph node dissection

Absolute

- Uncontrolled coagulopathy
- Severe chronic obstructive pulmonary disease
- Severe cardiovascular disease
- General peritonitis
- Abdominal wall infection
- Significant intestinal obstruction

Relative

- Obesity
- Abdominal aortic aneurysm
- Previous major intraperitoneal surgery
- Previous pelvic radiotherapy
- Moderate cardiovascular/cardiopulmonary disease

a lymph node dissection is to improve clinical staging of high-risk patients with prostate cancer and help them to avoid unnecessary morbidity and possible mortality associated with noncurative treatment. Removal of involved lymph nodes has not been associated with improved survival or cure and is believed to be of prognostic importance. Clinical staging has limitations; therefore, if prostate cancer could be staged accurately with 100% sensitivity and specificity, a lymph node dissection would be rendered unnecessary. Borley et al [1] reported on 55 patients with locally advanced prostate cancer who underwent either pelvic MRI or CT scan before L-PLND. MRI identified 3 (27%) but missed 8 patients with positive nodes detected pathologically. CT scan missed all 9 patients with documented lymph node involvement. Radiographic evaluation seems to have good specificity but poor sensitivity for detecting regional spread of disease to the pelvic lymph nodes.

To delineate better who is at risk for lymph node involvement of disease, many studies have used multivariant analysis to calculate which factors best predict high-risk disease. Partin et al [2] were instrumental in developing a nomogram that predicts the probability of nodal metastases based on three clinical factors: clinical stage (ie, digital rectal examination), preoperative serum prostate-specific antigen blood test, and tumor biopsy grade (Gleason score). This nomogram was later validated in a much larger population and proven to predict nodal metastases with 82.9% accuracy [3]. Using these three clinical characteristics, one can define patients as being "high risk" if they have more than a 3% chance of nodal involvement using the "Partin nomogram." This rate roughly correlates to patients with prostate-specific antigen more than 10, Gleason score more than 7, and clinical stage more than T1c. Another indication for performing a pelvic lymph node dissection is to stage accurately any patients who have failed radiotherapy before performing a salvage operation because of high risk of associated morbidities [4].

Once the decision to perform a lymph node dissection is made, one must decide if it will be performed via traditional laparotomy incision or laparoscopic technique. An early study by Parra et al [5] compared 24 patients who were alternately designated to have either a modified open or L-PLND. Patients shared comparable clinical characteristics in terms of age and clinical stage. No statistically significant difference was seen in the average number of nodes retrieved between the open laparotomy (11) and the laparoscopic (10.7) groups. A confirmatory study by Herrell [6] that compared 38 patients who underwent laparotomy versus 19 patients who had L-PLND found no statistically significant difference in the number of nodes harvested. Hospital stay was significantly longer in the open lymph node dissection cohort, as was a higher number of postoperative complications. Multiple studies have documented the safety of performing L-PLND. Longer term studies have not demonstrated any trocar site or abdominal wall tumor implantations after L-PLND [7]. Traditionally, an extended pelvic node dissection was performed that included the obturator, hypogastric, common, and iliac nodes. In the 1980s, the extended dissection largely was replaced with a modified template after several studies demonstrated little benefit and higher complication rates with the extended dissection [8]. The nodal package in the modified template compromises the obturator and hypogastric nodes only. A comparison of the extended and modified lymph node dissection was performed laparoscopically by Stone et al [9], who found that despite a slightly higher node positivity rate, the extended lymph node dissection offered no advantage over the modified template and was associated with a significantly higher complication rate.

Given that L-PLND is effective and safe, the unique situations in which a laparoscopic approach would be most preferable involve "high-risk" patients who are contemplating radiotherapy as primary therapy, undergoing perineal prostatectomy, and considering a salvage procedure.

Technique

Transperitoneal

In 1990, Schuessler [10] was the first to report the successful performance of a staging intraperitoneal L-PLND for patients with prostate cancer. L-PLND can be performed successfully by using general laparoscopic equipment without the need for any special tools. An operating room table with the ability to tilt 45° in right and left directions is helpful in allowing bowel to fall away from the field of interest. Ideally, two viewing monitors should be available and should be located just behind and below the surgeon and the assistant. If only one view screen is available, it is best placed at the foot of the table for optimal viewing. After the induction of anesthesia (avoiding nitrous oxide), an orogastric tube and Foley catheter are placed. The patient is positioned with his or her arms tucked comfortably at the sides, and they are well padded and secured. The prepared area should be from the xiphoid process down to the pubis. Compression boots are routinely recommended for deep venous thrombosis prophylaxis.

The procedure begins with placement of either a Veress needle or Hasson cannula just below the umbilicus with insufflation of the peritoneum using carbon dioxide. The abdomen is insufflated and maintained at a pressure of 15 mm Hg. The Veress needle is replaced with a 10-mm trocar and the abdominal compartment inspected with either a 0° or 30° lens to ensure that no injury occurs during insufflation or other abdominal pathology. In patients with a history of previous surgery, an open "bladeless" technique using the Hasson trocar may be used for initial port placement. Two more 5-mm trocars are then placed along the right and left mid-clavicular lines (Fig. 1). This "fan" positioning is our preferred technique, whereas other surgeons commonly place a fourth trocar midway between the umbilicus and pubis to form a small diamond configuration. We believe that this approach creates excess congestion within the pelvis and gains little advantage during the dissection. Important land marks to identify before dissecting are the inguinal ring, medial umbilical ligaments, bladder, and iliac vessels. The dissection begins by using either electrocautery or the harmonic scalpel and incising the posterior peritoneum just lateral to the medial umbilical ligament. Using blunt dissection, this plane can be developed to identify the external iliac artery and vein. The boundaries of the dissection are the external iliac vein laterally, the obturator nerve medially, the node of Cloquet inferiorly, and the iliac artery superiorly (Fig. 2). One should try to avoid dissection below the level of the obturator nerve to avoid troublesome bleeding. All lymphatic channels are ligated with hemostatic clips or electrocautery (Fig. 3). After the nodal package is

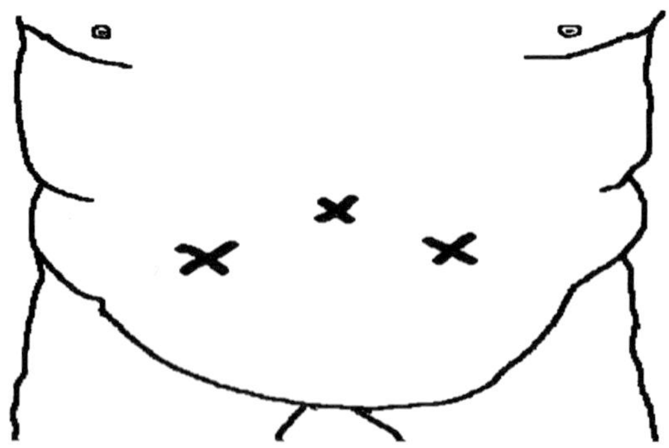

Fig. 1. Trocar placment for L-PLND.

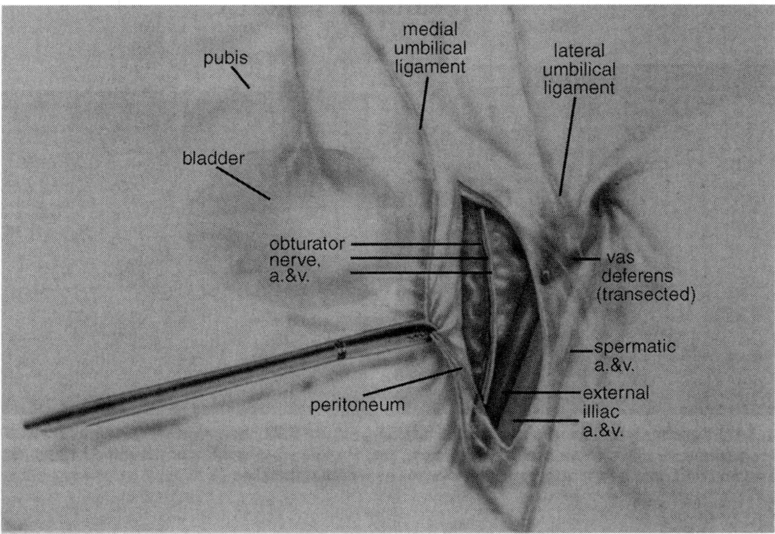

Fig. 2. Pelvic node dissection landmarks. (*From* Winfield NH. Laparoscopic pelvic lymph node dissection: application to genitourinary malignancies. In: Gomella LG, Kozminski M, Winfield HN, editors. Laparoscopic urologic surgery. New York: Raven Press, 1994; with permission.)

harvested completely, it is removed through the 10-mm port under direct vision. A laparoscopic entrapment sac can be used during extraction to avoid tearing of the specimen. This procedure is then duplicated on the contralateral side. After removing all nodal packages, only the fascia of the 10-mm port needs to be closed, and the skin incisions are reapproximated with a subcuticular suture.

Extraperitoneal (preperitoneal)

The traditional approach to pelvic lymph node dissection is via an extraperitoneal, retropubic approach. To better mirror the open approach, the extraperitoneal approach to laparoscopic lymph node dissection also was developed and first published by Ferzli et al in 1992 [11]. A small vertical incision is made just below the umbilicus. The anterior rectus and transverses abdominis fascias are incised. Using blunt finger dissection, the preperitoneal space is developed above the posterior rectus fascia, which ends at the arcuate line. Next, a balloon dilator is inserted down to the pubic bone and insufflated (Fig. 4). The remainder of the operation proceeds as described for the intraperitoneal approach.

The obvious advantage of this approach is that by avoiding the peritoneal cavity the risks of visceral injury and development of post-operative intra-abdominal adhesions are eliminated. Further advantages include obviating the need to remove existing adhesions to perform surgery and perhaps better exposure in obese patients. This approach also may offer

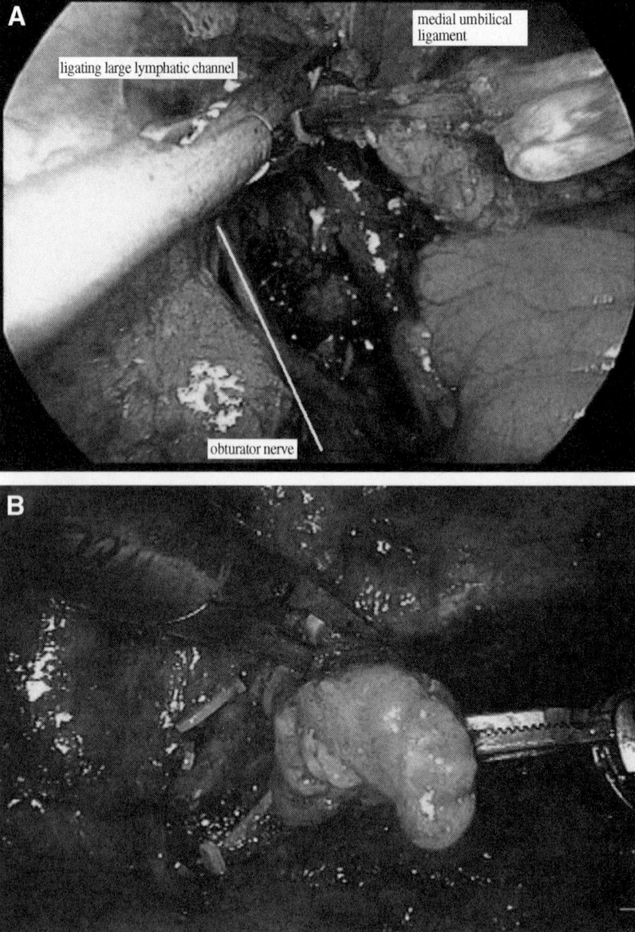

Fig. 3. (*A*) Ligating a large lymphatic channel while performing a left-sided L-PLND. (*B*) Nodal package from a laparoscopic/robotic lymph node dissection during a radical prostatectomy.

better visualization of the iliac vessels and obturator nerve, which are important landmarks during the dissection.

Several disadvantages of this approach also have been noted. First, the working space is significantly more limited than in the transperitoneal approach, which creates occasional congestion. Second, carbon dioxide absorption is significantly higher, which leads to more subcutaneous emphysema, hypercapnia, and acidemia [12]. The effects of the increased carbon dioxide absorption often can be overcome with hyperventilation, yet caution should be used in patients with pre-existing cardiopulmonary disease. Third, subsequent extraperitoneal pelvic surgery may be complicated by postoperative fibrosis and scarring.

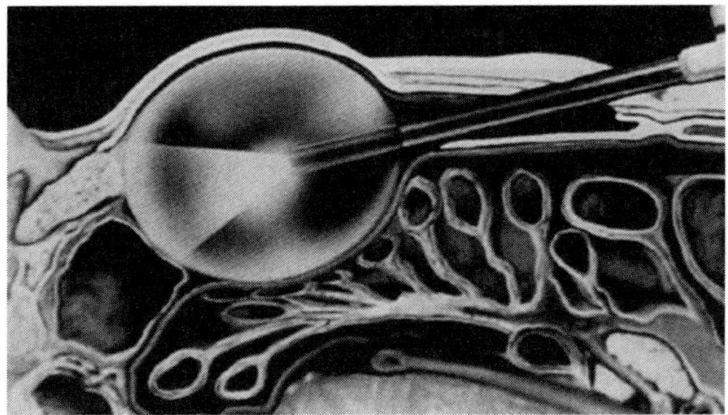

Fig. 4. Balloon dilatation for extraperitoneal pelvic lymph node dissection. (*From* Albala DM, Grasso M. Color atlas of endourology. Philadelphia: Lippincott-Raven; 1999. p. 120; with permission.)

Complications

Complications from L-PLND are low and seem to improve with the experience of the surgeon [13]. Overall complication rates vary from 9% to 15%, with most of these events occurring postoperatively [14,15]. Intraoperative complications can be a result of port placement or may occur during the dissection. Injuries to the epigastric vessels, iliac veins, and bowel are the most likely but are rare occurrences, with an incidence less than 1%. The most common postoperative complication is from ileus, and it is self-limiting. The other common postoperative complication is from lymphocele formation. A study that compared the radiographic frequency (routine use of CT scan) of asymptomatic postoperative lymphocele formation between open and laparoscopic lymph node dissection found a statistically significant lower incidence of lymphocele formation in the L-PLND group [16]. The overall frequency was 61% and 37%, respectively. More importantly, no clinically significant lymphoceles were found in the L-PLND group, but three were found in the open lymphadenectomy group. We could not find any studies that compared the incidence of lymphocele when comparing laparoscopic transperitoneal to extraperitoneal lymph node dissection. Other rare complications include seromas, deep venous thrombosis, wound infections, and nerve palsies. The mortality rate with L-PLND is less than 1%. In summary, L-PLND is safe and may add useful information in terms of prognosis or therapeutic interventions. Complications, although rare, are usually minor and can be managed conservatively. For surgeons with limited laparoscopic experience, however, serious bleeding can ensue if damage occurs to the major vascular structures nearby.

Bladder cancer

Recent studies have suggested significant clinical advantage in giving neoadjuvant chemotherapy to patients with invasive and metastatic bladder cancer [17,18]. Unlike for prostate cancer, preoperative nomograms have not been created to help predict the risk of extravesicular disease. Given the limitations of radiographic staging and understaging with transurethral resections of bladder tumors, a limited role for laparoscopic pelvic lymph node dissection exists. Candidates for this operation are patients who refuse radical cystectomy, desire definitive radiotherapy, and require accurate staging before starting treatment. Another population that may benefit from L-PLND includes patients with lymph node–positive squamous cell carcinoma or adenocarcinoma, in which case radical cystectomy would not be curative.

Penile cancer

Squamous cell carcinoma of the penis accounts for 0.4% to 0.6% of all malignancies in men. The presence and extent of metastasis to the regional lymph nodes are the key predictors for survival, even more so than grade or morphohistologic determinants [19]. Lymphatic drainage from the penile skin to the superficial and deep inguinal nodes and subsequently the pelvic nodes has been well established. Given the rarity of this disease, however, controversy regarding the type and timing of lymphadenectomy still exists. Once metastases are found in the pelvic nodes, the prognosis is dismal. Given this predictable pattern of metastases, Mukamel and deKernion [20] suggest performing bilateral pelvic lymphadenectomies as the initial staging procedure in patients with invasive penile cancer. If these nodes should prove to be positive, no further staging or therapeutic procedures would be warranted, sparing the patient unnecessary surgery with no additional benefit.

Urethral cancer

Urethral cancer is a rare disease with no definitive management recommendations. Distal tumors generally metastasize to superficial and deep inguinal nodes. Proximal urethral tumors usually metastasize to the external, internal, and obturator nodes. Node positivity professes a poor prognosis, and radical extirpative surgery offers little benefit. No published reports have examined the role of laparoscopic pelvic lymph node dissection for patients with urethral cancer.

Laparoscopic retroperitoneal lymphadenectomy

Testicular cancer

Testicular cancer is the most common malignancy in men aged 15 to 35 years. With early detection, accurate staging, and effective platinum-based chemotherapy, cure rates of more than 96% have been achieved. Surgical removal of involved localized nodes has been shown to have therapeutic benefit and is curative. The reliable and predictable landing pattern of metastatic testicular cancer to the retroperitoneum is an instrumental factor in achieving these high success rates. Right-sided testicular drainage includes the interaortocaval lymph nodes, followed by the precaval and paracaval nodes, whereas left-sided drainage includes the left para-aortic and preaortic lymph nodes [21]. These predictable patterns of metastases allow accurate staging and treatment of early and bulky metastatic disease.

Testicular cancer is generally divided into seminomatous and nonseminomatous germ cell tumors. Because seminomas have proved to be sensitive to external beam radiation and cisplatinum-based chemotherapy, the role of RPLND in this disease has been limited.

RPLND traditionally has played a major role after radical inguinal orchiectomy for high-risk nonseminomatous germ cell tumors because it is believed that the retroperitoneal lymph nodes are usually the first and often the only site of metastatic disease in approximately 90% of nonseminomatous germ cell tumors. Removal of these nodes is curative in most patients with pathologic stage I and low-volume stage II disease. The procedure does not come without potential risks, however. Open RPLND requires a large midline incision, extensive bowel dissection, and potential injury to the sympathetic chain. Weighing the risks and benefits, the real question becomes, when must a RPLND be performed? As in prostate cancer, radiographic studies are unable to detect retroperitoneal disease with 100% sensitivity and specificity. If they could, RPLND in stage I disease could be avoided safely. Fifteen percent to 40% of patients are clinically and radiographicly understaged, with a 30% incidence of pathologic stage II disease in clinical stage I patients [22,23]. Certain elements in the primary tumor place patients at higher risk of retroperitoneal disease, including a high proportion of embryonal carcinoma in the primary or evidence of lymphatic/vascular invasion. RPLND is recommended for high-risk stage I and stage II-a disease in patients with nonseminomatous germ cell tumors. The information gathered from the node dissection later becomes critical in deciding the need for and quantity of adjuvant chemotherapy.

Historically, the boundaries of the RPLND included bilateral suprahilar dissections and dissection of all the nodal tissue between both ureters down to the bifurcation of the common iliac arteries. Because of better radiographic staging and significant complications from the suprahilar dissection, however, a modified template was developed that does not compromise the efficacy of the lymph node dissection. The modified template uses the left renal vein as the cranial margin of dissection (Fig. 5). The modified template did not completely prevent the loss of antegrade ejaculation from injury to the sympathetic fibers, so this untoward side effect remains a significant problem. This subsequently led to even more limited templates for right- and left-sided RPLNDs to minimize contralateral dissection, particularly below the level of the inferior mesenteric artery, and the development of

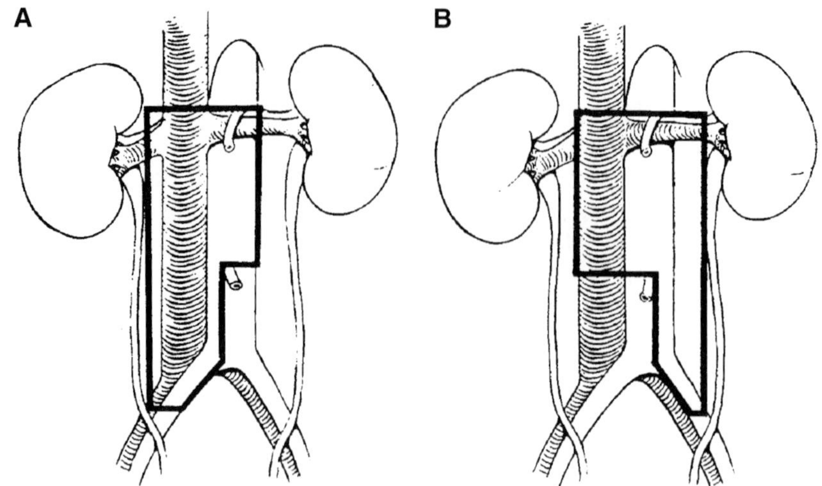

Fig. 5. Surgical templates for modified right- (*A*) and left-sided (*B*) RPLND. (*From* Gerber GS, Rukstalis DB. Retroperitoneal lymph node dissection. In: Smith AD, Badlani GH, Bagley DH, et al, editors. Smith's textbook of endourology. St Louis: Quality Medical Publishing; 1996. p. 1026; with permission.)

"nerve-sparing RPLNDs," in which the sympathetic chains, the post-ganglionic sympathetic fibers, and the hypogastric plexus are preserved.

Technique

Preoperative bowel preparation is crucial, as it is in open surgery. After giving prophylactic antibiotics, the patient is given general anesthesia. A nasogastric tube and Foley catheter are placed. The patient is then placed in 30° right or left oblique flank position, depending on the template being used. Pneumoperitoneum is created by using a Veress needle placed through an infraumbilical incision. A 10-mm trocar is then placed and the abdomen examined. Two additional 10-mm ports can be placed lateral to the rectus abdominus muscle, 5 cm above and below the umbilicus. The assistant can place additional 5-mm ports in the mid-axillary line to aid with retraction if needed. The procedure begins with mobilization of the colon by incising along the line of Toldt. All ligamentous attachments to the liver and spleen are divided. The peritoneal incision is carried caudally to the level of the internal inguinal ring to expose the spermatic vessels and a ligature that was placed at the time of radical orchiectomy. At this point, the spermatic vein can be traced proximally to the vena cava and left renal vein. The nodal packages over the vena cava are clipped and transected until the right and left renal veins are identified. The margins of dissection for a left-sided template are from the left renal vein to the bifurcation of the aorta and down to the bifurcation of the left common iliac artery to the left ureter. A right-sided template includes dissection from the right renal artery to the bifurcation of the vena cava and laterally to the right ureter. Meticulous hemostasis must be maintained throughout the operation with a combination of clipping and bipolar electrocautery. Any venous bleeding encountered usually can be controlled, either with direct pressure or the use of hemostatic agents such as oxidized cellulose. Identification and sparing of all sympathetic nerves, although tedious, should be attempted. After the nodal packages have been harvested, they are placed in an entrapment pouch and removed through one of the 10-mm ports. The fascia of the ports that are 10 mm or larger are closed. A closed suction drain can be placed and left through one of the port sites.

Outcomes

The L-RPLND experience began more than a decade ago. An early published series from Heidleberg, Germany described L-RPLND in 26 patients with clinical stage I and II disease [24]. The latter group contained 9 patients who had residual masses and negative markers after induction chemotherapy. The results were favorable with stage I disease, with surgery successfully completed in 16 of 17 patients. The average operative time was 290 minutes. Two complications were noted, including 1 patient with a delayed ureteral stenosis that required operative repair and another patient with an uneventful pulmonary emboli. The average length of hospital stay was 4.5 days. After a mean follow-up of 27 months, no patient had regional relapses, and 2 patients were successfully treated with chemotherapy for pulmonary metastases. Unfortunately, the experience with the stage II patients was not as encouraging. Only 2 of 9 cases were successfully completed laparoscopically because of difficulty with the desmoplastic reaction in the retroperitoneum. A more recent study reviewed the long-term outcomes of patients who underwent L-RPLND. Steiner et al [25] from Austria reviewed 185 patients who underwent a total of 188 L-RPLNDs. One hundred fourteen of these cases were performed for stage I NSGST, whereas 6 were performed for stage IIa disease. An additional 68 cases were performed after chemotherapy for residual retroperitoneal masses. The mean operative time and blood loss were 250 minutes and 119 mL, respectively. Mean hospital stay was 4 days. Antegrade ejaculation was preserved in 98.4% of patients. At a mean follow-up of 55.7 months, only 6 patients experienced disease relapse, but no patient died from the disease. The distribution of recurrences included one marker-only recurrence, three pulmonary metastases, and two retroperitoneal recurrences in the contralateral retroperitoneum outside the surgical template. The conclusion found in this and many other publications is that L-RPLND is safe and efficacious, with equivalent oncologic results as traditional open surgery for stage I and low volume stage II disease [26]. The clear benefits of L-RPLND include shorter hospital stays, less perioperative pain, and quicker convalescence. The quicker period of recovery can be important to young and active men afflicted with this disease. Critics of this procedure warn of the inadequate dissection around the lumbar vessels as a possible source of disease recurrence. They further point to the advanced laparoscopic skills needed to perform this operation and the ability to generalize this procedure to other urologists. In our opinion, this argument does not justify withholding the operation from men who may benefit from it. Increasing experience will help to shorten operative times and diminish complications.

Summary

Laparoscopic lymph node dissection plays a well-defined but limited role in urologic oncology. Laparoscopic lymph node dissection for prostate and testicular cancer represents the spectrum of expertise needed to perform these operations successfully. With adherence to the oncologic principles mandated in surgery, multiple studies have confirmed the feasibility, safety, and efficacy of these two procedures over the long term. The steep learning curve for laparoscopic surgery continues to be the largest obstacle to the permeation of these procedures to the general practice of urology. With time, refinement of techniques, and advancements in technology, these procedures may become easier and more common in the coming years.

References

[1] Borley N, Fabrin K, Sriprasad S, et al. Laparoscopic pelvic lymph node dissection allows significantly more accurate staging in "high risk" prostate cancer compared to MRI and CT. Scand J Urol Nephrol 2003;37(5):382–6.

[2] Partin AW, Yoo J, Carter HB, et al. The use of prostate specific antigen, clinical stage and Gleason score to predict pathologic stage in men with localized prostate cancer. J Urol 1993; 150:110–4.

[3] Partin AW, Kattan MW, Subong EN, et al. Combination of prostate specific antigen, clinical stage, and Gleason score to predict pathologic stage of localized prostate cancer: a multi-institutional update. JAMA 1997;277:1445–51.

[4] Lund GO, Winfield HN, Donovan JF, et al. Laparoscopic pelvic lymph node dissection following definitive radiotherapy for carcinoma of the prostate. J Urol 1997;157(2):548–51.

[5] Parra RO, Andrus C, Boullier J. Staging laparoscopic pelvic lymph node dissection: comparison of results with open pelvic lymphadenectomy. J Urol 1992;147:875–8.

[6] Herrell SD. Staging pelvic lymphadenectomy for localized carcinoma of the prostate: a comparison of 3 surgical techniques. J Urol 1997;157(4):1337–9.

[7] Cadeddu JA, Elashry OM, Snyder O, et al. Effect of laparoscopic pelvic lymph node dissection on the natural history of D1 prostate cancer. Urology 1997;50(3):391–4.

[8] Brendler CB, Cleeve LK, Anderson EF, et al. Staging pelvic lymphadenectomy for carcinoma of the prostate: risk versus benefit. J Urol 1980;124:849.

[9] Stone NN, Stock RG, Unger P. Laparoscopic pelvic lymph node dissection for prostate cancer: comparison of the extended and modified techniques. J Urol 1997;158(5):1891–4.

[10] Schuessler WW. Transperitoneal endosurgical lymphadenectomy in patients with localized prostate cancer. J Urol 1991;145(5):988–91.

[11] Ferzli G, Trapasso J, Raboy A, et al. Extraperitoneal endoscopic pelvic lymph node dissection. J Laparoendosc Surg 1992;2(1):39–44.

[12] Gloscock JM, Winfield HN. Pelvic lymphadenectomy: Intra- and Extraperitoneal access. In: Smith AD, Badlani GH, Bagley DH, et al, editors. Smith's textbook of endourology. St. Louis: Quality Medical Publishing; 1996. p. 870–92.

[13] Lang GS, Buckle HC, Hadley HR, et al. One hundred consecutive laparoscopic pelvic lymph node dissections: comparing complications of the first 50 cases to the second 50 cases. Urology 1994;44:221.

[14] Stone SN, Stock R. Laparoscopic pelvic lymph node dissection in the staging of prostate cancer. Mt. Sinai J Med 1999;66(1):26–30.

[15] Shingleton WB. Laparoscopic surgery. Surg Clin North Am 1996;76(3):585–93.

[16] Solberg A, Angelsen A, Bergan U, et al. Frequency of lymphocele after open and laparoscopic pelvic lymph node dissection in patients with prostate cancer. Scand J Urol Nephrol 2003;37(3):218–21.

[17] Grossman HB, Natale RB, Tangen CM, et al. Neoadjuvant chemotherapy plus cystectomy compared with cystectomy alone for locally advanced bladder cancer. N Engl J Med 2003; 349(9):859–66.

[18] Advanced Bladder Cancer Meta-analysis Collaboration. Neoadjuvant chemotherapy in invasive bladder cancer: a systematic review and meta-analysis. Lancet 2003;361(9373): 1927–34.

[19] Horenblas S, van Tinteren H. Squamous cell carcinoma of the penis: prognostic factors of survival. Analysis of tumor, nodes, and metastasis classification system. J Urol 1994;151: 1239.

[20] Mukamel E, deKernion JB. Early versus delayed lymph node dissection versus no lymph node dissection for carcinoma of the penis. American Urologic Association Update Series 1990;9(2):10–6.

[21] Weinstein M. Lymphatic drainage of the testes. Atlas of the Urologic Clinics of North America 1999;7:1–7.

[22] Hilton S, Herr HW, Teitcher JB, et al. CT detection of retroperitoneal lymph node metastases in patients with clinical stage I testicular nonseminomatous germ cell cancer: assessment of size and distribution criteria. AJR Am J Roentgenol 1997;169:521–5.

[23] Lashley DB, Lowe BA. A rational approach to managing stage I nonseminomatous germ cell cancer. Urol Clin North Am 1998;25:405–23.

[24] Rassweiler JJ, Seemann O, Henkel TO, et al. Laparoscopic retroperitoneal lymph node dissection for nonseminomatous germ cell tumors: indications and limitations. J Urol 1996; 156(3):1108–13.

[25] Steiner H, et al. Long term results of laparoscopic retroperitoneal lymph node dissection: a single center 10-year experience. Urology 2004;63(3):550–5.

[26] Bhayani SB, Ong A, Oh WK, et al. Laparoscopic retroperitoneal lymph node dissection for clinical stage I NSGCT: a long term update. Urology 2003;62(2):324–7.

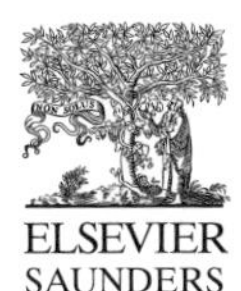
ELSEVIER
SAUNDERS

Surg Oncol Clin N Am
14 (2005) 367–379

SURGICAL
ONCOLOGY CLINICS
OF NORTH AMERICA

Standard Reconstruction Techniques: Techniques of Ureteroneocystostomy During Urinary Diversion

Murugesan Manoharan, MD, FRCS(Eng), FRACS*, Hari S.G.R. Tunuguntla, MD, MCh (Urol)

Department of Urology, University of Miami School of Medicine, PO Box 016960 (M814), Miami, FL 33101, USA

The principles of ureteric reconstruction during urinary diversion are not dissimilar from other reconstructive techniques used in the rest of the urinary tract. Excellent vascular supply, complete excision of devitalized tissue, good drainage, and a tension-free anastomosis are of paramount importance.

Various operative procedures have been described for replacement of the bladder after cystectomy or in conditions with severe bladder dysfunction (eg, in patients with neuropathic bladder). An important requirement after reconstruction of the lower urinary tract, such as with an ileal conduit or orthotopic bladder substitution, is that the reconstruction should not jeopardize the integrity of the upper urinary tract. The development of partial or complete obstruction of urine flow, the reflux of infected urine, and the formation of renal stones are factors that may adversely affect renal function.

Historical perspective

With the basic experiments of Coffey [1] in 1911, it became clear that the kidneys need protection from infection, reflux, and high pressure in the lower urinary tract. Protection of the kidneys is crucial and antireflux implantation by submucosal tunnel became the standard technique for most surgeons who performed ureterosigmoidostomies [2].

* Corresponding author.
E-mail address: mmanoharan@med.miami.edu (M. Manoharan).

doi:10.1016/j.soc.2004.11.015 ***surgonc.theclinics.com***

The first attempt at continent urinary diversion was reported by Simon [3] who performed the first ureterosigmoidostomy in 1852. He used a loop of silk thread to create a fistula between the ureter and rectum in a patient with bladder exstrophy. Early attempts at ureterosigmoidostomy were fraught with high mortality and morbidity rates related to sepsis and renal failure. Krynski [4] is credited as being the first to attempt to create an antirefluxing mechanism using a submucosal tunnel, but in 1911, Coffey [1] reported the first successful anastomosis of the ureters into the intact distal colon using a technique to tunnel the ureters through the bowel wall to prevent reflux of fecal flora. This success heralded the modern era of urinary diversion, and ureterosigmoidostomy became the predominant method used throughout the world for the next 40 years (Fig. 1A). A drawback of Coffey's ureterosigmoidostomy was that, instead of a direct mucosal anastomosis, the end of each ureter was left to hang free within the lumen of the bowel, which produced ureteral stenosis from inflammation and fecal contamination in some patients. To avoid this complication, Nesbit [5], in 1949, attempted a direct mucosal-to-mucosal ureterocolonic anastomosis (Fig. 1B) in which the ureteral edge was sutured directly to the colonic mucosa. Although the incidence of ureteral stenosis improved, the introduction of direct anastomosis did not improve the overall results of ureterosigmoidostomy, and this method was rapidly abandoned.

In 1951, Leadbetter and Clarke [6] described a technique with a long, extracolonic, seromuscular Coffey-type tunnel combined with Nesbit's direct mucosal anastomosis (Fig. 2). In 1953, Goodwin et al [2] described a similar combined technique but created a tunnel from within the bowel using an open, transcolonic ureterointestinal anastomosis (Fig. 3) that could

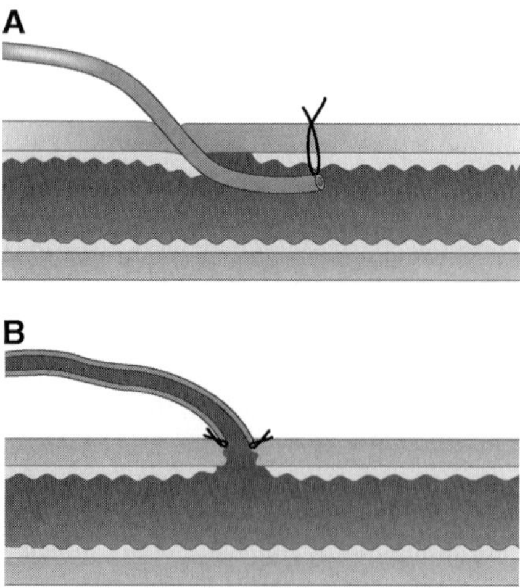

Fig. 1. (*A*) Coffey's tunneled free hanging anastamosis. (*B*) Nesbit's nontunneled end-to-side anastomosis.

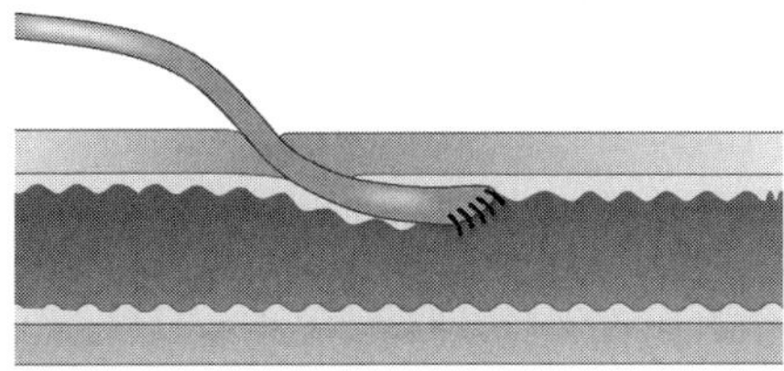

Fig. 2. Leadbetter's tunneled extracolonic anastomosis.

be performed under direct vision. Despite these elegant improvements in surgical technique, and with the additional safeguards of bowel preparations and antibiotics, reports continued to reveal a high incidence of complications secondary to ureterosigmoidostomy, including recurrent pyelonephritis, electrolyte imbalance, stone formation, secondary malignancy at the anastamotic site, and loss of renal function. The continent ureterosigmoidostomy was then almost abandoned and largely replaced by the ureteroileocutaneous diversion popularized by Bricker [7].

Furthermore, ureterosigmoidostomy did not address the problem of high-pressure storage, which was unrecognized at that time. The pressure in the intact sigmoid colon can reach up to 200 cm H_2O during defecation, and pressure waves that reach the distal colon with mass movements are approximately 60 to 80 cm H_2O [8]. More significantly, with increasing storage volumes, the resting basal pressure in the sigmoid rises. With volumes as little as 200 mL, basal pressure can begin to rise above 40 cm H_2O. The landmark study by McGuire et al [9] on myelodysplastic cases showed the deleterious effects of vesical storage pressures of more than 40 cm in terms of the development of hydronephrosis, reflux, and upper urinary tract deterioration. Intravesical pressures of more than 40 cm, even with sterile urine and without the presence of reflux, can predispose patients to renal deterioration. The necessity of creating a nonrefluxing ureteroenteric anastomosis in a low-pressure, continent reservoir remains controversial. The benefits of bowel detubularization to disrupt the circular

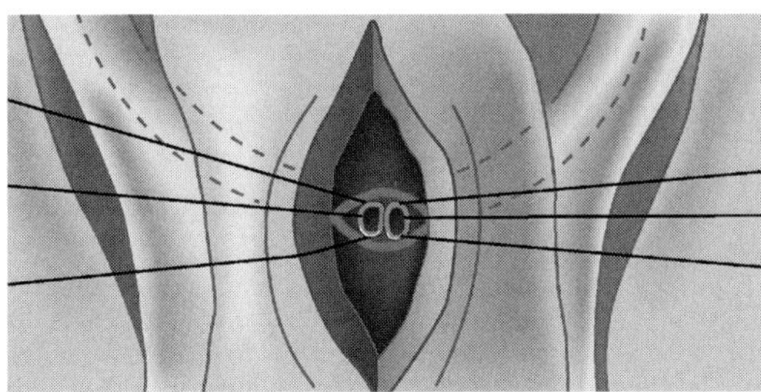

Fig. 3. Goodwin's tunneled transcolonic ureterosigmoidostomy.

muscle fibers and reorientation of the intestinal segments in opposite directions to interrupt high-pressure bowel peristalsis have been recognized since Goodwin et al [10] used the cup-patch technique for ileocystoplasty.

With the acceptance of the ileal conduit as the standard form of urinary diversion since the 1950s, the severe complications seen after ureterosigmoidostomy have become less common [11]. Long-term follow-up studies of patients with ileal conduits have shown that renal morbidity leading to functional deterioration develops in a significant number of patients, however [12,13]. The colonic conduit with an antireflux ureteric implantation was introduced in an attempt to preserve renal function [14]. Initial studies showed less renal damage with such a technique [15,16]. This finding was not confirmed in later reports, however [17,18].

Anatomic considerations

The ureters in adult humans are approximately 25 cm long. Variable lengths of the distal ureter are sacrificed during the cystectomy dependent on the oncologic margins, ease of dissection, and vascularity of the tissue. The main arterial supply comes from the renal artery (31%), vesical artery (26%), aorta (16%), iliac artery (9%), gonadal artery (8%), and others (10%). These vessels form the longitudinal periureteral plexus, which provides good collateral connection between the vessels. In approximately 15% to 25% of patients, these longitudinal collaterals are absent, which may result in ischemia of the ureteral anastamosis. Surgical removal of the bladder results in the deprivation of blood supply from the vesical and caudal vessels and its contribution to the longitudinal plexus.

Surgical techniques

Today, continent reconstruction (ie, orthotopic neobladder substitution and continent cutaneous diversion) is the standard diversion method in many centers. Ileal conduit still remains a popular diversion technique worldwide. Numerous techniques have been designed to achieve the goal of reflux prevention, reflecting the lack of a single method superior to any of the others. With the introduction of the principles of detubularizing and reconfiguring the intestinal segments, thus creating "low-pressure reservoirs," the concept of obligatory reflux protection has been challenged [19,20]. Stable renal function after direct ureteric implantation into detubularized reservoirs has been reported after short-term follow-up. The main argument of those who are against an antireflux mechanism is that the benefits of reflux prevention with the antireflux technique are lost because of a higher risk of stricture formation and upper urinary tract obstruction.

Is reflux prevention necessary during lower urinary tract reconstruction?

The need to incorporate an antireflux mechanism is supported by experimental findings, also in the low-pressure reservoirs/cystoplasties [21,22]. Others tested the hypothesis that under low pressure in an ileal cystoplasty there would be minimal effects on the kidneys with refluxing anastomosis at long-term follow-up [23]. Subtotal cystectomy and cup ileocystoplasty were performed on 13 dogs. Different methods of reimplantation were used: nine renoureteral units were refluxing, six were nonrefluxing, and 11 served as controls. Refluxing ureteric implantation was commonly associated with bacteriuria in the upper urinary tract and pyelonephritis. Antireflux ureteric implantation was beneficial for renal preservation in this setting. The findings are in accordance with other animal models in the setting of low-pressure reservoir/cystoplasty [21,24]. These findings are certainly alarming, although studies in humans are clearly needed to confirm this result in patients undergoing continent urinary reconstruction. High-pressure reflux with or without infection may lead to renal damage [9]. Antireflux procedures were therefore developed to reduce this risk following urinary diversion. Some of these techniques were developed before the introduction of orthotopic reconstruction, and their continued use with orthotopic reconstruction has been rather random and unscientific. Some surgeons with expertise in reconstruction have abandoned any form of antireflux procedure with orthotopic reconstruction [25].

Techniques of ureteric reimplantation

Techniques of ureteroneocystostomy during urinary diversion may be classified into three broad categories (Table 1): (1) refluxing, (2) nonrefluxing, and (3) combined.

Table 1
Types of ureteroneocystostomy during urinary diversion

Nonrefluxing	Refluxing	Combined
Leadbetter's ureterosigmoidostomy technique	Bricker's ureteroileal anastomosis	Studor's isoperistaltic limb
Goodwin's transcolonic technique	Wallace's technique	
Triple nipple extraluminal intussusception technique		
Split-cuff technique		
Le Duc technique		
Afferent nipple valve (used with Kock pouch)		
Hammock ureteroileal anastomosis		
Abol-Enein's serouslined extramural tunnel ureteroneocystostomy		

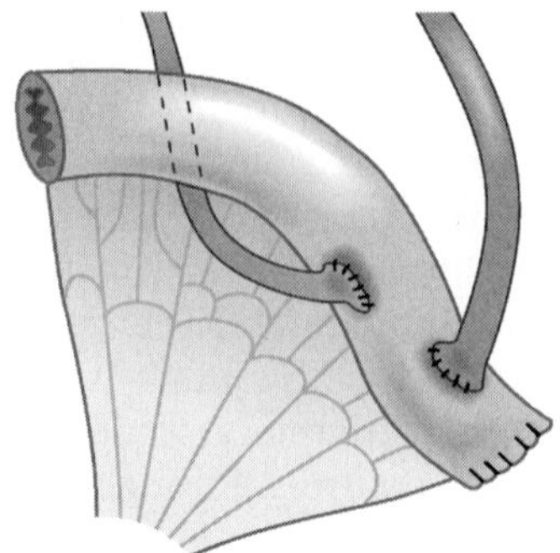

Fig. 4. Bricker's ureteroileal anastomosis.

Refluxing types of ureteral reimplantation

Obstruction, reflux, and bacteriuria are detrimental to renal function. An open refluxing technique (Bricker's and Wallace's techniques of ureteroileal anastomosis) (Figs. 4 and 5), however, is used for reimplantation of the ureter into the ileal conduit, although antirefluxing methods are available (eg, Le Duc and split-cuff ureteric nipple) [26,27]. The success of Bricker's ureteroneocystostomy depends on preservation of the vascular supply to the ileal segment and the ureters. Each ureter is spatulated and sutured to a small opening in the lateral aspect of the ileal conduit with absorbable sutures. The ureteroileal anastomosis by Wallace's technique differs from Bricker's method in that the spatulated ureters are anastomosed to each other before connecting the ureters to the open end of the isolated ileal segment. First, both ureters are trimmed to a convenient point so that the

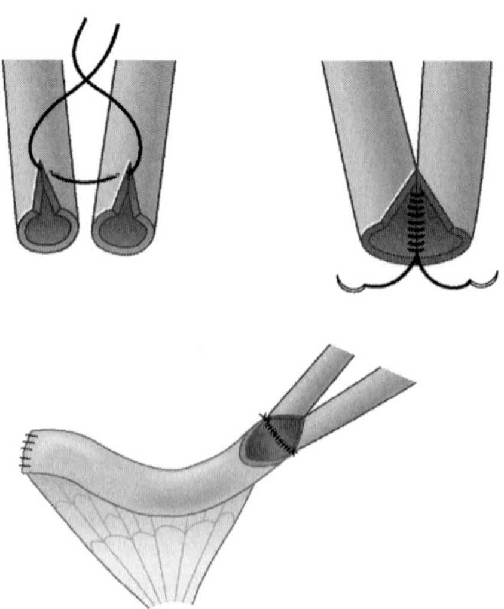

Fig. 5. Wallace's technique of ureteroileal anastomosis.

anastomosis is out of the pelvis in the event that radiation becomes necessary at a later date. Shortening of the ureters also prevents subsequent kinking. Both ureters are then spatulated along the anterior surface for approximately 1.5 cm, with care taken not to interfere with the blood supply, and joined together with interrupted 4-0 absorbable sutures. The conjoined ureters are then sutured to the proximal, open end of the isolated ileum. The conjoined ureters afford a larger anastomosis to the ileum, decreasing risks of ureteral anastomotic stenosis, and facilitate visualization of the ureteral orifice at the end of the isolated segment in case of retrograde instrumentation of the upper urinary tract at a later date.

Nonrefluxing types of ureteral reimplantation

For a colonic conduit, an antirefluxing submucous tunnel reimplantation (Leadbetter's and Goodwin's techniques; see Figs. 2 and 3) is used. With the introduction of continent diversion, new techniques for achieving non-refluxing units have become available. In the Le Duc technique, the ureter is placed in a 3- to 4-cm–long ileal mucosal trough, and the mucosal edges are sutured to the ureteric adventitia [26]. It may be used for reimplantation into the ileum or colon.

An afferent nipple valve is another antirefluxing mechanism and is an integral part of the Kock pouch urinary diversion. It is associated with complications, however, such as stone formation on staples and progressive fibrosis of the valve with urinary obstruction during follow-up [30]. In some centers, it has been replaced by the T-pouch [31]. An antirefluxing mechanism described by Abol-Enein and Ghoneim [32] is used during T-pouch urinary diversion. The Abol-Enein technique is a serous-lined extramural tunnel and can be used even for dilated ureters. A stricture rate of 3.8% has been reported with this technique [33].

A hammock anastomosis is another type of nonrefluxing ureteroileal anastomosis that prevents reflux caused by a retrograde peristalsis of the ileal conduit. It replaces the submucosal tunnel used in ureterocolonic anastomoses, which is not feasible in the thin wall of small bowel. The conjoined ureters are anastomosed to the side wall of the conduit at the proximal end of the ileal segment. The conjoined ureteral orifice is then buried into the intestinal wall, which is made elastic and supple by multiple longitudinal and transverse seromuscular incisions. The ureteroileal anastomosis is stented with polyethylene stents brought out through the abdominal stoma and removed on the fifth to seventh postoperative day, or it may be left unstented.

Combined technique

Studor et al [28] described an isoperistaltic afferent ileal loop technique (Fig. 4) that combines the reflux and antireflux mechanisms to obtain the best of both techniques. In this technique, the ureters are implanted directly end to side, thus in a refluxing manner, to the proximal part of an intact, tubular 20-cm–long ileal segment that opens into the pouch. The afferent limb is long and isoperistaltic and supposed to prevent reflux during voiding. Ureteric stenosis has been reported in 4 of 148 ureters following this method, and the loss of renal cortical thickness and function is less than 1% [29].

Outcomes following different techniques of ureteric reimplantation

The main problem with antireflux procedures is increased surgical complexity, which causes a higher complication rate. The renal deterioration that the surgeon is trying to avoid may be seen more frequently from obstruction at the ureteroileal junction.

Stricture rates with the Le Duc technique vary from 5% to 15% [34,35]. The split-cuff ureteric nipple was originally described for implantation into an ileal conduit. The technique has been used for reimplantation into ileal and colonic neobladders, however, with a stricture rate of 3 of 98 ureters [36].

Submucosal tunnel ureteral reimplantation into colonic segments causes strictures in 6% to 29% of patients [37,38].

Studer et al [39] prospectively randomized 70 patients undergoing orthotopic reconstruction to have either a freely refluxing end-to-side ureteroileal anastomosis into an afferent isoperistaltic ileal limb or an antirefluxing nipple valve. Ureteroileal stenosis resulting in severe upper tract dilation was seen in 13.5% of those ureterorenal units with antirefluxing nipple valves compared with only 3% of those with an afferent tubular segment. Although the follow-up period in this study was not very long, most patients were observed until death; the trial was abandoned because there were significantly more complications with intussuscepted nipple valves. Perhaps this form of antireflux mechanism has a particularly high complication rate, but other groups have reported high rates of stenosis using other forms of antireflux techniques as discussed later.

Longer term follow-up of 76 patients, with a mean of 84 months after afferent ileal limb bladder substitution, showed only 1% of ureterorenal units to have lost cortical thickness on ultrasound, which was associated with ureteroileal stenosis [29].

An afferent ileal limb does not prevent reflux altogether, but under normal voiding conditions, without an overfilled reservoir, reflux is minimal because the afferent tubular segment acts as a dynamic antireflux system. Videourodynamics do not show reflux of contrast medium during the Valsalva maneuver because pressure rises simultaneously in the bladder substitute and the upper tract [39]. Although measurement of renal cortical thickness and serum creatinine will not detect more minor degrees of renal deterioration that would be picked up with radioisotope measurement or glomerular filtration rate, it seems that the afferent ileal limb is safe in terms of renal function at 7 to 15 years.

Others therefore have now developed variations on this theme, such as the 3- to 5-cm chimney reported by Hautmann and Simon [40], who found a reduction in the ureteroileal stenosis rate of 9.5% in 363 consecutive patients with the Le Duc antireflux procedure to 1% in 195 subsequent patients with a freely refluxing anastomosis.

In a nonrandomized study of refluxing and nonrefluxing ureteroileal anastomoses in the Indiana pouch and ileal orthotopic bladder substitutes, Pantuck et al [41] also found a statistically significantly higher rate of benign ureteroileal stenosis with nonrefluxing anastomoses (13%) compared with a simple end-to-side anastomosis (1.7%) at a mean follow-up period of 41 months. They found no difference in the rate of hydronephrosis, pyelonephritis, upper tract stone formation, or serum creatinine between those patients with refluxing or nonrefluxing anastomoses.

In contrast, Kristjansson et al [42], in a randomized study of refluxing versus nonrefluxing ureteroenteric anastomoses with either an ileal or colonic conduit, found the ureteroileal stricture rate to be unrelated to the mode of implantation. The overall stricture rate was higher than expected, however, at 13.2% at a mean follow-up period of 10 years. (Since this report, they have modified antireflux techniques to a simpler submucosal tunnel.) The authors found no difference in reduction of glomerular filtration rate (GFR) between kidneys with and without reflux protection. If in a chronically infected conduit system no difference in GFR is detected with refluxing and nonrefluxing techniques, then it is unlikely that a difference would be seen with an orthotopic bladder substitute in which urine is usually sterile.

Surgeons should also remember that antireflux valves would not spare the upper tract from the effects of sustained high pressure in a bladder substitute. High pressure will close the valve, and, as urine production continues, pressure in the upper tract will increase until the bladder pressure reduces [39].

Bastian et al [43] compared the outcomes following different ureteric reimplantation techniques (Goodwin-Hohenfellner technique, Abol-Enein modification, and Le Duc procedure) during a follow-up period of 1 to 80 months (mean, 19 mo) in 41 patients (27 men and 14 women: median age, 56.3 y; range, 2–75 y). They concluded that different ureteric reimplantation techniques did not seem to be important. Ureteric stenosis requiring reimplantation occurred in two renal units (2%; one following the Goodwin-Hohenfellner technique and one following the Abol-Enein method). Le Duc et al [26] noted that strictures in the submucosal tunnel predominantly occurred during the first 2 years after surgery.

Causes of ureteroneocystostomy strictures

Causal factors suggested for strictures include the following: urine leak at the anastomosis, poor vascularity of the distal ureter, radiation, infection, poor surgical technique, inadequate spatulation of the ureter, and inadequate incision of the bowel at the ureteral entry site. Careful dissection and handling of the ureter is therefore extremely important. Anastomosis should be well vascularized, tension free, and water tight. The surgical technique should be meticulous. There is no clear consensus regarding what constitutes a stricture. Most studies on outcomes following various ureteroneocystostomy techniques are fraught with inadequacies, and the level of evidence is low.

Effects of ureteroneocystostomy on the urinary tract

The presumption that nonrefluxing ureteroneocystostomy techniques are associated with higher incidence of stricture and upper urinary tract obstruction led some to abandon these methods of reimplantation in continent urinary reconstructions using a low-pressure detubularized reservoir [41,44]. It is now believed that antirefluxing ureteroneocystostomy in low-pressure, high-capacity reservoirs is unnecessary [45]. Reflux prevention in neobladders is even less important than in a normal bladder [44]. Other authors [46], however, believe that prevention of reflux of urine from a bowel substitution urinary reservoir into the upper urinary tract is extremely important, with a rise in serum creatinine and pyelonephritis reported in patients who had ileal conduit converted to continent cutaneous diversion [47].

Gotoh et al [48] have reported intraluminal pressures of 80 to 115 cm H_2O at micturition in 44% of their patients with orthotopic bladder substitution. Studies have shown that neobladders are heavily colonized with potentially uropathogenic bacteria [49]. If a proper antireflux method is not used, or if there is an insufficiency in the antireflux mechanism, the micro-organisms might spread to the upper tract, even if the reservoir pressure is low. Whether such conditions are harmful to renal function is a matter of concern and long-term follow-up studies evaluating renal function are therefore warranted. Ghoneim [50] concluded that evidence from the current studies is neither sufficient nor convincing regarding the significance of antirefluxing ureteroneocystostomy. The potential advantage of reflux prevention, if it does not add a risk of obstruction, must also be considered.

Summary

A simple end-to-side freely refluxing ureteroenteric anastomosis into an afferent limb of a low-pressure orthotopic reconstruction, with regular voiding and close follow-up evaluation, is the procedure with the lowest overall complication rate. Continued peristalsis in the afferent ileal limb reduces but does not eliminate reflux. The potential benefit of "conventional" antireflux procedures in combination with orthotopic reconstruction seems outweighed by the higher complication and associated reoperation rates. There are no clear answers to the question of which is the better technique at present, however, and long-term randomized, prospective studies comparing the refluxing and nonrefluxing techniques are warranted.

References

[1] Coffey RC. Physiologic implantation of the severed ureter or common bile duct into the intestine. JAMA 1911;56:397–403.
[2] Goodwin WE, Harris AP, Kaufman JJ, Beal JM. Open transcolonic ureterointestinal anastomosis. A new approach Surg Gynecol Obstet 97:295–300.
[3] Simon J. Ectropia vesicae; operation for directing the orifices of the ureters into the rectum; temporary success; subsequent death; autopsy. Lancet 1852;2:568.
[4] Krynski L. Zur Technic der Ureterimplantation in der Mast Darm. Centralb I Chir 1896;23:73.
[5] Nesbit RM. Ureterosigmoid anastomosis by direct elliptical connection: a preliminary report. J Urol 1949;61:728.
[6] Leadbetter WF, Clarke BG. Five years' experience with uretero-enterostomy by the combined technique. J Urol 1955;73:67.
[7] Bricker E. Bladder substitution after pelvic evisceration. Surg Clin North Am 1950;30:1511.
[8] Fisch M, Wammack R, Steinbach F, et al. Sigma-rectum pouch (Mainz pouch II). Urol Clin North Am 1993;20:561.
[9] McGuire EJ, Woodside JR, Borden TA, et al. Prognostic value of urodynamic testing in myelodysplastic patients. J Urol 1981;126(2):205–9.
[10] Goodwin WE, Winter CC, Barker WF. Cup-patch technique of ileocystoplasty for bladder enlargement or partial substitution. Surg Gynecol Obstet 1959;108:370.
[11] Bricker EM. Bladder substitution after pelvic evisceration. Surg Clin North Am 1950;30: 1511–21.
[12] Madersbacher S, Schmidt J, Eberle JM, et al. Long-term outcome of ileal conduit diversion. J Urol 2003;169:985–90.
[13] Pernet FP, Jonas U. Ileal conduit urinary diversion: early and late results of 132 cases in a 25-year period. J Urol 1985;3:140–4.
[14] Turner-Warwick RT. Colonic urinary diversion. Proc R Soc Med 1960;53:56–8.
[15] Altwein JE, Jonas U, Hohenfellner R. Long-term follow-up of children with colon conduit urinary diversion and ureterosigmoidostomy. J Urol 1977;118:832–6.
[16] Starr A, Rose DH, Copper JF. Antireflux ureteroileal anastomoses in humans. J Urol 1975; 113:170–4.
[17] Elder DD, Moisey CU, Rees RW. A long-term follow-up of the colonic conduit operation in children. Br J Urol 1979;51:462–5.
[18] Husmann DA, Mclorie GA, Churchill BM. Nonrefluxing colonic conduits: a long-term life-table analysis. J Urol 1989;142:1201–3.
[19] Hohenfellner R, Black P, Leissner J, Alhoff EP. Refluxing ureterointestinal anastomosis for continent cutaneous urinary diversion. J Urol 2002;168:1013–7.
[20] Pantuck AJ, Ken-Ryu H, Perrotti M, Weiss RE, Cummings KB. Uretero-enteric anastomosis in continent urinary diversion: long-term results and complications of direct versus nonrefluxing techniques. J Urol 2000;163:450–5.
[21] Kock NG, Nilson AE, Norlén L, Sundin T, Trasti H. Changes in renal parenchyma and the upper urinary tracts following urinary diversion via a continent ileum reservoir. J Urol Nephrol 1978;49(Suppl):11–22.
[22] Kristjánsson A, Bajc M, Wallin L, Willner J, Mansson W. Renal function up to 16 years after conduit (refluxing or anti-reflux anastomosis) or continent urinary diversion. 2. Renal scarring and location of bacteriuria. Br J Urol 1995;76:546–50.

[23] Kristjánsson A, Abol-Enein H, Alm P, Mokhtar AA, Ghoneim MA, Mansson W. Long-term renal morphology and function following enterocystoplasty (refluxing or antireflux anastomosis): an experimental study. Br J Urol 1996;78:840–6.
[24] St. Clair SR, Hixon CJ, Richey ML. Enterocystoplasty and reflux nephropathy in the canine model. J Urol 1992;148:728–32.
[25] Hautmann RE. Urinary diversion: ileal conduit to neobladder. J Urol 2003;169:834–42.
[26] Le Duc A, Camey M, Teillac P. An original antireflux ureteroileal implantation technique: long-term follow-up. J Urol 1987;137:1156–8.
[27] Turner-Warwick RT, Ashken MH. The functional results of partial, subtotal and total cystoplasty with special reference to ureterocaecocysto-plasty, selective sphincterotomy and cystocystoplasty. Br J Urol 1967;39:3–12.
[28] Studer UE, Ackerman D, Casanova GA, Zingg EJ. A newer form of bladder substitute based on historical perspectives. Semin Urol 1988;6:57–65.
[29] Thoeny HC, Sonnenschein MJ, Madersbacher S, Vock P, Studer UE. Is ileal orthotopic bladder substitution with an afferent tubular segment detrimental to the upper urinary tract in the long term? J Urol 2002;168:2030–4.
[30] Jonsson O, Olofsson G, Lindholm E, Tomqvist H. Long-time experience with the Kock ileal reservoir for continent urinary diversion. Eur Urol 2001;40:632–40.
[31] Stein JP, Lieskovsky G, Ginsberg DA, Bochner BH, Skinner DG. The T-pouch: an orthotopic ileal neobladder incorporating a serosal lined ileal anti-reflux technique. J Urol 1998;159:1836–42.
[32] Abol-Enein H, Ghoneim MA. A novel uretero-ileal reimplantation technique: the serous lined extramural tunnel. A preliminary report. J Urol 1994;151(5):1193–7.
[33] Abol-Enein H, Ghoneim MA. Functional results of orthotopic ileal neobladder with serous-lined extramural ureteral reimplantation: experience with 450 patients. J Urol 2001;165: 1427–32.
[34] Mansson W, Davidsson T, Konyves J, Kiedberg F, Mansson A, Wullt B. Continent urinary tract reconstruction—the Lund experience. Br J Urol 2003;92:271–6.
[35] Shaaban AA, Gaballah MA, El-Daisty TA, Ghoneim MA. Urethral controlled bladder substitution: a comparison between the intussuscepted ileal nipple valve and the technique of Le Duc as antireflux procedures. J Urol 1992;148:1156–61.
[36] Sagalowsky AI. Further experience with split-cuff nipple ureteral reimplantation in urinary diversion. J Urol 1998;159:1843–4.
[37] Lampel A, Fisch M, Stein R, et al. Continent urinary diversion with the Mainz pouch. World J Urol 1996;14:85–91.
[38] Stein R, Fisch M, Beetz R, et al. Urinary diversion in children and young adults using the Mainz pouch I technique. Br J Urol 1997;79:354–61.
[39] Studer UE, Danuser H, Thalmann GN, Springer JP, Turner WH. Antireflux nipples or afferent tubular segments in 70 patients with ileal low pressure bladder substitutes: long-term results of a prospective randomized trial. J Urol 1996;156:1913–7.
[40] Hautmann RE, Simon J. Ileal neobladder and local recurrence of bladder cancer: patterns of failure and impact on function in men. J Urol 1999;162:1963–6.
[41] Pantuck AJ, Han KR, Perrotti M, Weiss RE, Cummings KB. Ureteroenteric anastomosis in continent urinary diversion: long-term results and complications of direct versus nonrefluxing techniques. J Urol 2000;163:450–5.
[42] Kristjansson A, Wallin L, Mansson W. Renal function up to 16 years after conduit (refluxing or anti-reflux anastomosis) or continent urinary diversion. 1. Glomerular filtration rate and patency of uretero-intestinal anastomosis. Br J Urol 1995;76:539–45.
[43] Bastian PJ, Albers P, Haferkamp A, et al. Modified ureterosigmoidostomy (Mainz pouch II) in different age groups and with different techniques of ureteric implantation. BJU Int 2004; 94:345–9.
[44] Hautmann RE. Urinary diversion: ileal conduit to neobladder. J Urol 2003;169:834–42.

[45] Hohenfellner R, Black P, Leissner J, Alhoff EP. Refluxing ureterointestinal anstomosis for continent cutaneous urinary diversion. J Urol 2002;168:1013–7.
[46] Turner-Warwick R, Chapple C. Functional reconstruction of the urinary tract and gynaeco-urology. Oxford, UK: Blackwell; 2002.
[47] Ahlering TE, Gholdoian G, Skarecky D, Weinberg AC, Wilson TG. Simplified technique with short and long-term follow-up of conversion of an ileal conduit to an Indiana pouch. J Urol 2000;163:1428–31.
[48] Gotoh M, Yoshikawa Y, Sahashi M, et al. Urodynamic study of storage and evacuation of urine in patients with a urethral Kock pouch. J Urol 1995;154:1850–3.
[49] Wullt B, Holst E, Steven K, et al. Microbial flora in ileal and colonic neobladders. Eur Urol 2004;45:233–9.
[50] Ghoneim MA. Editorial comment. J Urol 2002;168:1016–7.

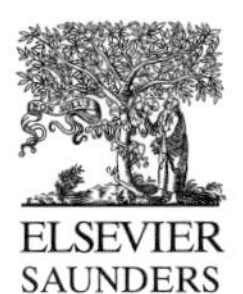
ELSEVIER
SAUNDERS

Surg Oncol Clin N Am
14 (2005) 381–396

SURGICAL
ONCOLOGY CLINICS
OF NORTH AMERICA

Internal Hemipelvectomy for the Management of Pelvic Sarcomas

Henry J. Mankin, MD*, Francis J. Hornicek, MD, PhD

Orthopaedic Oncology Service, Massachusetts General Hospital, Harvard Medical School, Gray 6 Orthopaedics, 55 Fruit Street, Boston, MA 02114, USA

Bone and soft-tissue sarcomas that arise in the pelvis are difficult to treat [1–31]. Tumors can be large and destructive before discovery, and they often involve vessels and nerves [1–7,21,32,33]. Achieving a wide or even a marginal surgical resection margin may be technically complex at times [34,35]. The adjuvant chemotherapy and radiation therapy are almost as difficult for patients as the extensive surgery, and a prolonged period of rehabilitation often is required [4,5,7,15,22,24,31,36–41]. The complication rate for the surgery is high, with excessive bleeding and infection as the most common problems. Bowel and bladder malfunction, requirements for vascular grafts, and especially issues related to skin closure often cause extraordinary difficulties for the patient and the care-taking team [1–4,11,15,21,24,26,30–32,36,42–44]. The outcomes as far as success of the surgery and patient survival are almost never as good as for similar pathologic lesions of the thigh, scapular, or arm regions or the more distal parts of the body [6,16,20,21,31,45,46].

Historically, patients with pelvic tumors were treated with hemipelvectomies. These operations not only were fraught with complications but also in most cases represented physical, functional, and psychological problems for the patients [47–54]. Several studies have described the difficulties patients have with such a procedure, and there is little doubt that regardless of the problems associated with the internal hemipelvectomies and reconstructions, such procedures are preferred to total limb ablation [51–54].

Neither of the authors has received any compensation or benefits as a result of this publication. No corporate entity is involved, and no pharmaceutical materials are defined as related to the presentation. Patient confidentiality has not been violated by this study, and the data system has been approved by the Institutional Review Board for the Massachusetts General Hospital.

* Corresponding author.

E-mail address: hmankin@partners.org (H.J. Mankin).

doi:10.1016/j.soc.2004.11.010

Internal limb-sparing hemipelvic surgeries are generally classified as partial resections, total resections and total resections and reconstructions [2,4,6,37]. The problems with partial resections vary with the site of the surgery, which may include the iliac wing, the ischial or pubic rami, the acetabular region, or some combination of them. The total resection without some form of reconstruction is simpler from the standpoint of the surgical procedure but can be disabling [5,17,33,42,43,45,47,55–57], whereas the pelvic reconstruction using allograft or other systems for restoration is fraught with complications but in many cases is much more successful in terms of function [15,35–38,58–60]. In deciding what sort of surgery to perform, the team must review carefully the type of tumor, its malignant potential, the possible response to adjuvant therapy, and the extent of the resection that is required to remove the tumor. Of considerable importance is the patient's age, the presence of metastases, and a clear definition of the patient's willingness to undergo the surgery [4,7,10,61].

Materials and methods

In consideration of the problems associated with pelvic surgery, one must evaluate the patient, determine the extent and character of the tumor, and introduce the most appropriate protocol that will render the patient free of disease and as functional as possible.

Patient evaluation

It is essential to obtain some key pieces of information about the patient. First, one must establish the age and health status, particularly in terms of other disorders, such as diabetes, cardiac disease, unexplained weight loss, distant metastases, functional status in terms of ambulation, pain control, and sleep-deprivation. Second, one must define the nature of the local complaints related to the pelvic neoplasm. The information required includes degree and character of the pain and methods used control it, the presence or absence of bladder or bowel symptoms, assessment of arterial or venous obstruction, presence or absence of atrophy, and determination of the presence and extent of neurologic disturbances in the region of the pelvis or lower extremity.

Tumor evaluation

The presence of a palpable mass and its location, size, increase in local warmth, pulsatile nature, and degree of tenderness should be assessed by physical examination and the information recorded. Routine roentgenograms are sometimes helpful (Fig. 1), but CT (Fig. 2) and especially MRI (Fig. 3) are essential. Such studies often help define the margins required for the surgery. Vascular studies of the lower extremity are sometimes useful in

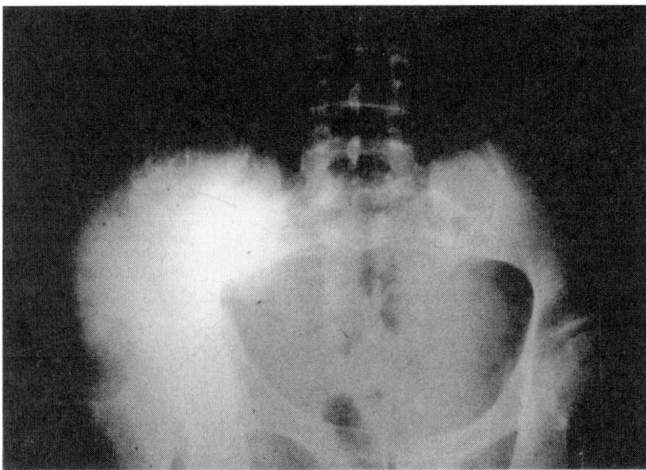

Fig. 1. A roentgenogram of the pelvis of a 55-year-old man with an enormous mass arising from the right ilium, which on biopsy was found to be a high-grade chondrosarcoma.

assessing the degree of partial occlusion, venous obstruction, or simply the proximity of the tumor to the vessels. An electromyography is sometimes useful in assessing the degree of damage to the nervous system; a CT of the chest and abdomen, a bone scan, and a positron emission tomographic scan frequently are helpful in determining the presence and extent of metastases. A biopsy is an essential part of the tumor evaluation and sometimes can be obtained by fine needle aspiration or with greater accuracy by CT-guided

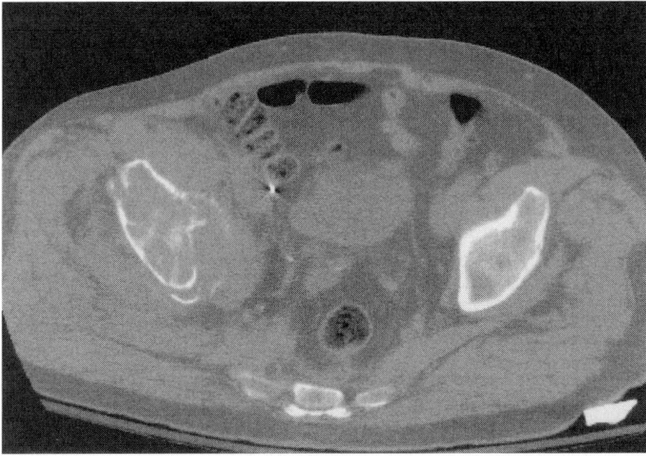

Fig. 2. A CT image of the pelvis of 62-year-old woman with complaints of pain in the left pelvis and hip disability. The malignant fibrous histiocytoma arose from the inner aspect of the pelvis and partially destroyed the supra-acetabular portion of the bone.

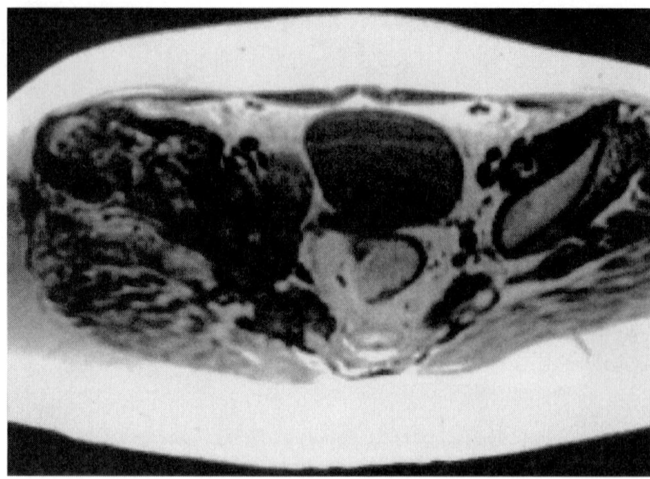

Fig. 3. An MRI of the pelvis in an 18-year-old man shows the enormous destructive mass arising from the ilium. The lesion was a high-grade osteosarcoma.

core needle biopsy. An open biopsy may be necessary, but it should be through the smallest possible incision, designed to be readily resectable at the time of definitive surgery.

Treatment planning

To provide the best possible treatment, the information obtained from the studies described previously must be reviewed carefully by a team that consists of the surgeon, a medical oncologist, a radiation oncologist, a pathologist, and a radiologist, all of whom have experience and knowledge regarding bone and soft-tissue tumors. Based on the size, location, and nature of the tumor, the presence or absence of metastases, and the patient's age and health status, a protocol must be established that could consist of one of the following [1–4,34,56]:

- Wide or marginal surgical resection
- Surgical resection followed by radiation or chemotherapy or both
- Neoadjuvant chemotherapy or radiation therapy followed by surgery and, if necessary, additional adjuvant therapy
- Palliative radiation or surgery as necessary to address metastatic spread and local tumor by appropriate measures

Surgical techniques

Surgical approaches and techniques vary depending on the location of the tumor and the planned resection. It should be apparent, however, that there are three different methods of tumor resection technology: (1) an intralesional procedure, which leaves gross tumor, (2) a marginal procedure, which uses the surrounding fibrous layer, known as a "psuedocapsule," as the margin and potentially leaves microscopic foci of tumor, and (3) a wide procedure, which removes sufficient material to completely remove the entire tumor and the surrounding psuedocapsule [1,2,7,34,37]. The last method is the least likely to allow a local recurrence but it is often the most difficult to achieve for pelvic tumors because of the proximity of the tumor to local major vessels and nerves.

For tumors of the iliac wing, the best approach is frequently along the iliac crest, which allows access to the anterior and posterior aspects of the tumor but may—if the tumor is large enough—cause some degree of skin vascular impairment. For tumors of the pubic rami, the longitudinal incision that runs along the pubis and extends to the ilium laterally and across the symphysis medially is often the simplest. For tumors of the ischium, an incision along the ischiopubic region that extends down the medial thigh and, if necessary, across the symphysis and into the region of the hip joint seems best. For tumors of the acetabular region, an anterior or lateral approach that extends into the thigh to add a hip replacement system is logical and relatively straightforward. For a total pelvic resection, either an extensive anterior approach (Smith-Petersen approach) or a long lateral incision starting at the crest and extending into the thigh is usually necessary.

Resection of the pubis often can be treated without any type of replacement (Fig. 4) or with an auto- or allograft insertion (Fig. 5). Resection of the ischium usually requires no replacement system. Resection of a portion of the ilium need not be replaced unless the lesional area lies in juxtaposition to the sacrum, in which case an auto- or allograft can be implanted to maintain structure and function (Fig. 6). Resection of the entire ilium and acetabulum can be treated by either resection and arthrodesis of the femoral head or trochanteric region to the sacrum (Fig. 7) or an allograft replacement without metallic femoral prosthesis (Fig. 8) or with a proximal femoral total joint (Fig. 9).

Over the past 32 years, the Orthopaedic Oncology Service has performed a large number of pelvic operative procedures and maintained information about them in an oncologic computerized database [60]. The system contains demographic, diagnostic, therapeutic, complication, and outcome information for more than 16,000 patients with benign and malignant tumors that affect the skeleton and adjacent soft tissues. The system has been approved by the hospital's institutional review board, is only available to members of the orthopedic oncology group, and is specifically designed to avoid violation of patient confidentiality. Information is recorded from the time of initial contact to the most recent visit. When the final outcome for the patient is not known, it is possible through several sources to gain information as to survival and sometimes the patient's life status and adjustments [61].

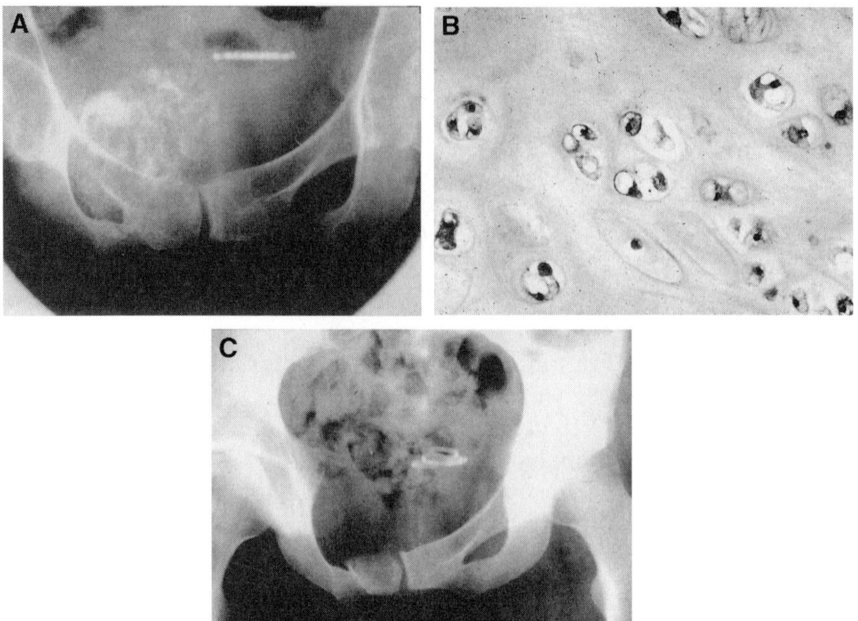

Fig. 4. A 36-year-old woman complained of a tender mass arising from the right pubic ramus. A radiograph showed the large mass (*A*), which histologically showed a low-grade cartilage tumor presumably arising in an osteocartilaginous exotosis (*B*). The lesion was completely resected and has not recurred (*C*).

Currently 344 patients in the computerized system are reported to have received treatment for malignant tumors of the pelvis. Of that group, 24 patients were excluded from this study because they had had no surgery, 20 were excluded because there was insufficient outcome information, and 94

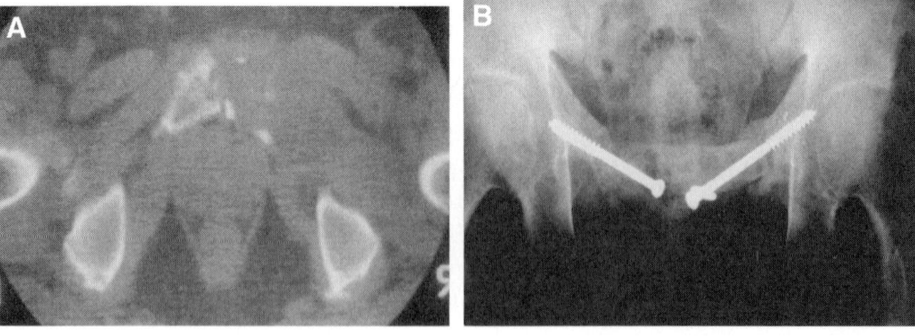

Fig. 5. A more destructive cartilaginous tumor of higher grade involved the right pubis and the symphysis pubis (*A*). The lesion was completely resected, and the symphysis and a portion of the ischial bones were removed. A segment of iliac bone was implanted and held in place with screws (*B*).

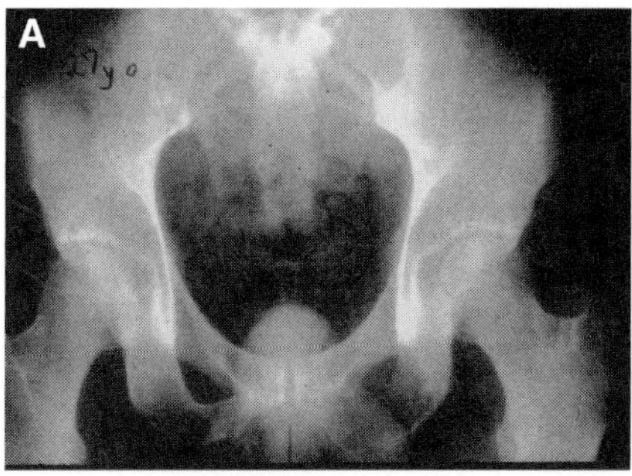

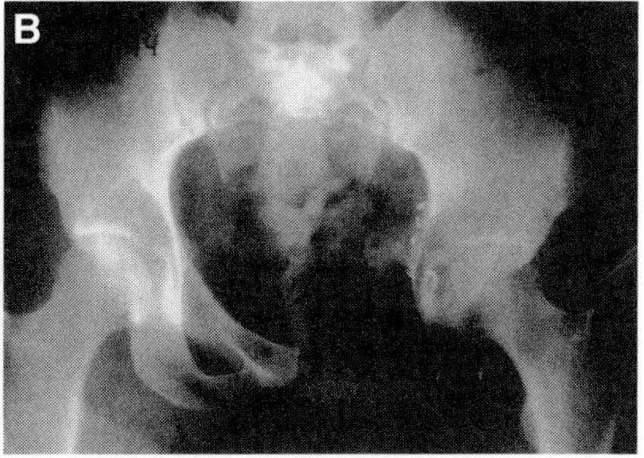

Fig. 6. A 27-year-old man complained of pain on sitting and was found to have a Ewing's sarcoma of the left ischium (*A*). A complete resection of the left ischium and pubis was performed and no reconstruction was required (*B*).

were excluded because the postoperative follow-up period was less than 3 years. The total group remaining for this study was 206 patients. The data provided information as to the types of procedures, the clinical success of the procedure, the complications, and the length of survival. It was also possible to compare the results for the different diagnoses, procedures, and age and gender of the patients. The data for this group of patients were further compared with data for patients with the same diagnoses but whose tumors were located in non-pelvic sites. The statistical analytic techniques used for this study included chi square calculations as assessed by Mantel-Haenszel and Fisher exact tests and Cox regression studies [62,63].

Results

Table 1 shows the demographic data for the 206 patients. The average age was 47 $\pm$ 20 years (range, 3–89 years), and there were 107 male patients

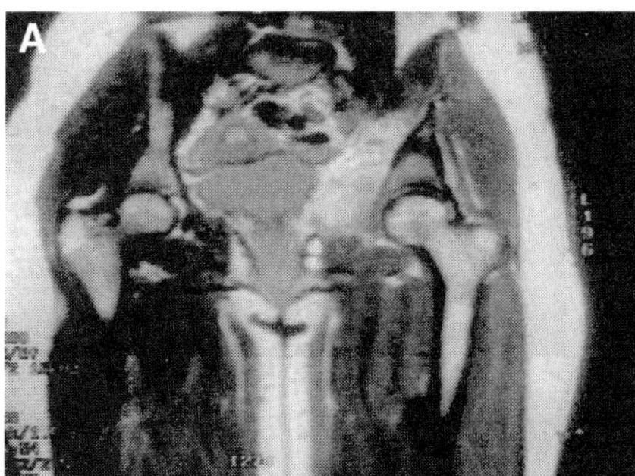

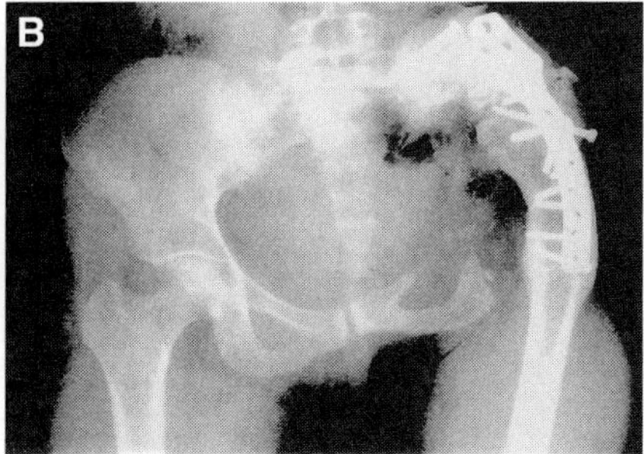

Fig. 7. A 25-year-old woman developed an osteosarcoma of the left pelvis (*A*). She and her family decided that they did not want an allograft. After the resection, a sacral-femoral arthrodesis was performed (*B*). The patient fared well and subsequently had a 2-inch segment from the right femur transplanted to the left to equalize her limb length.

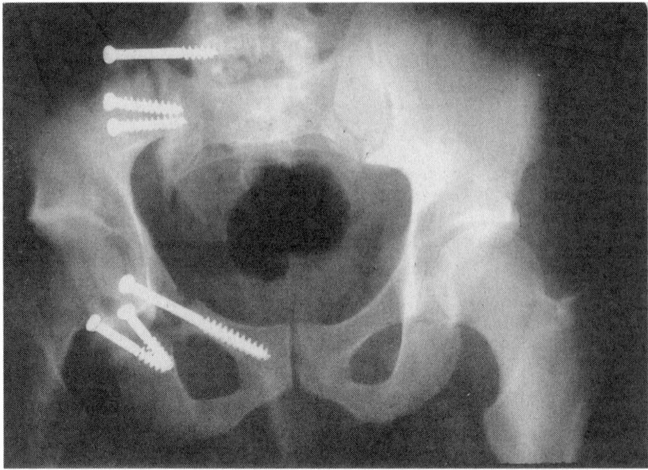

Fig. 8. An allograft pelvis was implanted in a man after resection of a chondrosarcoma. The patient's femoral head fit nicely into the new acetabulum so no metallic device was required.

and 99 female patients. The average length of follow-up for the patient group was 5.2 ± 5.2 years, with a range of 0.5 to 24 years. Forty-one of the patients had allografts implanted to replace the resected part of the pelvis; 144 had some form of resective surgery, sometimes with autograft replacement; and 21 patients had an external hemipelvectomy. The Musculoskeletal Tumor Society stages [34] are also shown in Table 1, and as can be noted, most sof the patients are classified as stages II or III. For the most part, the diagnoses for the patients are highly malignant tumors, including 46 chondrosarcomas, 45 osteosarcomas, 27 malignant soft-tissue tumors (mostly malignant fibrous histiocytomas), 22 Ewing's sarcomas, and 47 cases of metastatic carcinoma from various primaries, most often breast, prostate, and kidney.

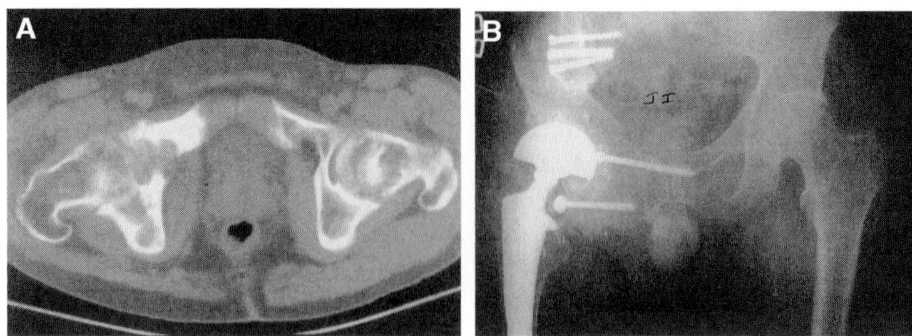

Fig. 9. A 65-year-old physician developed a chondrosarcoma of the pelvis that involved the acetabulum (*A*). The tumor was resected, an allograft was implanted, and a bipolar hip replacement was introduced (*B*). His disability was minimal.

Table 1
Demographic data for patients with pelvic tumors

Number of patients:		206
Gender:	men 107	women 99
Age:	average age 47 ± 20 (range, 3–89)	
Average duration of follow-up:		5.2 ± 5.2 y (range, 0.5–24 y)
MSTS stage		
O	0	
IA	5	
IB	26	
IIA	6	
IIB	99	
III	70	
Surgical procedures		
41 patients had allograft replacement of entire pelvis		
21 patients had formal complete hemipelvectomies		
144 patients had pelvic resective surgery		

Abbreviation: MSTS, Musculoskeletal Tumor Society.

Table 2 shows the survival data for the 206 patients to be approximately 50%. The mean figure for the time from beginning of treatment to demise for the 102 patients who died was 3 ± 3 years (range, 0.5–15 years). The survival time for the 104 survivors was 8 ± 6 years (range, 2–24 years).

The survival data for the patients with the various diagnoses are shown in Table 3. The overall figure is 50% survival rate, and most of the tumors show approximately equivalent values, with the exception of the 27 patients with malignant fibrous histiocytomas, who have a statistically significant reduced survival rate of only 30% ($P < 0.04$).

Gender had no effect on outcome. Age was a significant factor in outcome determination. The 101 patients over the age of 50 had a 44%

Table 2
Survival data for pelvic tumors

Diagnoses	Total	Dead	Percent surviving (%)
Total cases	206	102	50
Osteosarcoma	45	19	58
Chondrosarcoma	46	20	57
Ewing's	22	11	50
Malignant fibroushistiocytoma	27	19	30[a]
Metastatic carcinoma	47	24	49
Lymphoma	6	3	50
Myeloma	3	3	0
Liposarcoma	4	1	75
Chordoma	4	1	75
Leiomyosarcoma	2	1	50

[a] $P > 0.04$ chi square (Mantel-Haenszel).

Table 3
Effect of stage and treatment on survival

Stage and treatment	Number of patients	Number deceased	Percent surviving
MSTS stage			
Stage IA	5	0	100%
Stage IB	26	6	77%
Stage IIA	6	3	50%
Stage IIB	99	55	39%
Stage III	70	38	46%
Stage data are significant at $P < 0.007$			
Surgery			
Pelvic resection	144	77	54%
Hemipelvectomy	21	13	48%
Allograft	49	19	54%
Surgical data are not significant			
Adjuvant treatment			
Received neither	31	10	68%
Chemotherapy alone	26	8	69%
Radiation alone	15	7	47%
Received both	134	77	44%

Abbreviation: MSTS, Musculoskeletal Tumor Society.

Adjuvant data are significant at $P < 0.02$, but half of the patients not treated with either chemotherapy or radiation were MSTS stages IA or IB, whereas only three of the patients with chemotherapy alone were stage III and four were stage IA or IB.

survival rate compared with 105 patients under the age of 50 who had a 57% survival rate ($P < 0.02$).

Musculoskeletal Tumor Society stage also had a significant effect on outcome. The 31 patients classified as stages IA and IB had a high survivorship (81%), whereas 105 patients classified as stages IIA or IIB and 70 patients classified as stage III had a 45% rate of survival ($P < 0.007$) (Table 3). There was no significant difference between the outcome for stage II and stage III patients ($P < 0.91$).

Table 3 shows the effect of the type of surgery performed on survival data. The 21 patients who underwent an external hemipelvectomy and the 41 patients who received an allograft implant did not vary in their survival statistics from the 144 who underwent some type of resective surgery.

The effects of the use of adjuvant chemotherapy or radiation on survival are also shown in Table 3, and they disclose better survival data for patients who received no chemotherapy or radiation or who received chemotherapy alone. The statistical difference by Mantel-Haenzel test is $P < 0.02$. As noted in the Table 3, however, these data are presumed to be inaccurate based on the types of patients who comprised these groups. More than half of the 31 patients who received no adjuvant treatment were Musculoskeletal Tumor Society stages IA or IB, whereas only 3 of the 26 patients who received only chemotherapy were stage III and 4 were stage IA or IB.

Another area of concern involves the margins obtained at the time of surgery. Information regarding the margins was only available for 149 of the 206 patients. There was a marked decrease in survival for patients who had intralesional surgery compared with patients with either marginal or wide resection margins. The validity of this observation might be challenged on the basis that 18 of the 29 patients who had intralesional surgery had stage III metastatic carcinoma. Fewer patients who underwent marginal and wide resection had metastatic carcinomas, and the tumors were presumably smaller in size.

A second issue is related to the use of allografts in the pelvis. Table 4 compares the data for 41 pelvic allografts and 526 allografts introduced for high-grade malignancies but in other anatomic sites. The ages for the patients who underwent pelvic resection were higher, but the length of follow-up was similar. The patient survival data for the pelvic allografts were considerably lower ($P < 0.007$), as were the recurrence rate, frequency of metastasis, and infection. The likelihood of amputation was the same. For these two groups of patients, the current result for pelvic allografts was a score of 50% good or excellent, whereas for the non-pelvic allografts performed for stage II or stage III tumors it was 68% ($P < 0.02$).

Discussion

Although some authors have described reasonably good results for the treatment of some pelvic lesions [15,32,33], based on literature surveys there is little doubt that the treatment of patients with high-grade sarcoma and metastatic carcinoma of the pelvis is considerably more difficult than for other sites [1,6,11,19,43,51]. The failure rate is higher, the disability levels are greater, and, as noted in this effort and in many others, the survival rate is considerably poorer [1,8,12,14,18,33]. The question is not that it is so; all

Table 4
Comparison of results for patients with pelvic allograft surgery for high-grade tumors with those from other sites

Comparison data	Pelvic allografts	Other sites	Chi square P-values
Number	41	526	
Age	43 ± 19 (15–74)	35 ± 18 (2–86)	
Length of follow-up	5 ± 5 y (1–17)	7 ± 6 (2–28)	
Survival	54%	73%	$P < 0.007$
Recurrence	32%	9%	$P < 0.0009$
Metastases	66%	31%	$P < 0.00007$
Amputation	7%	8%	NS
Infection	20%	11%	$P < 0.03$

All statistical studies used Mantel-Haenzel and Fisher exact tests.

data support that. The two additional questions are why it is so and what can be done to make it better.

In terms of the causes for a poorer survival rate, there are several possible explanations.

1. The vascularity of pelvic tumors is significantly greater than in other more distal sites. Not only does this make the surgery more difficult in terms of blood loss but also it almost surely increases the likelihood of discharge of malignant tumor cells into the venous system at the time of surgery, which leads to an increased risk of metastasis. Another feature of the vascular issue is the internal body temperature at the site of the tumor, which is considerably higher than that for tumors in more distal sites. This may play a role in increasing the release of cytokines, such as the prostaglandins and others, which may increase the malignancy of the tumor and the risk of metastasis.
2. The size of the tumors is often much greater in the pelvis than in other sites. Although the pelvis has a collection of nerves passing through it, it is still possible for tumors at this site to grow much larger with less recognition by the patient or the examining physician as compared with other more distal sites or in the upper extremities. A lesion 10 cm in longest diameter in the calf or thigh—or especially in the foot or hand—is hard to ignore, but a similarly sized lesion in the pelvis can exist without patient awareness as long as fracture or neural or vascular compression does not occur.
3. Surgical resection is often much more complex for pelvic tumors based on the proximity of blood vessels and nerves. Avoiding viscera and trying to save the femoral, sciatic, or obturator nerves or the internal iliac and femoral vessels and even some of the smaller arteries and veins can lead to not only a marginal resection but also an intralesional resection. As noted in the previous data, intralesional surgical resection has a high mortality for pelvic lesions compared with marginal or wide resections.
4. Reconstructive surgery about the pelvis is complex and sometimes difficult. Restoring anatomy for the hip, maintaining the length of the limb, and retaining the function for the muscles are hardly simple tasks and sometimes require far more time and ingenuity than procedures in other anatomic sites. The duration of surgery increases the likelihood of infection and anesthetic complications. Most patients who receive pelvic surgery for high-grade tumors spend several days in a special care unit at our institution and frequently remain intubated and on intravenous fluids for a much longer period of time than patients who are treated for lesions in other anatomic sites.
5. Insertion of a pelvic allograft has some advantages in comparison with autograft reconstruction or metallic inserts, but it also has the highest rate of failure of any allograft procedure [2,11,15,35,38,55,58]. At times,

dealing with the complex complications may exceed the potential value of the procedure for the patient. It is also likely that the pelvic allograft has the highest rate of donor bacterial contamination, and many tissue banks treat their pelvic components with radiation to reduce the likelihood of an infection in the host [55,59]. These devices are presumably less likely to be infective but are perhaps more fragile mechanically because of the exposure to radiation or are less likely to be revascularized by the host bone tissue.

6. Radiation and chemotherapy were given to most patients in this series and presumably were partly responsible for the continued survival of half of the patients. The patients who did not receive such adjuvant care were too few in number to assess the role of these measures, but one must presume on the basis of our understanding of the treatment protocols for at least osteosarcoma, Ewing's sarcoma, and malignant fibrous histiocytoma that the outcome would have been far poorer had they not received the medication [8,14,15,22,25,29,39,40,41]. Radiation and chemotherapy treatment may be life saving, but it decreases the rate of rapid healing of tissues and incorporation of the allograft or autograft components [59].

Summary

There are some interesting and fascinating issues raised by this research effort. First, it seems that the mean figure for survival for patients with pelvic tumors is approximately 50%, and that figure includes patients with metastatic carcinoma and patients with an array of bone sarcomas. The malignant fibrous histiocytomas fared less well, presumably because of the invasion of viscera, nerves, and blood vessels that made resection more difficult.

Second, gender had no effect and age had only a moderate effect on outcome. Men fared as well as women, and although older patients fared less well, the difference was probably related to the increased frequency of metastatic disease in the older age group. Third, it seems remarkable that the choice of surgical treatment seems to make little difference in outcome. Patients with hemipelvectomies and allograft replacements survived just as well or poorly as patients with partial resections. Fourth, marginal and wide margins at surgery had almost identical outcomes at the same 50% level, whereas the 29 patients with intralesional margins fared less well.

It seems that the critical comment regarding all this is that almost no matter what the tumor is and how it is treated, 50% of the patients survive, particularly if the margins are marginal or wide and adjunctive treatment is administered. That level of success is not as good as we would like, but it is certainly a baseline start to see if some efforts will help improve the outcome. Based on the data reported in this article, the approaches must include improved surgical techniques, altered adjuvant therapy protocols, and better mechanical restoration systems. These are clearly the directions we must take if we are to improve the status and outlook for these patients.

References

[1] Campanacci M, Capanna R. Functional results of reconstruction for peri-acetabular pelvic resections requiring sacrifice of the hip joint. In: Enneking WF, editor. Limb salvage in musculoskeletal oncology. New York: Churchill-Livingstone; 1987. p. 187–91.

[2] Campanacci M, Capanna R. Pelvic resection: the Rizzoli experience. Orthop Clin North Am 1991;22:65–86.

[3] Capanna R, Guernelli N, Ruggieri P, et al. Periacetabular pelvic resections. In: Enneking WF, editor. Limb salvage in musculoskeletal oncology. New York: Churchill-Livingstone; 1987. p. 141–6.

[4] Conrad EU III, Springfield D, Peabody T. Pelvis. In: Simon MA, Springfield DS, editors. Surgery for bone and soft tissue tumors. Philadelphia: Lippincott-Raven; 1998. p. 323–41.

[5] Eilber FR, Grant TT, Sakai O. Internal hemipelvectomy: excision of the hemipelvis with limb preservation. An alternative to hemipelvectomy. Cancer 1979;43:806–9.

[6] Eilber RF, Eckardt JJ, Grant TG. Resection of malignant bone tumors of the pelvis: evaluation of local recurrence, survival and function. In: Enneking WF, editor. Limb salvage in musculoskeletal oncology. New York: Churchill-Livingstone; 1987. p. 136–41.

[7] Enneking WF, Dunham WK. Resection and reconstruction for primary neoplasms involving the innominate bone. J Bone Joint Surg Am 1978;60A:731–46.

[8] Fahey M, Spanier SS, Vander Giriend RA. Osteosarcoma of the pelvis. J Bone Joint Surg Am 1992;74A:321–30.

[9] Johnson JT. Reconstruction of the pelvic ring following tumor resection. J Bone Joint Surg Am 1978;60A:747–51.

[10] O'Connor MI, Sim FH. Salvage of the limb in the treatment of malignant pelvic tumors. J Bone Joint Surg 1989;71:481–94.

[11] O'Connor MI. Malignant pelvic tumors: limb-sparing resection and reconstruction. Semin Surg Oncol 1987;13:49–54.

[12] Patterson FR, Peabody TR. Operative management of metastases to the pelvis and acetabulum. Orthop Clin North Am 2000;31:623–31.

[13] Prewitt TW, Alexander HR, Sindelar WF. Hemipelvectomy for soft tissue sarcoma: clinical results in fifty-three patients. Surg Oncol 1995;4:261–9.

[14] Pring ME, Weber KL, Unni K, et al. Chondrosarcoma of the pelvis: a review of sixty-four cases. J Bone Joint Surg Am 2001;83A:1630–42.

[15] Scully SP, Temple HT, O'Keefe RJ, et al. Role of surgical resection in pelvic Ewing's sarcoma. J Clin Oncol 1995;13:2336–41.

[16] Shin KH, Rougraff BT, Simon MA. Oncologic outcomes of primary bone sarcomas of the pelvis. Clin Orthop 1994;304:207–17.

[17] Stephenson RB, Kaufer H, Hankin FM. Partial pelvic resection as an alternative to hindquarter amputation for skeletal neoplasms. Clin Orthop 1989;242:201–11.

[18] Tomeno B, Languepin A, Gerber C. Local resection with limb salvage for the treatment of periacetabular bone tumors: functional results in nine cases. In: Enneking WF, editor. Limb salvage in musculoskeletal oncology. New York: Churchill-Livingstone; 1987. p. 147–55.

[19] Windhager R, Karner J, Kutschera HP, et al. Limb-salvage in periacetabular sarcomas: a review of 21 consecutive cases. Clin Orthop 1989;331:265–76.

[20] Donati D, Giacomini S, Gozzi E, et al. Osteosarcoma of the pelvis. Eur J Surg Oncol 2004;30:332–40.

[21] Rodl R, Gosheger G, Ledinger B, et al. Correction of leg-length discrepancy after hip transposition. Clin Orthop 2003;416:271–7.

[22] Wunder JS, Ferguson PC, Griffin AM, et al. Acetabular metastases: planning for reconstruction and review of results. Clin Orthop 2003;415(Suppl):S187–97.
[23] Wolf RE. Sarcoma and metastatic carcinoma. J Surg Oncol 2000;73:39–46.
[24] Ozaki T, Flege S, Kevric M, et al. Osteosarcoma of the pelvis: experience of the Cooperative Osteosarcoma Study Group. J Clin Oncol 2003;21:334–41.
[25] Schwameis E, Dominkus M, Kepler P, et al. Reconstruction of the pelvis after tumor resection in children and adolescents. Clin Orthop 2002;402:220–35.
[26] Somville J, Van Bouwel S. Surgery for primary bone sarcomas of the pelvis. Act Orthop Belg 2001;67:442–7.
[27] Lewis SJ, Wunder JS, Couture J, et al. Soft tissue sarcomas involving the pelvis. J Surg Oncol 2001;77:8–14.
[28] Bergh P, Gunterberg B, Meis-Kindblom JM, et al. Prognostic factors and outcome of pelvic, sacral and spinal chondrosarcomas: a center-based study of 69 cases. Cancer 2001;91: 1201–12.
[29] Sucato DJ, Rougraff B, McGrath BE, et al. Ewing's sarcoma of the pelvis: long-survival and functional outcome. Clin Orthop 2000;373:193–201.
[30] Ham SJ, Kroon HM, Koops HS, et al. Osteosarcoma of the pelvis: oncological results of 40 patients registered by the Netherlands Committee on Bone Tumours. Eur J Surg Oncol 2000; 26:53–60.
[31] Grimer RJ, Carter SR, Tillman RM, et al. Osteosarcoma of the pelvis. J Bone Joint Surg Br 1999;81B:796–802.
[32] Aboulafia AJ, Malawer MM. Surgical management of pelvic and extremity osteosarcoma. Cancer 1989;71(Suppl 10) 3358–66.
[33] Lane JM, Duane K, Glasser DAB, et al. Periacetabular resections for malignant sarcomas. In: Enneking WF, editor. Limb salvage in musculoskeletal oncology. New York: Churchill-Livingstone; 1987. p. 156–66.
[34] Enneking WF, Spanier SS, Goodman MA. A system for the surgical staging of musculoskeletal sarcoma. Clin Orthop 1980;153:106–20.
[35] Vaughan L, Tomford WW, Mankin HJ. Pelvic and proximal femoral resective surgery and allograft replacement. In: Evarts CM, editor. Surgery of the musculoskeletal system. 2nd edition. London: Churchill Livingstone; 1990; p. 3185–3210.
[36] Apfellstaedt JP, Zhang PJ, Driscoll DL, et al. Various forms of hemipelvectomy for soft tissue sarcomas: complications, survival and prognostic factors. Surg Oncol 1995;4: 217–22.
[37] Enneking WF. Pelvis. In: Musculoskeletal tumor surgery. New York: Churchill-Livingstone; 1983. p. 483–90.
[38] Verma NN, Kuo KN, Gitelis S. Acetabular osteoarticular allograft after Ewing's sarcoma resection. Clin Orthop 2004;419:149–54.
[39] Bacci G, Ferrri S, Mercuri M, et al. Multimodal therapy for the treatment of nonmetastatic Ewing sarcoma of pelvis. J Pediatr Hematol Oncol 2003;25:118–24.
[40] Groff DB. Pelvic neoplasms in children. J Surg Oncol 2001;77:65–71.
[41] Rodl RW, Hoffmann C, Gosheger G, et al. Ewing's sarcoma of the pelvis: combined surgery and radiation therapy. J Surg Oncol 2003;83:154–60.
[42] Hillmann A, Hoffman C, Gosheger G, et al. Tumors of the pelvis: complications after reconstruction. Arch Orthop 2003;123:340–4.
[43] Damron TA, Sim FH. Surgical treatment for metastatic disease of the pelvis and the proximal end of the femur. Instr Course Lect 2000;49:461–70.
[44] Patterson FR, Peabody TD. Operative management of metastases to the pelvis and acetabulum. Orthop Clin North Am 2000;31:623–31.
[45] Satcher RL Jr, O'Donnell RJ, Johnston JO. Reconstruction of the pelvis after resection of tumors about the acetabulum. Clin Orthop 2003;409:209–17.
[46] Minard-Colin V, Kalifa C, Guinebretiere JM, et al. Outcome of flat bone sarcomas (other than Ewing's) in children and adolescents: a study of 25 cases. Br J Cancer 2004;90:613–9.

[47] Ariel IM, Shah JP. The conservative hemipelvectomy. Surg Gynecol Obstet 1977;144: 406–13.

[48] Douglass HO, Razack M, Holyoke D. Hemipelvectomy. Arch Surg 1975;110:82–5.

[49] Higinbotham NL, Marcove RC, Casson P. Hemipelvectomy: a clinical study of 100 cases with a five-year follow-up on 60 patients. Surgery 1966;59:706–8.

[50] Mankin HJ. History of the treatment of musculoskeletal tumours. In: Klenerman L, editor. Evolution of orthopaedic surgery. London: Royal Society of Medicine Press; 2002. p. 191–210.

[51] Materson EL, Davis AM, Wunder JS, et al. Hindquarter amputation for pelvic tumors: the importance of patient selection. Clin Orthop 1998;350:187–94.

[52] Pringle JH. The interpelvic-abdominal amputation with notes on two cases. Br J Surg 1916; 194:283–7.

[53] Steel HH. Partial or complete resection of the hemipelvis: an alternative to hindquarter amputation for periacetabular chondrosarcoma of the pelvis. J Bone Joint Surg Am 1978; 60A:719–30.

[54] Baliski CR, Schachar NS, McKinnon JG, et al. Hemipelvectomy: a changing perspective for a rare procedure. Can J Surg 2004;47:99–103.

[55] Alho AJ, Ekfors T, Dean PB, et al. Incorporation and clinical results of large allografts of the extremities and pelvis. Clin Orthop 1991;307:200–13.

[56] Enneking WF, Menendez LR. Functional evaluation of various reconstructions after periacetabular resection of iliac lesions. In: Enneking WF, editor. Limb salvage in musculoskeletal oncology. New York: Churchill-Livingstone; 1987. p. 117–35.

[57] Natarajan MV, Bose JC, Mazhavan V, et al. The Saddle prosthesis in periacetabular tumours. Int Orthop 2001;25:107–9.

[58] Harrington KD. The use of hemipelvic allografts or autoclaved grafts for reconstruction after wide resections of malignant tumors of the pelvis. J Bone Joint Surg Am 1992;74A: 331–41.

[59] Yoshida Y, Osaka S, Mankin HJ. Hemipelvic allograft reconstruction after periacetabular bone tumor resection. J Orthop Sci 2000;5:198–204.

[60] Mankin HJ. A computerized system for orthopaedic oncology. Clin Orthop 2002;399: 252–61.

[61] Refaat Y, Gunnoe J, Hornicek FJ, et al. Comparison of quality of life after amputation or limb salvage. Clin Orthop 2002;397:298–305.

[62] Cox DR. Regression models and life tables. J R Stat Soc 1972;34:187–220.

[63] Bailar JC, Mosteller F. Guidelines for statistical reporting in articles for medical journals: amplifications and explanations. Ann Intern Med 1988;108:258–65.

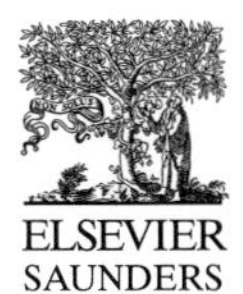
ELSEVIER
SAUNDERS

Surg Oncol Clin N Am
14 (2005) 397–417

SURGICAL
ONCOLOGY CLINICS
OF NORTH AMERICA

Extended Pelvic Resection for Sarcoma or Visceral Tumors Invading Musculoskeletal Pelvis

Lloyd A. Mack, MD, FRCSC[a,b],
Walley J. Temple, MD, FRCSC, FACS[a,b,*]

[a] *Tom Baker Cancer Centre, 1331-29th Street NW, Calgary, Alberta, Canada T2N 4N2*
[b] *University of Calgary, Calgary, Alberta, Canada T2N 4N2*

Locally extensive primary or recurrent pelvic cancer invading the musculoskeletal pelvis is one of the most challenging problems in oncology. Often, these patients are offered only palliative therapy, such as external beam radiation or a defunctioning colostomy, instead of a potentially curative procedure [1]. Pain, bleeding, intestinal or urinary fistulae or obstruction, and neurologic symptoms are frequently inevitable [2,3]. The consequences of no treatment are commonly worse than the disability secondary to surgery and result in immeasurable suffering [2,3]. A major principle of oncologic surgery is that any tumor, even extensive tumors that are locally confined and resectable, must be considered potentially curable; this concept forms the basic premise for this article.

The biology of tumors of the rectum, anus, bladder, cervix, uterus, and prostate and retroperitoneal sarcoma includes invasion of the adjacent visceral and bony confines of the pelvis. Similarly, primary pelvic sarcoma can invade visceral organs. Recurrent disease is usually more extensive than are primary tumors and much more difficult to control, perhaps because of its biology or contamination at the primary surgery [4–6]. Although there are several studies addressing the role of pelvic exenteration, there are fewer data on the role of extended pelvic resection or composite resection,

* Corresponding author. Tom Baker Cancer Centre, 1331-29th Street NW, Calgary, Alberta, Canada T2N 4N2.

E-mail address: walleyte@cancerboard.ab.ca (W.J. Temple).

doi:10.1016/j.soc.2004.11.002 ***surgonc.theclinics.com***

including sacrectomy, internal hemipelvectomy, and external hemipelvectomy for tumors invading the musculoskeletal pelvis [1,7–16].

Epidemiology shift

Advanced pelvic malignancy invading the musculoskeletal pelvis is becoming more infrequent. Screening programs for cervical cancer, colorectal cancer, and prostate cancer have either significantly decreased the incidence of these diseases or led to increased detection of more treatable primary disease [17–26]. The appropriate multimodality therapy of primary cancers also has reduced the number of patients burdened with recurrent pelvic malignancy invading the musculoskeletal pelvis. This situation is most dramatically shown in the reduction of the local recurrence rates of rectal cancer from more than 40% to less than 10% over the last two decades as a result of redefining the appropriate rectal cancer operation, total mesorectal excision [27,28]. Randomized trials evaluating multimodality preoperative therapy, adjuvant 5-fluorouracil, and radiotherapy confirm downstaging of large (T4) tumors and decreased local recurrence rates [29,30]. Because isolated and locally advanced pelvic malignancies become less frequent, these patients will need to be handled in specialized centers where subspecialty training and experience are available. This surgery is best done by teams that include expert surgical oncologists, colorectal surgeons, gynecology oncologists, urologists, plastic surgeons, and neurosurgeons.

Patient selection, preoperative assessment, indications, and contraindications

Appropriate patient selection is crucial. Physiologic age and adequate cardiopulmonary reserve are the most important factors. In addition, a well-motivated, fully informed patient with a well-developed social support system is mandatory. The patient must want an operation (convincing a reluctant patient of the need for a significant, potentially disabling procedure will lead to unsatisfactory outcomes).

Clinical assessment focuses on symptoms such as hematuria, pneumaturia, rectal bleeding, tenesmus, central pelvic pain, or, more concerning, radicular pain, which indicates major nerve involvement. Constitutional symptoms, such as weight loss or fatigue, which suggest distant disease, are worrisome and should intensify the search for systemic disease. On physical examination, clinically suspicious nodes outside the abdomen (eg, neck, axilla, or groin) should be inspected by means of a biopsy. Rectal and pelvic examination will determine whether the tumor is fixed and give an impression of tumor extent.

Evidence of rapid tumor growth, growth during primary treatment, or early recurrence after primary treatment are likely to be important, although to date these findings have not been well-documented prognostic factors in extended pelvic resections. It is the current authors' impression that early recurrence, after fewer than 6 to 12 months despite adequate primary therapy, is a relative contraindication to extended pelvic resection unless the primary surgery was poorly performed. Similarly, patients with significant nodal burden at primary presentation usually have more biologically aggressive disease. In rectal cancer, recurrence following low anterior resection is more likely to be resectable and improve median survival compared with recurrence following abdominoperineal resection [31]. This finding may reflect a differing biology of primary anastomotic recurrence versus diffuse seeding after abdominoperineal resection.

With the previously described concepts in mind, preoperative imaging may determine whether disease is potentially curable with an extended pelvic resection. A CT scan of the head, chest, abdomen, and pelvis plus a bone scan are necessary to rule out distant disease in visceral cancers regardless of patient symptoms. CT chest and abdominal scans are performed to rule out distant disease in primary pelvic bony or retroperitoneal sarcoma. Recurrent rectal cancer is at especially high risk of bony metastases or marrow involvement [32]. An MRI scan of the pelvis is necessary in determining the extent of pelvic disease, sidewall involvement, and regional metastases [33,34]. Bilateral hydroureter secondary to tumor obstruction or proximal tumor growth above S2 (sciatic notch) is generally considered incurable in recurrent rectal cancer [1,6]. Although positron emission tomography is not routinely used, it is a promising test for more precise assessment of disease outside of the pelvis [18,35]. The principle of avoiding radical surgery if there is any evidence of systemic disease cannot be overstated.

Adjuvant radiation therapy

Before proceeding with surgical intervention, pre- or postoperative radiation therapy is a critical component of obtaining local control for most tumors in the pelvis. Patients have often had "full-dose" radiation therapy for their primary treatment, and further radiation is not recommended in recurrent disease [36,37]. Reirradiation should be considered, however, and may have less toxicity than traditionally believed [38–40]. Mannaerts et al used a reirradiation dose of 30 Gy in 7 patients with locally recurrent rectal cancer who had previous full-dose radiation therapy before sacropelvic resection [39]. Intraoperative electron beam radiotherapy (IOERT; 10–17.5 Gy) was also delivered if there was an area at high risk of residual tumor following resection. Complications included grade 1 to 2 neuropathy in five patients, radiation cystitis in one patient, and ureter stenosis in one patient [40]. Other specialized centers are reporting similar results of IOERT [38,40,41].

A neoadjuvant approach has been particularly successful in the present authors' center for local control of sarcoma [42]. Three days of continuous adriamycin (30 mg/d) as a radiosensitizer and a subsequent 10 days of radiation (300 cGy/d) has been used for soft tissue and bony pelvic sarcomas where bowel is not included in the radiation field. For tumors with a retroperitoneal or intrapelvic component where significant small bowel will be radiated, an intraperitoneal, saline-filled silastic spacer is placed at laparotomy to displace small bowel out of the pelvis [43]. A dexon mesh is sutured to the peritoneum to hold the spacer in place. This step allows 50 to 60 Gy of radiation therapy to be given with minimal small bowel toxicity. Definitive surgery occurs approximately 4 to 6 weeks after radiation with the removal of spacer and tumor. In a pilot study of 15 patients with unresectable tumors (ie, R0 resection not possible) treated in this manner, there were no complications from prosthesis placement or radiation therapy, even though this treatment required very large fields (11 × 16 cm to 17 × 23 cm; Temple WJ, unpublished data, 1990). Eleven patients went on to definitive resection, three developed metastases before planned resection, and one refused further surgery. Significant tumor shrinkage was identified in eight patients with retroperitoneal sarcoma, in four with recurrent colon cancer, and in one patient with transitional cell carcinoma, suggesting sterilization of the margins. Two patients with renal cell cancer had no response. Local control has been maintained in nine survivors who have had 12- to 48-month follow-up evaluations. Since this pilot experience, the present authors have continued to use intraperitoneal spacers to deliver full-dose radiation in more than 40 patients with minimal toxicity and infrequent interruption of radiation treatment or decrease of dose. With this approach, the authors routinely use preoperative radiation therapy because there are few tumors in the pelvis for which it does not improve resectability and local control.

Extended pelvic operations

In keeping with cancer surgery principles, advanced primary or recurrent pelvic cancer invading the musculoskeletal pelvis must be excised en bloc. When such an operation involves the bony pelvis, the terms *composite resection* or *extended pelvic resection* have been used [1,12]. In general, primary connective tissue sarcoma of the pelvis represents the most straightforward scenario, especially if other pelvic organs are not involved. Visceral cancers invading the musculoskeletal pelvis are approached by means of pelvic exenteration plus extended pelvic resection as necessary.

Sacral composite resection

Several operative approaches to sacral composite resection have been described [1,6,7,37]. Wanebo et al [6,31,32] described a two-stage approach, beginning with an anterior procedure, followed by a posterior sacral procedure after 1 to 2 days. All patients undergo complete laparotomy to rule out distant metastatic disease, including liver metastases, serosal seeding, or extrapelvic nodal metastases such as para-aortic nodes; all sites of suspected involvement should be examined by frozen section before proceeding or abandoning the procedure. Dissection begins along the lower aorta and iliac arteries. The involvement of common iliac pelvic nodes precludes curative resection, and the procedure is terminated. An en bloc formal pelvic lymphadenectomy is performed with the tumor resection. Posterior or total pelvic extenteration proceeds, depending on extent of disease. If the ureter or bladder is involved then these are divided and a urinary diversion is performed. Internal iliac arteries and veins are divided. An end sigmoid colostomy is performed, with the stapled rectal stump left in the pelvis. The tumor and involved organs are maximally mobilized anteriorly and laterally without disruption of the posterior tumor–sacrum interface. Finally, the abdomen is closed, and the patient is prepared for the second stage of the procedure.

The patient is positioned prone for the dorsal sacral resection. The procedure begins with a midline incision over the sacrum, curving inferolaterally around the buttocks to allow subcutaneous flaps exposing the gluteus maximus. The muscle is split to identify the sciatic nerve. The gluteal musculature is then dissected from the sacrum, and the sacrotuberous and sacrospinous ligaments are incised from the ischium. A finger is inserted through the endopelvic fascia inferior and medial to the sciatic nerve to palpate the pelvic floor at the level of resection. Sacral laminectomy occurs just above the planned level of resection. The dural sac is ligated, and the proximal sacral nerve roots are preserved under direct vision. An osteotome or oscillating saw is then used to transect the sacrum, and the specimen, including sacrum, pelvic sidewalls, and tumor with attached viscera (previously dissected from the anterior approach), is removed. Once hemostasis is achieved, the pelvic defect is closed with local gluteus flaps or distant myocutaneous flaps, commonly from the rectus abdominus. Although Wanebo and Marcove [6] described a 2-day procedure (abdominal, posterior), Bakx et al [7] performed the sacropelvic resection in one operative session with a combination of abdominal and dorsal approaches (Salam position).

An alternate one-stage approach with the patient in one position is similar [1,37]. The main difference is the use of a combined abdominal and perineal approach occurring with the patient in the lithotomy position, with a pad placed under the lower lumbar spine to elevate the sacrum off the operating table. Initial laparotomy and staging are identical to the two-stage approach. The isolation and control of the aorta are important early because temporary cross-clamping is performed during the sacral transaction [1,44]. Again, the pelvic sidewall is mobilized at the level of the endopelvic fascia. Involved pelvic fascia or musculature, including obturator internis or pyriformis, may be resected to obtain clear margins. Pelvic lymphadenectomy is included with tumor excision, and sacral nerve roots are preserved unless directly invaded. The key is anterior and lateral mobilization of the tumor, with no attempt at separating the tumor mass from the sacrum. The sacrum is cleared for resection 1 to 2 cm proximal to the tumor [1,44].

The perineal dissection is started with a skin and subcutaneous incision similar to the perineal portion of a standard abdominoperineal procedure. An excision margin of 2.5 to 3 cm is maintained around the tumor. Attachments of the gluteus maximus to the sacrum are divided superiorly to the level of intended sacral transaction. Aortic cross-clamping just above the common iliac arteries is temporarily performed, without the use of intravenous heparin at the present authors' center [1]. Others have described the used of heparin followed by rapid reversal with protamine [44]. This maneuver has been used safely for 20 to 25 minutes without complication and decreases blood loss by half during this portion of the operation [1]. The sacrum is divided with an osteotome, and remaining soft tissue attachments are quickly divided by heavy curved scissors to allow specimen removal. Hemostasis is now easily obtained with the improved exposure following exenteration, and the aortic cross-clamp can be removed. It is important to check for leaking cerebrospinal fluid and repair any defect in the dural sac. Urinary diversion, including an ileoconduit, a continent pouch, or an ileo-neobladder, is created as necessary; an end sigmoid colostomy is created and a transabdominal myocutaneous rectus flap is universally used to fill in the large pelvic/perineal defect [45]. In the authors' initial experience of 15 consecutive rectus myocutaneous flaps for coverage of pelvic defects, all flaps survived with no necrosis (Temple WJ, unpublished data, September 1995). This finding has dramatically improved their results from local infection or breakdown, from 30% to 12% [1]. No patient developed pelvic abscess, although one had an enterocutaneous fistula that closed in 3 weeks. The skin of the myocutaneous flap was tubularized to reconstruct the vagina in three women, as described by other authors [46].

Difficult pelvis

Although cross-clamping the aorta without heparinization is routine for the sacral transection portion of the resection at the current authors' center, the surgeon must be prepared to do this at any stage of the operation where uncontrolled blood loss is possible. In a particularly difficult pelvis with severe radiation fibrosis, cross-clamping the aorta and using an osteotome to carve endopelvic fascia surrounding the tumor at the pelvic sidewall have been necessary. Once complete, hemostasis can be achieved and the aorta unclamped. The only difficulty found with cross-clamping the aorta has been in one patient with atherosclerosis of the aorta in whom bilateral occlusion of the external iliac arteries was used, and thrombus on one side requiring thrombectomy occurred.

A useful maneuver to improve exposure in the narrow pelvis or a large tumor is to open the symphysis pubis. This procedure is performed with a Gigli saw passed right on the inferior surface of the pubis to avoid urethra injury. A rib spreader can spread the pubic gap up to 5 cm, which often changes a difficult procedure into an easy one. Bone wax is used for hemostasis. Patients do well without reconstruction; the pubis can simply be allowed to scar together. The authors' initial attempts at reconstruction using wires or plates resulted in early hardware breakdown at the hardware–bone interface and have been abandoned.

Internal/modified hemipelvectomy

Traditionally, internal hemipelvectomy consists of removal of the innominate bone and adjacent muscles but with preservation of the ipsilateral extremity. It is generally used for bony or soft tissue sarcomas, although at times also for locally advanced visceral tumors. The procedure has been well described by Karakousis [47] and Eilber et al [48]. Briefly, the incision is started near the sacroiliac joint and along the iliac crest to the anterior superior iliac spine (ASIS). Anteriorly, it follows the inguinal ligament to the pubis and posteriorly at the level of the greater trochanter. Dissection continues to divide the abdominal wall musculature (external oblique aponeurosis, internal oblique and transversus abdominis), and the peritoneum is reflected medially to expose the external iliac vessels and ureter. The inguinal ligament is divided at the ASIS and pubic tubercle, and the anterior rectus sheath is divided at the pubic crest. The pubic symphysis is cleared of fibrofatty tissue, and urethral injury is avoided by staying on the inferior surface of the pubis with a Gigli saw. The pubis is then divided.

Posteriorly, the femoral nerve is exposed and preserved between the psoas and iliacus. The psoas is preserved, if possible. The iliac/femoral vessels are isolated with vessel loops or an umbilical tape. The iliacus muscle is divided at the level of the sacroiliac joint, and the adductor musculature is divided near their origin on the pubic bone. Laterally, the origins of the sartorius, tensor fascia lata, rectus femoris, and insertions of gluteus medius/minimus are divided. The hip capsule is incised and the femur neck transected with an oscillating saw.

The sciatic nerve is identified coursing from the greater sciatic notch between the greater trochanter and the ischial tuberosity. Pyriformis, gemelli, and quadratus femoris are then divided as they attach to the greater trochanter. The sacroiliac joint is then transected, again with an oscillating saw or a Gigli saw, although the transection can be through the sacral ala depending on tumor extension. The lumbosacral nerve trunk that runs medially needs to be protected. The remaining musculature is then detached from the specimen, including levator ani and the posterior hamstrings attached to the ischial tuberositates, and then the sacrospinous and sacrotuberous ligaments are divided to allow removal of the specimen. At the end of the procedure, the iliofemoral vessels, femoral nerve, psoas, sciatic nerve, and undivided posteromedial subcutaneous tissue and skin are left attached to the trunk and lower extremity.

If a portion of the innominate bone is not involved and can be spared, the operation is classified as a partial or modified internal hemipelvectomy. The preservation of the pubic bone allows preservation of the adductor musculature and the accompanying obturator nerve [47]. If the acetabulum can be preserved, functional impairment is dramatically decreased [49].

Reconstruction options include allograft prosthesis with total hip replacement, saddle prosthesis, or covering the exposed femoral neck and simply closing the wound in layers [8,47,50]. In the latter option, the leg has significant shortening (~3 cm), with the neck of the femur resting against scar tissue, and is the simplest reconstruction method [47]. Currently, all reconstruction methods for hip reconstruction are far from ideal but are preferable to the alternative of external hemipelvectomy.

External hemipelvectomy

External hemipelvectomy is an uncommon procedure performed for a range of pelvic neoplasms. The most common indications include primary neoplasm of the bony pelvis or soft tissue sarcoma involving the pelvis. Much less commonly, advanced melanoma, squamous cell carcinoma (SCC), cervix or other gynecologic cancers, bladder cancer, and locally advanced or recurrent rectal cancer may be treated in this manner [8,51,52]. The operation has two well-described operative approaches, by Karakousis and Vezeridis [10] and Kulaylat et al [53]. This operation is conceptually easier than internal or modified hemipelvectomy. The lower limb is completely prepared and draped to allow manipulation and improve exposure during the procedure. The incision is similar to the internal hemipelvectomy incision but is completed along the medial leg and inguinal crease. Also, the incision is modified to allow either a posterior or anterior myocutaneous flap, depending on tumor location, to fill in the large defect [10,53]. In addition to the dissection described for internal hemipelvectomy, the iliac vessels are controlled early to prevent blood loss and are ligated once tumor resectability is confirmed. The sciatic and femoral nerves are sharply transected. The final specimen includes the innominate bone and entire lower extremity. Care must be taken to protect the ureter and pelvic viscera during the pelvic dissection.

The posterior flap is subject to partial necrosis in 40% or more of cases because the superior gluteal vessels are usually taken, leaving a random-pattern blood supply from the lumbar vessels to perfuse it. Leaving the gluteus muscle as part of the flap is reported to be helpful [53]. If the posterior flap is at risk, it is prudent to cover the bowel with omentum in case of skin tissue loss. If the buttock is involved with tumor, the anterior thigh myocutaneous flap based on the femoral artery provides excellent coverage [54,55].

Results

Short-term outcomes

Sacral composite resection

Sacral composite resection is a difficult operation and is best performed by a team of surgeons skilled in exenterative and reconstructive techniques. Operative mortality ranges from 0% to 10% in experienced centers (Table 1) [1,12,16,31]. Perioperative complications are frequent (see Table 1) [12,16,31]. Wanebo et al [31], with the largest experience in sacral composite resection, reported on a series of 61 patients who underwent extended resection for locally recurrent rectal cancer invading the sacrum. Perioperative mortality was 5.4% overall (8% in curative resections), and main complications included sepsis (38%), acute renal failure (13%), acute respiratory distress syndrome (10%), and posterior wound infection or flap breakdown (28%). Operating times (two-stage procedure) were as follows: 18.5 hours in their first 27 patients, 20.13 hours in the next 20 patients, and 23.2 hours in their last 7 patients. Mean estimated blood loss was > 7900 mL, 11,700 mL, and 8470 mL in the first 27 patients, the next 20, and the last seven respectively. With a one-stage approach, Temple and Saettler [1] described a mean operating time of 8 hours and median blood loss of 9 units. Cross-clamping the aorta when dividing the sacrum seems to significantly decrease mean blood loss from 10 to 5 units [1,44].

Bakx et al [7] described a different approach to avoiding intraoperative hemorrhage. A vascular Endo gastrointestinal anastomosis stapler (GIA) (US Surgical, Norwalk, Connecticut) is used to staple and transect the anterior branches of the internal iliac vessels between the obturator fossa and the presacral plane. Tension on the posterior sacral veins is released by this maneuver, and it is believed that risk of hemorrhage decreases. In their series of 26 procedures using a combined abdominal and dorsal approach, the mean operating time was 6 hours (2.5–10 h), the median blood loss was 3600 mL (420–11,500 mL), and the median hospital stay was 20 days (5–202 d) [7]. There were 27 operation-related major complications in this series: five patients required relaparatomy for the following conditions: pelvic blood loss (two patients), small bowel obstruction (one patient) or perforation (one patient), and necrosis of the ileoconduit.

Mannaerts et al [39] reported on a series of 50 patients with either locally advanced primary (13 patients) or locally recurrent (37 patients) rectal cancer who underwent composite abdominosacral resection. All patients with primary tumors and 25 patients with recurrent disease had neoadjuvant external beam radiation therapy (50.4 Gy if not previously irradiated and 30 Gy for reirradiation). Twelve patients did not have reirradiation. Patients had additional intraoperative electron beam radiotherapy (10–17.5 Gy) for areas at risk for residual tumor. The median operating time (including intraoperative radiation) was 390 minutes (210–590 min), the median blood

Table 1
Short-term outcomes in patients undergoing extended pelvic resection with curative intent

Procedure/first author	No. patients	Cancer type	Median estimated blood loss (cc)	Mortality (%)	Common morbidity	
					Type	%
Sacropelvic resection						
Wanebo [31]	61	Recurrent rectal cancer	>7900, 27 pts	5.4	Sepsis	38
			11,700, 20 pts		Flap infection/breakdown	28
			8470, 7 pts			
Temple [1]	20	Mainly recurrent rectal cancer	9000, cross-clamping decreased blood loss from 10 to 5 units	10	Perineal wound infection/breakdown	
					Before rectus flap	30
					After	12
					Relaparotomy	19
Bakx [7]	26	Majority rectal cancer	3600	3.8	Perineal wound infection/breakdown	30
Mannaerts [39]	50	Rectal cancer	3500	4	Overall	82
					Wound complications	48
					Relaparotomy	8
Lopez [12]	34	Majority rectal cancer	1500	0	Overall	68
					Relaparotomy	26
Touran [56]	17	Primary sacral/advanced anorectal	1600	0	Wound complication	25
					Urinary retention/incontinence	35

Zacherl [57]	12	Recurrent rectal cancer	4250	0	Overall	42
Weber [40]	23	Recurrent anorectal cancer	4371	0	Overall	78
					Wound infection/ breakdown	48
Magrini [38]	16	Recurrent anorectal cancer	3400	0	Overall	50
					Flap reoperation	17
Maetani [13]	35	Recurrent rectal cancer	NR	5.7	Wound infection/ impaired healing	10
Modified/internal/external hemipelvectomy						
Baliski [8]	16	7 sarcoma	2730	8	Overall	77
		6 carcinoma			Skin-flap necrosis	38
Apffelstaedt [49]	32	Majority sarcoma, IH	2300	9.4	Wound infection	47
					Skin-flap necrosis	12
Apffelstaedt [51]	68	Majority sarcoma, EH	4200, mean	6	Overall	53
					Wound infection	35
					Skin-flap necrosis	16
Zeifang [58]	50	All pelvic bone tumors	NR	0	Overall	76

Abbreviations: EH, external hemipelvectomy; IH, internal hemipelvectomy; NR, not reported; pts, patients.

loss was 3500 mL (400–10,000 mL), and the median length of stay was 19 days (9–129 d); there were two treatment-related mortalities. Complications occurred in 82% of patients, the most common being wound complications (48%), urinary retention (18%), and relaparatomy for small bowel injury (8%). In addition, five patients had late grade 1–2 neuropathies. This approach seems to have an unacceptable level of toxicity. Pearlman et al [37] reported on 19 patients (7 sacropelvic extenterations; 12 total pelvic exenterations) where operating time ranged from 8 to 16 hours and estimated blood loss was 3000 to 10,000 mL (mean, 5000 mL). In a series of 34 patients who underwent an extended pelvic resection, Lopez and Luna-Perez [12] described 18 patients who underwent one-stage sacropelvic resection. The operating time ranged from 7 to 20 hours (mean, 11.4 h), and estimated blood loss ranged from 750 to 4250 mL (mean, 1500 mL). In addition, 67% of patients had perioperative complications with infection; the most frequent complications included wound infection, pelvic abscess, and pneumonia. Reoperation to control sepsis was required in 26% of the patients.

Additional small to moderate-sized series of sacropelvic resection have described similar overall operative times, mean estimated blood loss, length of stay, and perioperative complications (see Table 1) [13,38,40,56,57]. Magrini et al [38] described 16 patients who received IOERT in addition to sacropelvic resection. All patients had received previous external beam radiation therapy, six with their primary therapy, six following detection of their first local recurrence, and 13 patients had received external beam radiation therapy before sacral resection. A single procedure with four stages, including an anterior approach, posterior approach, IOERT, and pelvic reconstruction, was used. The median operative time was 12.5 hours, and the median estimated blood loss was 3.4 L. There were no perioperative deaths, but there was a major complication rate of 50%, including perineal wound infections, dehiscence, urinary leaks, and an ileal fistula.

It is the current authors' impression that there is a significant learning curve in this operation. The associated morbidity has significantly improved by applying a team approach, routinely using myocutaneous rectus flaps to fill in dead space, and using newer antibiotics with broad-spectrum coverage.

Limb composite resection

Pelvic resections, including modified, internal, or external hemipelvectomy, are associated with a 5% to 10% mortality rate depending on case mix and extent of surgery [8,13,49,51]. Perioperative complications should be anticipated and occur in most patients [8,13,49]. When pelvic viscera do not require resection, it is uncommon to have intestinal complications. Baliski et al [8] described an 8% mortality rate among 13 patients (9 external hemipelvectomy, 4 internal hemipelvectomy); 77% of patients had at least one complication. Of significance, 38% of the patients developed skin-flap necrosis, which required one to three operations per individual for debridement and tissue coverage. Other in-hospital complications included the following: cellulitis, prolonged ileus, pneumonia, urinary retention, intra-abdominal abscess, and bowel obstruction [8]. The mean length of stay was 30 days (14–70 d).

Apffelstaedt et al [49] described a perioperative mortality rate of 9.4% and a 35-day mean length of stay (6–116 d) among 32 patients following partial or complete internal hemipelvectomy. The most common complications were wound infections (47%) and skin-flap necrosis (12.5%), although only half of these required operative debridement. A review of 68 patients by the same group noted a 6% perioperative mortality rate, a 53% complication rate with flap necrosis in 16% of patients, and wound infection in 35% of patients following external hemipelvectomy [51]. The mean hospital stay was 39 days versus 24 days for curative versus palliative resections, respectively.

Zeifang et al [58] treated 50 consecutive patients. Complications occurred in two thirds of limb-sparing operations and in 75% of external hemipelvectomies. Wound-related complications were the most common, but removal of reconstruction hardware was required in four patients.

Long-term outcomes

In Wanebo et al's [31] series of 61 patients undergoing sacropelvic resection for recurrent rectal cancer, 53 of these operations were performed with curative intent. The median disease-free survival time was 22 months, and the 5-year disease-free survival rate was 23%. The overall median survival time was 36 months, and the 5-year survival rate was 31%. Patients with prior anterior resection had a 53-month median survival time and a 41% 5-year survival rate compared with a 22-month median survival time and an 18% 5-year survival rate in those with prior abdominoperineal resection ($P = 0.001$). Preoperative carcinoembryonic antigen (CEA) levels and Dukes' B versus C stage were not significant in predicting overall survival time or outcome.

A preoperative CEA level of less than 10 ng/mL was associated with better disease-free survival, with a median disease-free survival time of 48 months and 5-year disease-free survival rate of 34%, versus a CEA level of more than 10 ng/mL, which had a median disease-free survival time of 16 months and 5-year disease-free survival rate of 10%. Patients with bone marrow invasion, positive margins, or peripelvic nodal metastases had a poor outcome, with a median survival time of 10 months, which was comparable to those undergoing surgery with palliative intent. Of note, short-term relief of symptoms occurred in almost all patients in Wanebo's series.

Several coincident or subsequent studies have confirmed overall survival rates of approximately 30% in well-selected patients (Table 2) [1,12,51,59]. In the present authors' center, 20 composite resections were performed

Table 2
Long-term outcomes in patients undergoing extended pelvic resection with curative intent

Procedure/first author	No. patients	Cancer type	Local control	Median disease-free survival	Median overall survival	Long-term overall survival
Sacropelvic Resection						
Wanebo [31]	61	Recurrent rectal cancer	NR	22 mo	36 mo	31% 5-y
Temple [1]	20	Mainly recurrent rectal cancer	50% at death or last F/U	NR	24 mo, mean 38 mo	10% 10-y
Bakx [36]	40	Recurrent rectal cancer	55% at 100 mo	18 mo	25 mo	28% 5-y overall 26% DFS 5-y
Mannaerts [39]	50	Rectal cancer	61% 3-y	NR	NR	41% 3-y 31% DFS 3-y
Lopez [12]	34	Majority rectal cancer	68%	38 mo, rectal cancer 32 mo, squamous	NR	44% 5-y
Maetani [59]	59	Recurrent rectal cancer	39%	NR	27 mo	25% 5-y 15% 10-y
Modified/internal/external hemipelvectomy						
Baliski [8]	16	7 sarcoma 6 carcinoma	100%	NR	9 mo, cervix carcinoma	86% at 1-y, sarcoma
Apffelstaedt [49]	32	Majority sarcoma, IH	75%	NR	NR	51% 5-y 45% 10-y
Apffelstaedt [51]	68	Majority sarcoma, EH	65%	NR	33 mo, bone 20 mo, soft tissue sarcoma	52% 2-y 21% estimated 5-y
Kawai [11]	50	All pelvic bone tumors	66%	NR	NR	55% 5-y 10% 5-y with positive margin
Wirbel [62]	93	Pelvic sarcoma	81%	NR	21.5 mo, mean	5-y survival 86% LG bone 42% HG bone 25% soft tissue sarcoma
Pring [63]	64	Pelvic chondrosarcoma	81%	NR	NR	80% 10-y 14% 10-y if dedifferentiated

Abbreviations: DFS, disease-free survival; EH, external hemipelvectomy; F/U, follow up; HG, high grade; IH, internal hemipelvectomy; LG, low grade; NR, not reported/median not reached.

mostly for recurrent rectal cancer. Half of these patients had transection at the S1–S2 level and the remainder at the S2–S3 level [1]. Local control was achieved in 50% of patients at time of death or last follow-up. The mean and median survival time was 38 and 24 months, respectively. Two patients survived 12 to 15 years, which gave a long-term cure rate of 10%. Bakx et al [36] reported a median overall survival time of 25 months (95% confidence interval [CI], 13–37 mo) and 5-year survival rate of 28% (95% CI, 12%–45%) among 40 patients. Similarly, in a large-scale series of 50 patients, Mannaerts et al [39] reported a 3-year overall survival rate and disease-free survival and local control rates of 41%, 31%, and 61%, respectively. Negative final margins were predictive of survival, disease-free survival, and local control.

Lopez and Luna-Perez [12] noted a 5-year overall survival rate of 44% in 34 patients undergoing the following types of extended pelvic or composite resections: sacral resection (18 patients), ischial resection (5 patients), pubis (4 patients), rami (4 patients), and external hemipelvectomy (3 patients). Primary tumors included the following: cervix (6), vaginal (3), penile (1), rectal (19), anal (4), and sarcoma (1), and correlated with 5-year survival. Of note, five of six patients with cervical cancer subsequently had either recurrent local or systemic disease, whereas 8 of 19 patients with rectal cancer had recurrence at 37-month median follow-up.

Baliski et al [8] reported their experience with 13 patients who required internal (4 patients) or external (9 patients) hemipelvectomy. Primary tumors included seven sarcomas (four bone, three soft tissue) and six carcinomas (five genital tract, one unknown primary). Survival was better in patients with sarcomas (86% cancer-specific survival at 12-mo median follow-up [9–108 mo]) compared with those with carcinoma (median survival, 9 mo [4–20 mo]). Kawai et al [11] reported a 5-year survival rate of 55% for patients with bony sarcoma of the pelvis. Positive margins are associated with a 10% 5-year survival rate, however, even in this group [60]. The poor long-term prognosis of genital tract malignancies requiring hemipelvectomy has been reported by others [16,61]. Most patients develop recurrent distant disease, although there were no local recurrences in the series by Baliski et al [8], suggesting a possible role in short-term disease control.

Affelstaedt et al's [49] series of 32 patients who underwent internal hemipelvectomy, including 29 bone or soft tissue sarcomas, reported estimated 71%, 51%, and 45% 2-year, 5-year, and 10-year survival rates, respectively, among those patients who underwent resection for cure. Of these patients, 25% developed a local recurrence. The 2-year survival rate was 29% among eight patients resected for palliation. Apffelstaedt et al [51] also reported a large review of 68 patients undergoing external hemipelvectomy; pathology included bone tumors (11 patients), soft tissue sarcoma (39 patients), melanoma (7 patients), SCC (10 patients), and giant neurofibroma (1 patient). Forty-seven patients had resections with curative intent, and estimated the 5-year survival rate was 21%, with a 35% local recurrence rate. Median survival times of 33 months, 20 months, 10 months, and 12 months were described for bone tumors, soft tissue sarcoma, SCC, and melanoma, respectively.

Grade of tumor predicts long-term survival in patients who have sarcoma. In their series of 93 patients with consecutive pelvic sarcomas, Wirbel et al [62] reported 5-year survival rates of 86%, 42%, and 25% in low-grade bone tumors, high-grade bone tumors, and high-grade soft tissue sarcomas, respectively. Similarly, Pring et al [63] noted a 69% overall survival rate in 64 patients with chondrosarcoma of the pelvis at a median follow-up of 140 months. Patients with high-grade chrondrosarcoma (grade 3, dedifferentiated) had a significantly worse outcome with a 10-year survival rate of 14%.

Functional results

Functional deficits following internal or external hemipelvectomy vary depending on the extent of resection. Functional results, especially bladder control, are improved if sacrectomy can be limited to S3 or lower. In those resections at the S1 or S2 level (on one side), very few motor deficits ensue. Approximately two thirds of patients return to their previous lifestyle, and 50% return to work following judicious physiotherapy and rehabilitation. Most patients are able to ambulate without mechanical aids unless more extensive resections were performed [13]. The injury of S1 nerve roots causes loss of plantar flexion [31]. The bilateral transection of S1 nerve roots also leads to complete denervation of the bladder [6]. The bilateral transaction of S2 roots causes poor detrusor tone and increased residuals [6]. Combined abdominal wall contraction and external abdominal wall pressure (Crede maneuver) may provide satisfactory function, however [6].

In a series of 32 patients, 34% were able to ambulate without assistance, 59% required a cane or crutches, and 7% required a wheelchair following partial or complete internal hemipelvectomy at time of hospital discharge [49]. As expected, long-term follow-up confirmed that ongoing deficits correlated with the initial extent of surgery. The resection of the pubis and rami did not affect ambulation after a short period of rehabilitation. The resection of the iliac bone with preservation of the acetabulum caused leg shortening; this condition initially requires a cane, but at 1 year, a shoe lift is usually sufficient. This result may be prevented by replacing the iliac bone with an allograft femur strut. The resection of the entire innominate bone requires the long-term use of crutches, a walker, or, in the older patients, a wheelchair. No patient in this series had specialized reconstruction. Most patients use crutches following external hemipelvectomy; a small number can tolerate a prosthesis, although most find the bulky prosthesis an impediment to mobility, and older patients require a wheelchair [51].

Quality of life

In general, loss of function secondary to surgery is preferable to progressive disease. It is important that patients with curable disease at least have a choice of surgery or nonoperative palliation. The present authors would not expect quality of life (QOL) to be ideal with surgery; however, studies suggest that QOL is reasonable.

In a retrospective questionnaire, all patients undergoing hemipelvectomy in the authors' series stated they did not regret extended surgery and would repeat surgical intervention, if necessary [8]. Merimsky et al [64] reported improved functional status in 19 of 21 patients and improved QOL in two thirds of patients after major amputation. Global QOL and psychosocial functioning was assessed by the quality of life core questionnaire 30 instrument of the European Organization for Research and Treatment of Cancer in 15 survivors (of a total of 36 patients) of pelvic Ewing's sarcoma following modified internal hemipelvectomy [65]. Global QOL scores in patients (70% $\pm$ 16%) were comparable to the general population (75% $\pm$ 24%). Similarly, in a retrospective cohort study, women undergoing pelvic exenteration for gynecologic or urologic cancers reported similar levels of emotional functioning and general QOL compared with the healthy population despite changes in physical, sexual, and social functioning [66].

There is a definite need for prospective QOL studies comparing pre- and post-treatment status with appropriate assessment instruments. It is the current authors' impression that health care professionals often deny patients the opportunity of extended pelvic surgery because they feel it is too morbid a procedure and results in unacceptable QOL. Physicians have a much more positive attitude toward paraplegics following trauma, even though these individuals have less overall physical function than in those who undergo exenteration or hemipelvectomy.

Role of palliative resection?

Extended pelvic resection is not recommended for palliation. In those patients who eventually experience recurrence following their operation, however, effective palliation by means of local control is impressive. This area remains to be defined but currently is not an indication for extended pelvic resection.

Summary

Current literature clearly supports composite pelvic resections for most cancers invading the musculoskeletal pelvis or primary pelvic sarcoma invading visceral organs. Patient selection and preoperative imaging are critical to avoid surgery if there is any evidence of systemic disease. New techniques of delivering preoperative radiotherapy, including IOERT or the use of intraperitoneal silastic spacers to protect small intestine, will likely improve resectability and local control rates. The morbidity and mortality associated with these procedures are significant but improving. The use of a team approach in a specialized center, improving exposure by dividing and spreading the pubis as necessary, decreasing blood loss with temporary cross-clamping of the aorta or endovascular staplers, and routine use of myocutaneous flaps will continue to decrease perioperative morbidity. New urinary diversion techniques have improved continence rates, and continued research in reconstruction options following internal hemipelvectomy will improve functional outcomes and decrease the need for external hemipelvectomy.

Composite pelvic resections improve disease-free survival and provide an overall cure rate better than with other malignancies, such as pancreatic or esophageal cancer. QOL is reasonable and generally better than the alternative of progressive disease, although prospective studies are needed in this area. In summary, it is critical that all individuals are given a choice of surgery versus nonoperative palliative options in potentially curative yet locally advanced pelvic cancers.

References

[1] Temple WJ, Saettler EB. Locally recurrent rectal cancer: role of composite resection of extensive pelvic tumors with strategies for minimizing risk of recurrence. J Surg Oncol 2000; 73:47–58.

[2] Gunderson LL, Sosin H. Areas of failure found at reoperation following curative surgery for adenocarcinoma of the rectum. Clinicopathologic correlation and implications for adjuvant therapy. Cancer 1974;34:1278–92.

[3] Temple WJ, Ketcham AS. Surgical palliation for recurrent rectal cancers ulcerating in the perineum. Cancer 1990;65:1111–4.

[4] Turk PS, Wanebo HJ. Results of surgical treament of nonhepatic recurrence of colorectal carcinoma. Cancer 1993;71:4267–77.

[5] Wanebo HJ, Koness RJ, Vezeridis MP, et al. Pelvic resection recurrent rectal cancer. Ann Surg 1994;220:586–97.

[6] Wanebo HJ, Marcove RC. Abdominal sacral resection of locally recurrent rectal cancer. Ann Surg 1981;194:458–71.

[7] Bakx R, van Lanschot JB, Zoetmulder FAN. Sacral resection in cancer surgery: surgical technique and experience in 26 procedures. J Am Coll Surg 2004;198:846–51.

[8] Baliski CR, Schachar NS, McKinnon JG, et al. Hemipelvectomy: a changing perspective for a rare procedure. Can J Surg 2004;47:99–103.

[9] Crowe PJ, Temple WJ, Lopez MJ, et al. Pelvic exenteration for advanced pelvic malignancy. Semin Surg Oncol 1999;17:152–60.

[10] Karakousis CP, Vezeridis MP. Variants of hemipelvectomy. Am J Surg 1983;145:273–7.

[11] Kawai A, Healey JH, Boland PJ, et al. Prognostic factors for patients with sarcomas of the pelvic bones. Cancer 1997;82:851–9.

[12] Lopez MJ, Luna-Perez P. Composite pelvic exenteration: is is worthwhile? Ann Surg Oncol 2004;11:27–33.

[13] Maetani S, Nishikawa T, Iijima Y, et al. Extensive en bloc resection of regionally recurrent carcinoma of the rectum. Cancer 1992;69:2876–83.

[14] Temple WJ, Ketcham AS. Sacral resection for control of pelvic tumors. Am J Surg 1992;163: 370–4.

[15] Wanebo HJ, Koness RJ, Turk PS, et al. Composite resection of posterior pelvic malignancy. Ann Surg 1992;215:685–95.

[16] Wanebo HJ, Whitehill R, Gaker D, et al. Composite pelvic resection: an approach to advanced pelvic cancer. Arch Surg 1987;122:1401–6.

[17] De Koning HJ, Auvinen A, Sanchez AB, et al. Large-scale randomized prostate cancer screening trials: program performances in the European Randomized Screening for Prostate Cancer trial and the Prostate, Lung, Colorectal and Ovary Cancer trial. Int J Cancer 2002;97: 237–44.

[18] Huebner RH, Park KC, Shepherd JE, et al. A meta-analysis of the literature for whole-body FDG PET detection of recurrent colorectal cancer. J Nucl Med 2000;41:1177–89.

[19] Kewenter J, Bjork S, Haglind E, et al. Screening and rescreening for colorectal cancer. A controlled trial of fecal occult blood testing in 27700 subjects. Cancer 1988;62:645–51.

[20] Kronborg O, Fenger C, Olsen J, et al. Randomised study of screening for colorectal cancer with faecal-occult-blood test. Lancet 1996;348:1467–71.

[21] Liberman DA, Weiss DG, Bond JH, et al. Use of colonoscopy to screen asymptomatic adults for colorectal cancer. N Engl J Med 2000;343:162–8.

[22] Mandel JS, Church TR, Ederer F, et al. Colorectal cancer mortality: effectiveness of biennial screening for fecal occult blood. J Natl Cancer Inst 1999;91:434–7.

[23] Sasieni PD, Cuzick J, Lynch-Farmery E. Estimating the efficacy of screening by auditing smear histories women with and without cervical cancer. The National Co-ordinating Network for Cervical Screening Working Group. Br J Cancer 1996;73:1001–5.

[24] Smith RA, Cokkinides V, Eyre HJ. American Cancer Society guidelines for the early detection of cancer. CA Cancer J Clin 2003;53:27–43.

[25] US Preventive Services Task Force. Screening for cervical cancer: recommendations and rationale. Am Fam Phys 2003;67:1759–66.

[26] Winawer ST, Stewart ET, Zauber AG, et al. A comparison of colonoscopy and double-contrast barium enema for surveillance after polypectomy. N Engl J Med 2000;342:1766–72.

[27] Enker WE, Kafka NJ, Martz J. Planes of sharp pelvic dissection for primary, locally advanced, or recurrent rectal cancer. Sem Surg Oncol 2000;18:199–206.

[28] Heald RJ, Ryall RD. Recurrence and survival after total mesorectal excision for rectal cancer. Lancet 1986;1:1479–82.

[29] Gastrointestinal Tumor Study Group. Prolongation of the disease-free interval in surgically treated rectal carcinoma. N Engl J Med 1985;312:1465–72.

[30] Kapiteijn E, Kranenbarg EK, Steup WH, et al. Total mesorectal excision (TME) with or without preoperative radiotherapy in the treatment of primary rectal cancer: prospective randomised trial with standard operative and histopathological techniques. Eur J Surg 1999; 165:410–20.

[31] Wanebo HJ, Antoniuk P, Koness RJ, et al. Pelvic resection of recurrent rectal cancer: technical considerations and outcomes. Dis Colon Rectum 1999;42:1438–48.

[32] Wanebo HJ, Gaker DL, Whitehill R, et al. Pelvic recurrence of rectal cancer: options for curative resection. Ann Surg 1987;205:482–95.

[33] Popovich MJ, Hricak H, Sugimura K, et al. The role of MR imaging in determining surgical eligibility for pelvic exenteration. AJR Am J Roentgenol 1993;160:525–31.

[34] Wallis F, Gilbert FJ. Magnetic resonance imaging in oncology: an overview. J R Coll Surg Edinb 1999;44:117–25.

[35] Goldberg MA, Lee MJ, Fischman AJ, et al. Fluorodeoxyglucose PET of abdominal and pelvic neoplasms: potential role in oncologic imaging. Radiographics 1993;13:1047–62.

[36] Bakx R, van Tinteren H, van Lanschot JJB, et al. Surgical treatment of locally recurrent rectal cancer. Eur J Surg Oncol 2004;30(8):857–63.

[37] Pearlman NW, Donohue RE, Stiegmann GV, et al. Pelvic and sacropelvic exenteration for locally advanced or recurrent anorectal cancer. Arch Surg 1987;122:537–41.

[38] Magrini S, Nelson H, Gunderson LL, et al. Sacropelvic resection and intraoperative electron irradiation in the management of recurrent anorectal cancer. Dis Colon Rectum 1996;39: 1–9.

[39] Mannaerts GHH, Rutten HJT, Martijn H, et al. Abdominosacral resection for primary irresectable and locally recurrent rectal cancer. Dis Colon Rectum 2001;44:806–14.

[40] Weber K, Nelson H, Gunderson LL, et al. Sacropelvic resection for recurrent anorectal cancer: a multidisciplinary approach. Clin Orthop 2000;1:231–40.

[41] Mannaerts GHH, Martijn H, Crommelin MA, et al. Intraoperative electron beam radiation therapy for locally recurrent rectal carcinoma. Int J Radiat Oncol Biol Phys 1999;45:297–308.

[42] Temple WJ, Temple LF, Arthur KA, et al. Prospective cohort study of neoadjuvant treatment in conservative surgery of soft tissue sarcomas. Ann Surg Oncol 1997; 4:586–90.

[43] Mack LA, Temple WJ, DeHaas WG, et al. Groin soft tissue tumors—a challenge for local control and reconstruction: a prospective cohort analysis. J Surg Oncol 2004;86(3):147–51.

[44] Eisenkop SM, Spirtos NM, Lin WM, et al. Reduction of blood loss during extensive pelvic procedures by aortic clamping—a preliminary report. Gynecol Oncol 2003;88:80–4.

[45] Shukla HS, Hughes LE. The rectus abdominis flap for perineal wounds. Ann R Coll Surg Engl 1984;66:337–9.

[46] D'Souza DN, Pera M, Nelson H, et al. Vaginal reconstruction following resection of primary locally advanced and recurrent colorectal malignancies. Arch Surg 2003;138:1340–3.

[47] Karakousis CP. Internal hemipelvectomy. Surg Gynecol Obstet 1984;158:279–82.

[48] Eilber FR, Grant TT, Sakai D, et al. Internal hemipelvectomy—excision of the hemipelvis with limb preservation. Cancer 1979;43:806–9.

[49] Apffelstaedt JP, Driscoll DL, Karakousis CP. Partial and complete internal hemipelvectomy: complications and long-term follow-up. J Am Coll Surg 1995;181:43–8.

[50] Renard AJS, Veth RPH, Schreuder HWB, et al. The saddle prosthesis in pelvic primary and secondary musculoskeletal tumors: functional results at several postoperative intervals. Arch Orthop Trauma Surg 2000;120:188–94.

[51] Apffelstaedt JP, Driscoll DL, Spellman JE, et al. Complications and outcome of external hemipelvectomy in the management of pelvic tumors. Ann Surg Oncol 1996;3:304–9.

[52] Malawer MM, Buch RG, Thomson WE, et al. Major amputations done with palliative intent in the treatment of local bony complications association with advanced cancer. J Surg Oncol 1991;47:121–30.

[53] Kulaylat MN, Froix A, Karakousis CP. Blood supply of hemipelvectomy flaps: the anterior flap hemipelvectomy. Arch Surg 2001;136:828–31.

[54] Temple WJ, Mnaymneh W, Ketcham AS. The total thigh and rectus abdominis myocutaneous flap for closure of extensive hemipelvectomy defects. Cancer 1982;50:2524–8.

[55] Mazeron J, Suit HD. Lymph nodes as sites of metastases from sarcomas of soft tissue. Cancer 1987;60:1800–8.

[56] Touran T, Frost DB, O'Connell TX. Sacral resection: operative technique and outcome. Arch Surg 1990;125:911–3.

[57] Zacherl J, Schiessel R, Windhager R, et al. Abdominosacral resection of recurrent rectal cancer in the sacrum. Dis Colon Rectum 1999;42:1035–9.

[58] Zeifang F, Buchner M, Zahlten-Hinguranage A, et al. Complications following operative treatment of primary malignant bone tumours in the pelvis. Eur J Surg Oncol 2004;30(8): 893–9.

[59] Maetani S, Onodera H, Nishikawa T, et al. Significance of local recurrence of rectal cancer as a marker of disseminated disease. Br J Surg 1998;85:521–5.

[60] Apffelstaedt JP, Zhang PJ, Driscoll DL, et al. Various types of hemipelvectomy for soft tissue sarcomas: complications, survival and prognostic factors. Surg Oncol 1995;4:217–22.

[61] King LA, Downey GO, Savage JE, et al. Resection of the pubic bone as an adjunct to management of primary, recurrent, and metastatic pelvic malignancies. Obstet Gynecol 1989;73:1022–6.

[62] Wirbel RJ, Schulte M, Mutschler WE. Surgical treatment of pelvic sarcomas: oncologic and functional outcome. Clin Orthop 2001;390:190–205.
[63] Pring ME, Wever KL, Unni KK, et al. Chondrosarcoma of the pelvis. A review of sixty-four cases. J Bone Joint Surg Am 2001;83:1630–42.
[64] Merimsky O, Kollender Y, Inbar M, et al. Palliative major amputation and quality of life in cancer patients. Acta Oncol 1997;36:151–7.
[65] Rodl RW, Hoffman C, Gosheger G, et al. Ewing's sarcoma of the pelvis: combined surgery and radiotherapy treatment. J Surg Oncol 2003;83:154–60.
[66] Roos EJ, de Graeff A, van Eijkeren MA, et al. Quality of life after pelvic exenteration. Gynecol Oncol 2004;933:610–4.

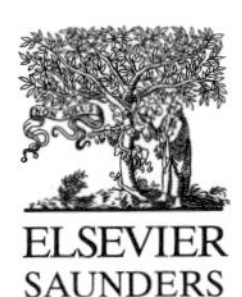
ELSEVIER
SAUNDERS

Surg Oncol Clin N Am
14 (2005) 419–431

SURGICAL
ONCOLOGY CLINICS
OF NORTH AMERICA

Image-Guided Ablative Techniques in Pelvic Malignancies: Radiofrequency Ablation, Cryoablation, Microwave Ablation

Caroline J. Simon, MD, Damian E. Dupuy, MD*

Department of Diagnostic Imaging, Brown Medical School, Rhode Island Hospital, 593 Eddy Street, Providence, RI 02903, USA

Pelvic malignancy refers to any cancer of the pelvic organs, including the following: gastrointestinal tract cancers, such as those of the colon and rectum; genitourinary cancers, such as those of the prostate and bladder; and gynecologic cancers, such as those of the cervix, endometrium, and ovary. Although surgical resection, with or without adjuvant chemotherapy and radiation therapy, remains the mainstay in the treatment of pelvic malignancies, local recurrences and metastases pose a common and difficult clinical problem. Recurrent pelvic surgery and radiation therapy are the primary methods currently used in the treatment and management of local pelvic tumor recurrences and metastases; however, few options exist for patients who fail to obtain adequate pain relief following radiation. Frequent failure of these treatment options often result in ineffective pain management, with the recurrent tumor causing pain by means of infiltration of the lumbosacral plexus. Surgery is not always an option, especially when patients present with advanced disease and poor functional status. For these patients, opioid analgesics remain the only alternative treatment option, and for some patients, the side effects, such as constipation, nausea, and sedation, can be significant.

Newer, minimally invasive treatment options in the management of pelvic recurrences and metastases include percutaneous cryoablation, radiofrequency (RF) ablation, and microwave (MW) ablation. This article

* Corresponding author.
E-mail address: ddupuy@lifespan.org (D.E. Dupuy).

1055-3207/05/$ - see front matter
doi:10.1016/j.soc.2004.11.005 **surgonc.theclinics.com**

focuses on the principles of therapy, methods of treatment, and current uses and experiences with these percutaneous modalities.

Cryoablation

The actual concept of tissue destruction through freezing has been in use over the past century [1]. Although cryotherapy has been selectively used in the treatment of a wide variety of disorders, its use in in situ tumor destruction was initially applied in the treatment of skin cancers. The development of a closed, pressurized liquid nitrogen delivery system in the early 1960s led the way in expanding the uses of cryotherapy. Cryoablation, with the local application of liquid nitrogen, as an adjuvant to resection and curettage in the treatment of bone tumors was first introduced more than three decades ago. Cryoablation of metastatic disease has been well documented in the liver, with most previous experiences coming from open or laparoscopic approaches.

In the past, experiences with percutaneous cryoablation have been limited, secondary to the large cryotherapy applicator diameters and the high incidence of associated postprocedural bleeding. These results reflected a lack of understanding of the potentially destructive effects of liquid nitrogen. More controlled cryotherapy applications and a better understanding of the destructive effects of liquid nitrogen have significantly reduced these early postprocedural complications. Despite these limitations, however, a search of the current literature shows a fairly large and growing clinical experience with ultrasound (US-)-guided percutaneous treatment of prostate cancer following the first publication describing this technique in 1993 [2].

With the development of the argon-based cryoablation system, now widely available, cryotherapy applicator diameters have decreased significantly, making the use of this technique to other sites of disease more feasible than ever before. Recent literature has been published on the successful use of the percutaneous cryoablation technique in treating hepatic, renal, and extra-abdominal metastatic disease [3–6].

Liquid nitrogen stored below -197°C can be used for the cryogenic preservation and destruction of viable tissue. Cryogenic tissue preservation is achieved by first performing a slow freeze followed subsequently by a quick thaw, whereas a quick freeze followed by a slow thaw results in cryogenic tissue destruction. Bone necrosis occurs with local temperatures of less than -21°C. The cryogenic destruction of living tissue occurs by means of several mechanisms, all of which depend on the rate of the initial freeze. The most important of these mechanisms are as follows: cryoablation-induced protein denaturation; osmotic shifts in intracellular and extracellular water; and subsequent membrane destabilization, cellular rupture, and tissue ischemia.

Different tissue-freezing patterns are achieved with different cryotherapy applicator cooling rates. A fast cryoprobe will have a tissue cooling rate of approximately 500°C/minute, whereas a slower cryoprobe will display cooling rates of between 200°C to 300°C/minute. As expected, the closer the proximity to the cryoprobe, the higher the recorded freezing rates. As cryotherapy freezing begins, minute ice crystals form in the intracellular and extracellular space. The apparent structural architecture of the treated tissue is therefore maintained. With the presence of ice in the extracellular space, intracellular ice begins forming when the targeted cells are rapidly "supercooled" to between −5°C and −15°C.

Intracellular ice is lethal to cells because cellular proteins denature and condense around ice crystals. Damage also occurs during the slow thaw phase as the intracellular ice crystals thaw and then reform, causing shearing disruption of cellular organelles and surrounding cellular membranes. As expected, slower cooling rates are present at the periphery of the cryogenic freeze zone. As the intra- and extracellular tissue temperature decreases, ice crystals form in the vascular space, preferentially beginning along the small vascular channels because cellular membranes pose a barrier to the formation and propagation of ice. As the minute ice crystals form, solutes are concentrated in the surrounding intracellular fluid. This relative hyperosmolarity causes an osmotic shift of intracellular water to the extracellular and vascular spaces. This process subsequently leads to cellular dehydration, intracellular hyperosmolarity, and a resultant denaturation of cellular proteins. The targeted tissue architecture becomes grossly distorted as the vascular space expands up to 4 times its normal volume with contiguous ice crystals, resulting in damage to the vascular endothelium and basement membrane.

During the thawing phase, edema, vessel disruption, and thrombosis cause significant ischemic necrosis of the treated region. Also, as the ice crystals melt, a significant osmotic gradient develops between the extracellular and intracellular spaces. Because cell membranes already have been destabilized, extracellular water rushes into the cells, causing rapid cellular swelling and subsequent rupture. This process occurs during the slow cool phase at the periphery of the freeze zone.

The middle region of the freeze zone is characterized by a variable intermediate rate of freezing. There can be any combination of intracellular and extracellular ice formation and cell dehydration. This freeze zone has the highest rate of cell survival. Tumors seem to freeze differently when compared with normal tissue, which is very sensitive to freezing. It has been suggested that differences in tissue architecture and vascularity, close cellular packing, and less permeable cellular membranes account for the altered freezing patterns between tumor and normal tissue. Tumor tissue is more resistant to cellular dehydration at slower cooling rates, thus expanding the intermediate freeze rate zone. Approximately 10% of cells remain viable following one freeze–thaw cycle.

At the current authors' institution, percutaneous cryoablation is performed under CT guidance using an argon-based cryoablation system (Endocare, Irvine, California) and 2.4-mm–diameter percutaneous cryotherapy applicators (Fig. 1). Pretreatment placement of the cryoablation applicators is

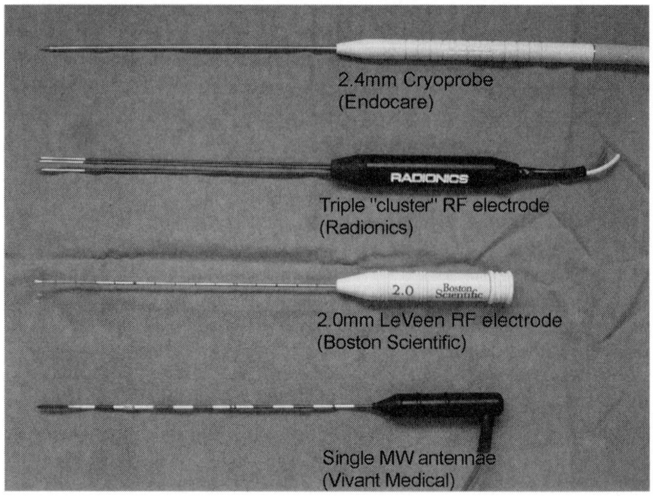

Fig. 1. A collection of various percutaneous ablation devices available in the United States. All the devices come in varied lengths, with the Vivant MW and Radionics RF ablation applicators available in different active tips as well.

planned according to the site and size of the tumor, the tumor margins, and involved surrounding structures to achieve pain palliation. Typically, each patient undergoes a 10-minute freeze, followed by a 5-minute active helium thaw, followed by another 10-minute freeze. The number of freeze–thaw–freeze cycles depends on the individual clinical case. A post-treatment CT scan is typically performed, with the low-density changes within the targeted tumor tissue measured and approximated to the size of the ablated region. Because the margin of the freeze zone is variable and cytotoxic temperatures may not have been achieved, a 1-cm margin is subtracted from the diameter of the low-density–ablated region to better approximate the true volume of tissue necrosis [6].

Cryosurgery was first used to treat prostate cancer in the early 1970s, but it was not until 1993, when the results from percutaneous US-guided cryosurgery were published, that the potential advantages of this treatment became apparent. Changes in cryotherapy equipment and techniques have greatly improved the results of cryosurgery, in both tumor control and lower morbidity [7]. US-guided percutaneous transperineal placement of the cryoprobes allows for real-time monitoring of tissue freezing. In addition, monitoring the targeted tissue temperature at critical locations, separating the rectum and prostate by saline injection, and using argon gas instead of the liquid nitrogen–based equipment have improved results and lowered complication rates [7]. The advantages of cryosurgery include the ability to re-treat patients without the added morbidity and to treat patients after radiation therapy with acceptable results and morbidity rates.

Giant cell tumors of the sacrum remain a difficult clinical problem. Wide local excision (total sacrectomy) is associated with high morbidity and pelvic instability rates. In a long-term follow-up study, Malawer et al [8] treated 102 patients who had giant cell tumors with cryotherapy and followed up these patients for a minimum period of 4 years. These patients were shown to achieve a high cure rate with an accompanying low complication rate. These patients also had a less than 6% incidence of developing pathologic fractures. These data showed cryosurgery to be a safe and excellent adjunct in the treatment of this locally aggressive tumor. Cryosurgery also enables pelvic and spinal joint preservation, excellent functional outcome, and low recurrence rates when compared with other joint preservation procedures.

In addition, cryoablation can be considered a viable adjuvant treatment option in the management of patients who have rectal cancer with pelvic recurrences (Fig. 2).

Radiofrequency ablation

In 1920, Harvey Cushing was the first to use RF ablation to create small lesions within the central nervous system. Since then, the technique has been refined such that precise control of lesion size can now be achieved by measuring the local temperature and electrical resistance within the targeted tissues being treated. Successful RF ablations of neural tissue have been used in the treatment of pain from trigeminal neuralgia [9], facet osteoarthritis, and failed back syndrome [10]. The established ability of RF ablation in creating localized necrotic lesions makes it the treatment of choice for many symptomatic cardiac arrhythmias [11] and small, painful, benign osteoid osteomas [12]. The clinical efficacy of RF ablation in these areas has been clearly established.

RF ablation is a technique whereby an alternating electrical current operating in the frequency of radio waves (460–480 kHz) is emitted from the tip of an electrode or needle placed directly into targeted tissues. The alternating RF current causes the local ions in targeted tissues to vibrate, thus giving rise to heat. This tissue heating consequently induces coagulative necrosis and cell death in a controlled and predictable manner. The cellular cytotoxic temperature threshold is 50°C, but with RF ablation techniques, the intratumoral ablated temperatures usually far exceed this. A major limitation of RF ablation used to be the small thermocoagulation sizes created. Recently, technical advances in RF ablation systems have greatly improved the size of the ablation zone such that ablated heat lesions larger than 5 cm in diameter can now be created with a single treatment [13].

There are currently three RF systems that are being used for treating tumors. Two of the systems (RITA Medical Systems, Inc., Mountain View, California; Boston Scientific, Natick, Massachusetts) use a deployable array RF electrode which consists of 10 to 16 small wires that are deployed through a 15- to 17-gauge needle. The third RF system (Radionics, Inc., Burlington,

Massachusetts) uses either single nonperfused or single and triple "cluster" perfused electrodes (see Fig. 1). The nonperfused conventional thermistor electrodes are approximately 18 gauge and have a small 5-mm exposed tip. These smaller electrodes can ablate tissue with a treatment diameter of approximately 10 to 16 mm and are used for the ablation of osteoid osteomas, nervous tissue, and small tumors. The internally cooled RF electrode can increase the volume of induced coagulation necrosis up to 4 to 7 cm in diameter, as reported in the liver [14], but may be greater in soft tissue malignancies because of the diminished cooling effect of regional blood flow. Perfusion at the RF electrode tip reduces tissue charring, thus allowing for a greater radius of RF energy deposition. A single or triple cluster RF

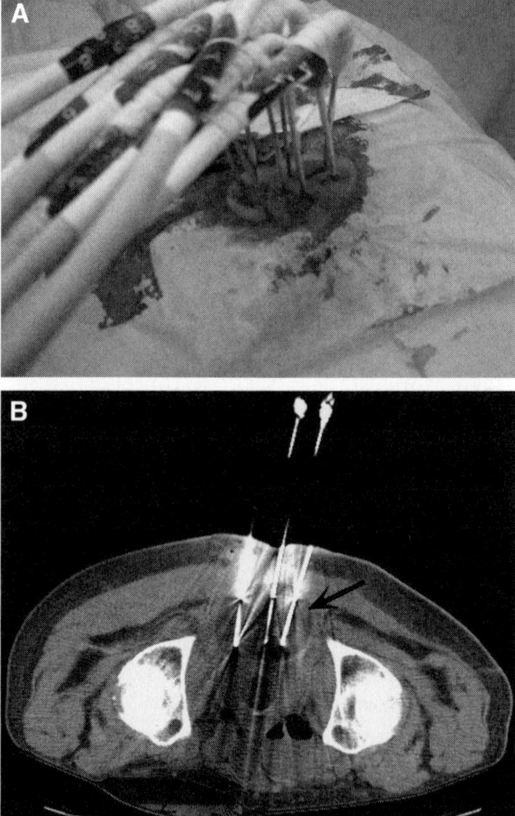

Fig. 2. CT-guided percutaneous cryoablation in a 56-year-old man with recurrent rectal cancer in the presacral and coccygeal region who was previously treated with external beam radiation therapy and chemotherapy. (*A*) Eight 2-mm cryotherapy probes were inserted percutaneously into the 7-cm soft tissue mass. Two 10-minute freezes to −136°C followed by a 5-minute thaw in between were performed. (*B*) Ice ball visualization (*arrow*) confirmed appropriate coverage of most of the soft tissue mass.

electrode is currently available. The electrode has a 1 to 3 cm uninsulated tip. Each needle contains an RF electrode with a thermocouple embedded in the tip to measure temperature. Circuitry incorporated within the generator and needle permits continuous measurement of tissue impedance. Two internal lumens extend to each electrode tip. One is used to deliver chilled perfusion fluid (sterile saline or water) to the electrode tip, whereas the second returns the perfusion effluent to a collection unit located external to the patient. An external peristaltic pump is used to infuse the perfusion fluid into the cooling lumen of the RF electrode at 80 mL/minute.

A grounding pad (or pads) is placed on the patient. If a single RF treatment probe is used, at least two grounding pads (96-cm^2 surface area each) or the equivalent (minimum total surface area of ~200 cm^2) must be used. If a triple cluster electrode is used, at least four grounding pads or their equivalent (~400-cm^2 surface area) must be used. The pads must be placed horizontally to maximize the grounding effect and prevent thermal injury to the skin. The grounding pad or pads and electrode are connected to the RF generator. When the RF generator is activated, current flows between the conductive electrode tip and the grounding pad (or pads) or "dispersive electrode." The increase in the tissue temperature is proportional to the current density. Because the current density is highest near the conductive electrode tip, coagulation is induced in the tissue surrounding the treatment probe. When performing an RF treatment, the coagulation depth is controlled by means of the length of the uninsulated "active" electrode tip. The diameter of coagulation necrosis produced around the tip of the treatment electrode depends on the current, duration of treatment, and local tissue blood flow.

In the pelvis, RF ablation mainly has been used in the treatment of pelvic metastases and recurrences from colorectal carcinoma and painful metastases involving bone. Ohhigashi et al [15], in 2003, reported their experience in treating pelvic recurrences of rectal carcinoma with the treatment of 14 lesions in 10 patients. Four patients with a solitary recurrent tumor were treated curatively, whereas the 10 lesions in the remaining six patients with distant metastases were treated mainly for pain palliation. The reported complications following RF ablation included abscess formation, neuralgia, and bleeding.

Recently, Goetz et al [16] published a large multicenter study involving the use of percutaneous image-guided RF ablation in the treatment of painful bone metastases. Of the 43 patients treated, 24 had painful bone metastases in the pelvis (n = 12) and sacrum (n = 12). Common tumor types treated were from colorectal, renal, and lung carcinoma primaries. Most patients had received prior radiation therapy or were considered to be poor candidates for radiation. Most patients were receiving prescription opioid analgesics for pain control. This study reported highly significant reductions in pain scores and improvement in the quality of life following RF ablation of these painful metastases involving bone. These findings were significant, not just because of the magnitude of the benefit but because the findings were achieved in a cohort of patients traditionally considered refractory to most conventional treatments. In total, 95% of the patients experienced at least a rapid 2-point drop in their recorded worst pain score (10-point numeric rating scale) following the RF ablation. This study shows that RF ablation provides effective palliation of localized, painful osteolytic metastases involving bone. Patient who have cancer are thus provided an additional method to relieve their symptoms of refractory bone pain, when standard treatment options have failed (Figs. 3 and 4).

Microwave ablation

MW ablation refers to the use of all electromagnetic methods for inducing tumor destruction using devices with frequencies of 900 MHz or greater. MW ablation offers many advantages of RF ablation, but has several other theoretic advantages that may increase its effectiveness in the treatment of tumors. These advantages include the following: an improved heat convection profile with larger ablation volumes and shorter ablation times when compared with existing RF technologies; the ability for the simultaneous use of multiple antennae, yielding synergistically larger

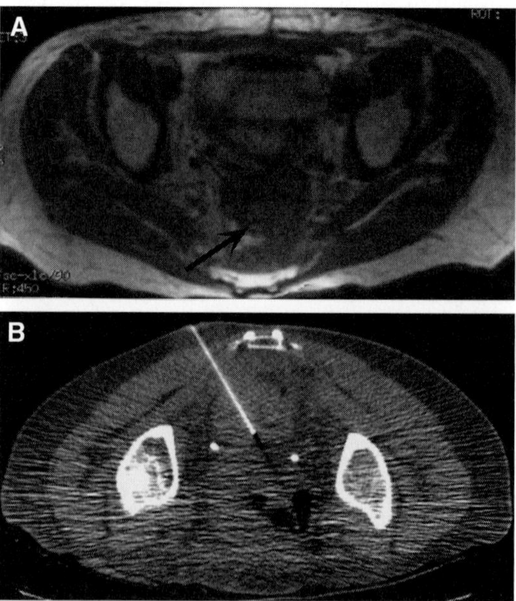

Fig. 3. A 63-year-old woman with endometrial carcinoma who had a history of surgery and external beam radiation therapy to the pelvis presented with recurrent rectal bleeding. (*A*) An axial T1-weighted MRI showed the soft tissue mass to be consistent with the patient's known metastatic pelvic endometrial carcinoma invading the rectum (*arrow*). (*B*) A 3-cm active-tip single RF electrode was introduced into the center of the lesion, and two treatments were administered. The patient's symptoms improved and bleeding was controlled by the procedure.

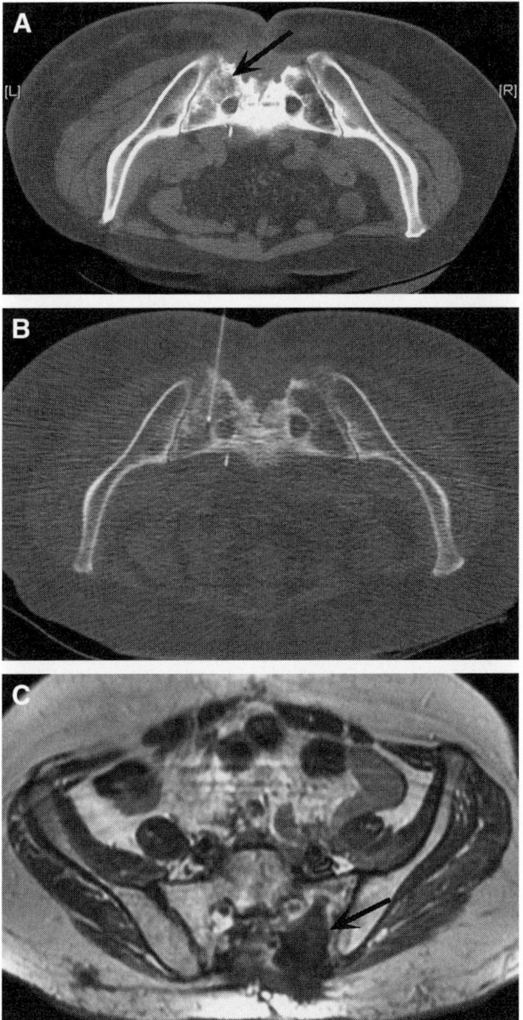

Fig. 4. A 39-year-old man with a history of rectal cancer status after surgical resection, chemotherapy, and radiation therapy presented for RF ablation of a biopsy-proven, painful left sacral recurrence. (*A*) A noncontrast CT examination showed a 2.5-cm soft tissue sacral mass consistent with the patient's known metastasis (*arrow*). With the patient placed in the prone position, a 14-gauge Ackermann needle was introduced into the center of the lesion. (*B*) A 20-cm RF probe with a 3-cm active tip was introduced into the lesion by means of the Ackermann sheath. Three RF ablations were performed. The patient's pain resolved after treatment. (*C*) At 6-week follow-up, gadolinium-enhanced T1-weighted MRI shows tumor thermocoagulation with a thin rim of enhancement (*arrow*).

ablation zones, and the elimination of grounding pads. MW ablation, like RF ablation, results in direct thermocoagulation of the tumor mass.

Although intraoperative MW ablation has been reported [17,18], usually performed in combination with intra-arterial chemotherapy or low-dose

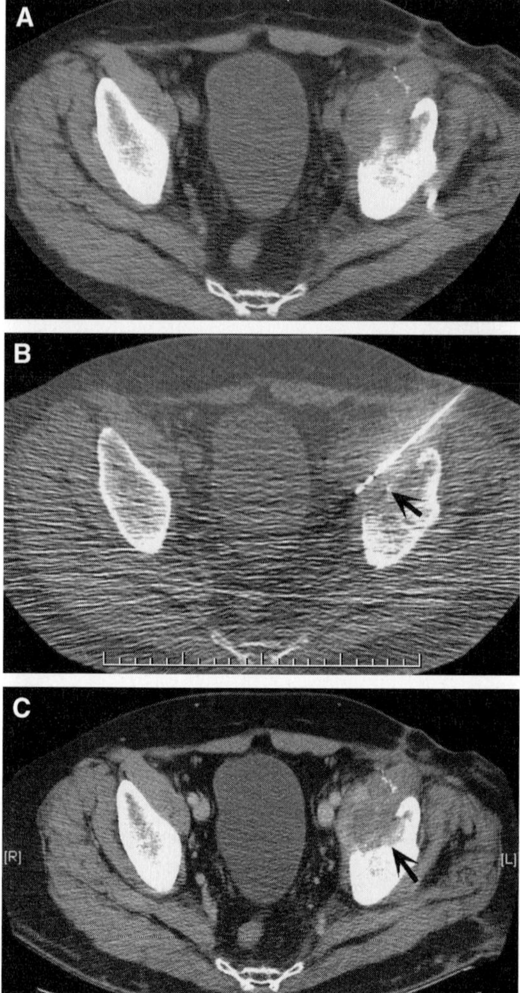

Fig. 5. This 57-year-old man with renal cell carcinoma presented with metastatic disease in his left acetabulum. He had failed previous RF ablation because of tumor hypervascularity. He now presents for MW ablation of his painful bony metastasis. (*A*) Preliminary CT imaging shows a 4-cm soft tissue mass with associated bony destruction of the left acetabulum. A single MW antenna was advanced into the center of the metastasis. (*B*) Six MW ablations were performed. A thermocouple (*small arrow*) placed next to the MW antennae was used throughout the entire procedure to monitor the maximum temperature achieved. The patient tolerated the procedure well with no immediate complications. (*C*) A postprocedure CT revealed no contrast enhancement in the bony metastasis (*arrow*).

interstitial radiotherapy or external beam radiation, percutaneous MW ablation is still in its infancy. Although percutaneous MW ablation for hepatic tumors has been performed [19–22], the present authors have found no published reports using this technique in the treatment of pelvic tumors.

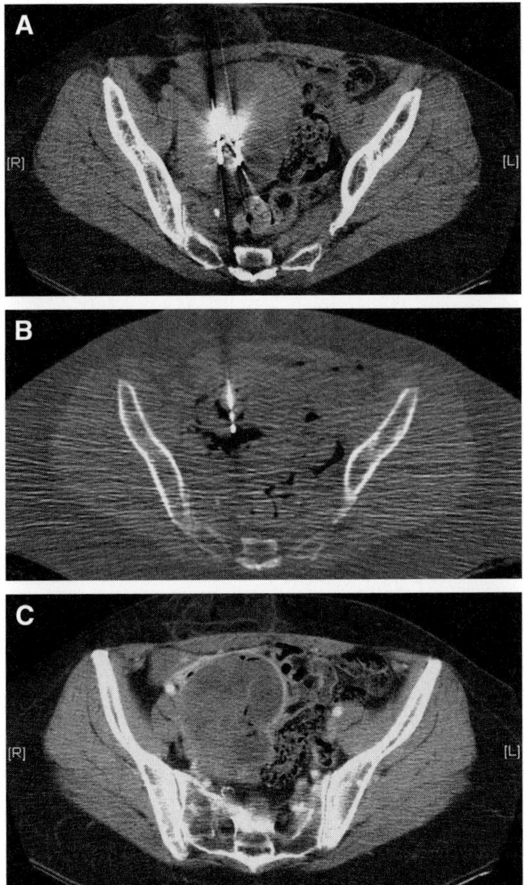

Fig. 6. Percutaneous MW ablation was performed on this 42-year-old woman with a history of metastatic breast carcinoma and an enlarging right pelvic mass despite chemotherapy. Initial noncontrast CT images through the pelvis show a large (10 × 8 × 10 cm) heterogeneous soft tissue mass centered within the right lower pelvis. (*A*) Under CT fluoroscopic guidance, three single 3.5-cm active-tip MW antennae were inserted into the mass in a cluster configuration, spaced approximately 2 cm apart. Two MW ablations were performed. (*B*) During the MW ablation procedure, expected gas formation was noted within the large heterogeneous mass. (*C*) Immediately post procedure, a contrast-enhanced CT of the pelvis showed complete thermocoagulation of the mass.

Currently, there is one percutaneous MW ablation system (see Fig. 1) available in the United States (Vivant Medical, Mountain View, California). The technique for performing percutaneous MW ablation involves CT-guided placement of an appropriately sized microwave antennae (either single or triple cluster) into the center of the tumor. Depending on the site and size of the tumor, the tumor margins, and involved surrounding structures, single or multiple 10-minute ablations are then performed with a power of 45 W to achieve adequate local tumor control and pain palliation. Remote thermocouple measurements can be recorded adjacent to the MW antennae along the tumor margin by separate placements of the thermocouple (Figs. 5 and 6).

Summary

Surgery, in combination with radiation therapy or chemotherapy, remains the mainstay in the treatment of pelvic malignancies. Upcoming percutaneous ablation techniques, such as RF ablation, cryoablation, and MW ablation, however, present a valid treatment alternative. These techniques exhibit all the advantages of a minimally invasive procedure, including the following: the ability to be performed in the outpatient setting, which reduces the need for overnight hospital admissions, saving time and cost for both the patient and the health care system; the avoidance of surgery and general anesthetic, with its accompanying associated reduction in morbidity and mortality; the ability to perform multiple retreatment procedures, either in single or multiple sessions; the ability to target patients who would otherwise be deemed surgically inoperable; and the proven efficacy of these techniques in local tumor control and pain palliation management.

Technical advances in percutaneous tumor ablation give rise to the ability for better targeting of tumors and a more accurate control over and prediction of ablation sizes, with the accompanying larger ablation volumes and faster ablation times.

References

[1] Gage AA. History of cryosurgery. Semin Surg Oncol 1998;14(2):99–109.

[2] Onik GM, Cohen JK, Reyes GD, Rubinsky B, Chang Z, Baust J. Transrectal ultrasound-guided percutaneous radical cryosurgical ablation of the prostate. Cancer 1993;72(4): 1291–9.

[3] Silverman SG, Tuncali K, Adams DF, et al. MR imaging-guided percutaneous cryotherapy of liver tumors: initial experience. Radiology 2000;217(3):657–64.

[4] Shingleton WB, Sewell PE Jr. Percutaneous renal cryoablation of renal tumors in patients with von Hippel-Lindau disease. J Urol 2002;167(3):1268–70.

[5] Mala T, Edwin B, Samset E, et al. Magnetic-resonance-guided percutaneous cryoablation of hepatic tumours. Eur J Surg 2001;167(8):610–7.

[6] Beland MD, Dupuy DE, Mayo-Smith WW. Percutaneous cryoablation of extra-abdominal metastatic disease: initial results. AJR 2005;184. In press.

[7] Onik G. Image-guided prostate cryosurgery: state of the art. Cancer Control 2001;8(6): 522–31.

[8] Malawer MM, Bickels J, Meller I, Buch RG, Henshaw RM, Kollender Y. Cryosurgery in the treatment of giant cell tumor. A long-term followup study. Clin Orthop 1999;(359):176–88.

[9] Sweet WH, Wepsic JG. Controlled thermocoagulation of trigeminal ganglion and rootlets for differential destruction of pain fibers. 1. Trigeminal neuralgia. J Neurosurg 1974;40(2): 143–56.

[10] Cho J, Park YG, Chung SS. Percutaneous radiofrequency lumbar facet rhizotomy in mechanical low back pain syndrome. Stereotact Funct Neurosurg 1997;68(1–4 Pt 1):212–7.
[11] De Giovanni JV. Treatment of arrhythmias by radiofrequency ablation. Arch Dis Child 1995;73(5):385–7.
[12] Rosenthal DI, Hornicek FJ, Wolfe MW, Jennings LC, Gebhardt MC, Mankin HJ. Percutaneous radiofrequency coagulation of osteoid osteoma compared with operative treatment. J Bone Joint Surg Am 1998;80(6):815–21.
[13] Goldberg SN, Gazelle GS, Solbiati L, Rittman WJ, Mueller PR. Radiofrequency tissue ablation: increased lesion diameter with a perfusion electrode. Acad Radiol 1996;3(8): 636–44.
[14] Goldberg SN, Solbiati L, Hahn PF, et al. Large-volume tissue ablation with radio frequency by using a clustered, internaliy cooled electrode technique: laboratory and clinical experience in liver metastases. Radiology 1998;209(2):371–9.
[15] Ohhigashi S, Watanabe F. Radiofrequency ablation is useful for selected cases of pelvic recurrence of rectal carcinoma. Tech Coloproctol 2003;7(3):186–91.
[16] Goetz MP, Callstrom MR, Charboneau JW, et al. Percutaneous image-guided radiofrequency ablation of painful metastases involving bone: a multicenter study. J Clin Oncol 2004;22(2):300–6.
[17] Estes NC, Morphis JG, Hornback NB, Jewell WR. Intraarterial chemotherapy and hyperthermia for pain control in patients with recurrent rectal cancer. Am J Surg 1986; 152(6):597–601.
[18] Seegenschmiedt MH, Sauer R, Miyamoto C, Chalal JA, Brady LW. Clinical experience with interstitial thermoradiotherapy for localized implantable pelvic tumors. Am J Clin Oncol 1993;16(3):210–22.
[19] Murakami R, Yoshimatsu S, Yamashita Y, Matsukawa T, Takahashi M, Sagara K. Treatment of hepatocellular carcinoma: value of percutaneous microwave coagulation. AJR Am J Roentgenol 1995;164(5):1159–64.
[20] Seki T, Tamai T, Nakagawa T, et al. Combination therapy with transcatheter arterial chemoembolization and percutaneous microwave coagulation therapy for hepatocellular carcinoma. Cancer 2000;89(6):1245–51.
[21] Lu MD, Chen JW, Xie XY, et al. Hepatocellular carcinoma: US-guided percutaneous microwave coagulation therapy. Radiology 2001;221(1):167–72.
[22] Shibata T, Iimuro Y, Yamamoto Y, et al. Small hepatocellular carcinoma: comparison of radio-frequency ablation and percutaneous microwave coagulation therapy. Radiology 2002;223(2):331–7.

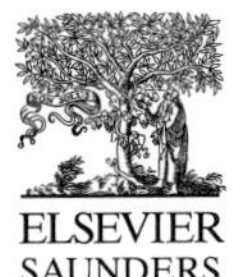

ELSEVIER
SAUNDERS

Surg Oncol Clin N Am
14 (2005) 433–439

SURGICAL
ONCOLOGY CLINICS
OF NORTH AMERICA

Index

Note: Page numbers of article titles are in **boldface** type.

1055-3207/05/$ - see front matter
doi:10.1016/S1055-3207(05)00017-7

Q

R

S

T

U

V

Changing Your Address?

Make sure your subscription changes too! When you notify us of your new address, you can help make our job easier by including an exact copy of your Clinics label number with your old address (see illustration below.) This number identifies you to our computer system and will speed the processing of your address change. Please be sure this label number accompanies your old address and your corrected address—you can send an old Clinics label with your number on it or just copy it exactly and send it to the address listed below.

We appreciate your help in our attempt to give you continuous coverage. Thank you.

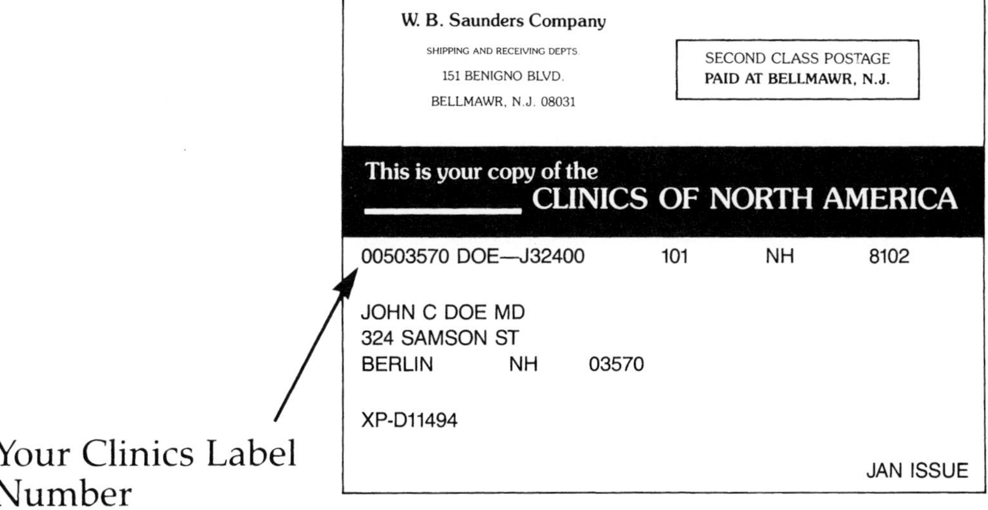

Your Clinics Label Number

Copy it exactly or send your label along with your address to:
W.B. Saunders Company, Customer Service
Orlando, FL 32887-4800
Call Toll Free 1-800-654-2452

Please allow four to six weeks for delivery of new subscriptions and for processing address changes.

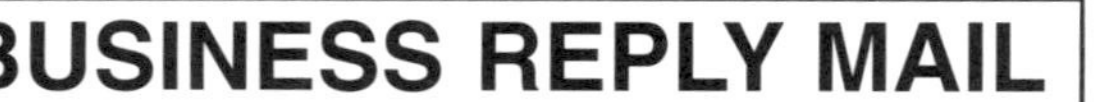